Concise Chinese Materia Medica

Compiled by Zheng Guili
Zhang Chengbo
Translated by Yang Huiqin

Shandong Science and Technology Press

First Edition 1997
ISBN 7－5331－1841－3

Concise Chinese Materia Medica

Compiled by Zheng Guili
Zhang Chengbo
Translated by Yang Huiqin
Editor in Charge Ma Wannian

Published by Shandong Science and Technology Press
16 Yuhan Road, Jinan, China 250002
Printed by Shandong Binzhou Xinhua Printing House
Distributed by China International Book Trading Corporation
35 Chegongzhuang Xilu, Beijing 100044, China
P.O. Box 399, Beijing, China
Printed in the People's Republic of China

Preface

Concise Chinese Materia Medica is one volume of *The Series of Traditional Chinese Medicine for Foreign Readers.*

This book consists of 2 parts: general information and classified introduction. General information deals with the basic theory of Chinese materia medica including the characteristics and processing of the drugs as well as their compatibility, contraindication, dosage, administration, etc. Classified introduction makes a detailed description of 197 commonly-used drugs in clinical practice which are stated in 18 categories according to their nature and indications. Each drug, in turn, is expounded in 6 respects: description, characteristics, action, indications, administration and precautions.

With the emphasis of this book laid on action and indications, the compilers made an effort to write the content concisely and clearly in simple words so as to meet the needs of foreign readers.

Such drugs as Hu Gu (Os Tigris), Chuan Shan Jia (Squama Manitis) and Xi Niu Jiao (Cornu Rhinocerotis) which are under protection are still included in this book with a view to presenting truly Chinese materia medica.

Compilers

Contents

GENERAL INFORMATION

Medicinal Properties of Chinese Materia Medica

Medicinal properties of Chinese materia medica include nature and flavor, the action of lifting, lowering, floating and sinking, meridian tropism and toxicity of the drugs. The reason that Chinese medicine has a curative function lies in the therapeutic elements it contains in correcting the Excess or Deficiency of Yin and Yang in the body so that a balanced physiological condition is restored and thus the illness is cured. The characteristics of the drugs are summarized from clinical practice based on the theories of Yin-Yang, Zang-Fu, Channels and Collaterals as well as principles of treatment, which, in turn, serve as a guide to clinical application of Chinese materia medica.

1. Nature and Flavor

Also called four natures and five flavors. Each drug has its nature and flavor which constitute an important basis for clinical application of the drug, for they are significant signs of the drug's properties.

Nature here includes cold, hot, warm and cool natures of the drug and it is generalized from various responses the patients have after the drug enters the body and also from other therapeutic effects it produces. Drugs capable of treating Heat syndromes are cold-natured or cool-natured, while those capable of treating Cold syndromes are hot-natured or warm-natured.

Cold and cool are different in nature from warm and hot, whereas cold and cool differ in degree in the same way as warm and hot. Cool is milder than cold just as warm is milder than hot. Cool or cold-natured drugs are usually used in treating Heat syndromes as they are capable of purging Heat and Fire, detoxicating and nourishing Yin; while warm or hot-natured drugs are mainly used to treat Cold syndromes as they can eliminate Cold, warm the Middle-jiao, strengthen Yang and suppress the adverse flow of Qi.

Apart from the four natures mentioned above, there is a kind of in-between (neutral) drugs which can be applied to both Cold and Hot syndromes as they do not manifest obvious cold or hot nature. Nevertheless, such drugs also show bias toward either hot or cold nature, for that reason, drugs are habitually divided into four natures.

Flavor refers to taste of a drug which includes acrid, sweet, sour, bitter, salty, insipid and astringent. Because sweet and insipid are mentioned together, and sour and astringeny have the same function, it is an accepted classification to have the drugs devided into five flavors, namely: acrid, sweet, sour, bitter and salty. Different flavors show different pharmacodynamics and therapeutic function, while the same flavor manifests similar function. Flavor here does not necessarily mean the real taste of the drug, sometimes it is summarized from the function of the drug. Therefore, some drugs may taste different from what are recorded in medical books. The following are descriptions of the five flavors:

(1) Acrid. Inducing sweat and promoting the circulation of Qi and Blood, generally used in treating superficies-syndromes due to attack of exogenous pathogens and stagnation of both Qi and Blood.

(2) Sweet. Invigorating and regulating the Middle-jiao, relieving pain, moderating the potency of drugs, etc. Generally, drugs with

sweet flavor are capable of treating Deficiency syndromes, dry cough, constipation, incoordination between the Spleen and Stomach, pain and so on. Besides, some of the sweet-flavored drugs can counteract toxicity.

(3) Sour. Astringent. Usually used to treat night sweat, prolonged cough, long-time diarrhea, nocturnal emission, enuresis, frequent urination, protracted metrorrhagia, etc.

(4) Bitter. Clearing away Heat and purging Fire, lowering the adverse rising of Qi to arrest cough and vomiting, promoting the bowel movement, eliminating Dampness, etc. Usually used in treating Fire-Heat syndromes, cough and adverse flow of Qi, vomiting, constipation due to sthenic Heat, Damp-Heat and Damp-Cold, etc.

(5) Salty. Relaxing the bowels, softening the hard lumps and dispelling the nodes, usually applied to scrofula, subcutaneous nodule, goiter and tumor, constipation due to accumulation of pathogenic Heat, etc.

(6) Insipid. Promoting diuresis. Usually used for edema, dysuria and so on.

(7) Astringent. Similar in function to sour.

Each drug has its own nature and flavor. generally, drugs with the same nature and flavor show similar functions while those with different nature and flavor manifest marked difference in function. Drugs same in nature but different in flavor or vice versa may have part of the function in common. For instance, Huang Qin (Radix Scutellariae) and Sheng Di (Radix Rehmannia) are both cold in nature, yet the former is bitter in flavor and the latter is sweet in flavor; the former is used for Damp-Heat syndromes, as it can purge Heat and eliminate Dampness, while the latter for febrile diseases due to damage to Yin as it can eliminate Heat and tonify Yin. Another example can be found in acrid-flavored Gui Zhi (Ramulus Cinnamoni) and Bo He (Herba Menthae), the former is warm in nature and used for superficies-syndromes due to Wind-Cold, as it can eliminate Wind-Cold; while the latter is cool in nature and used for superficies-syndromes due to Wind-Heat as it can dissipate Wind-Heat. Therefore, only by a combined analysis of the drugs' nature and flavor can it be possible to understand and apply the drugs accurately.

2. The Action of Lifting, Lowering, Floating and Sinking

Lifting, lowering, floating and sinking refer to upward, downward, outward and inward directions in which drugs tend to act in the body. Generally speaking, drugs with lifting and floating tendencies are responsible for upward and outward flow and they are capable of raising Yang, promoting perspiration, eliminating pathogenic Wind and Cold, emetic, inducing resuscitation, etc.; while drugs with lowering and sinking tendencies are responsible for downward and inward movement and they are capable of purging Heat, purgation, promoting diuresis, suppressing Yang, lowering the adverse flow of Qi to stop vomiting, relieving cough and dyspnea, promoting digestion by removing stasis, tranquilizing the mind, etc.

Different locations of the illness such as upper or lower parts, exterior or interior make a variation of different tendencies such as upward (like vomiting), downward (like metrorrhagia, prolapse of anus), outward (like spontaneous perspiration, night sweat) and inward (like invasion of exopathogenic factors). That is to say, there exists a corresponding relation between lifting, lowering, floating and sinking of the drugs and location and tendency of illness, usually with the same location but against the tendency of the illness. When pathological changes occur in the upper and superficial part, lifting and floating are needed as in invasion by exopathogenic factors, while lowering and sinking are used for those in the lower and interior part as in constipation. For adverse rising of illness trend, lowering is needed, e.g. headache and vertigo due to hyperactivity of Liver-Yang should be treated with lowering and sinking drugs to calm the Liver and suppress Yang; while downward trend of illness such as collapse of Middle-jiao, prolapse of anus due to prolonged diarrhea, should be treated with drugs for promoting Qi circulation to raise Yang.

Lifting, lowering, floating and sinking are closely related to the nature and flavor of the drug. Generally, drugs acrid or sweet in flavor and warm or hot in nature have lifting or floating function, on the other hand, drugs bitter or sour or salty in flavor, cool or cold in nature have lowering and sinking function. There are also relations between lifting, floating, lowering, sinking and the texture of the drug. Usually drugs with loose texture are capable of lifting and floating, while drugs of close texture are capable of lowering and sinking. But there are exceptions.

Besides, lifting, floating, lowering and sinking can be influenced by preparation and compatibility of the drugs. e. g. Drugs with lowering and sinking function are capable of lifting and floating after being prepared with wine; in the same way, drugs with lifting and floating function can be capable of lowering and sinking once they are prepared with salt water. Drugs with lifting and floating function can become lowering and sinking ones when used together with many lowering and sinking drugs, and vice versa.

3. Meridian Tropism

This refers to certain drugs' main or special therapeutic action on certain viscera, Channels and Collaterals, or pathological changes in them, when the same drugs may have little or no action on other viscera, Meridians or pathological changes in them. For example, some Heat-clearing drugs may act on Lung Heat, others may act on Heart Heat; some tonics may function on Lung, some on Spleen, others may on Kidney.

Meridian tropism is summarized from the theory of Zang-Fu and Meridians and from various cases. Human body is an organic whole in which Channels and Collaterals connect interiorly and exteriorly. When pathological changes take place, the diseased superficies may affect the internal organs and vice versa. e. g. in the case of inhibited Lung-Qi, cough and dyspea can be seen; in the case of depression of the Liver-Qi and stagnation of Qi, hypochondriac pain is always seen. As Xing Ren (Semen Armeniacae Amarum) can relieve cough and dyspnea, Chai Hu (Radix Bupleuri) can cure hypochondriac pain, so the former is attributive to the Lung Meridian, the latter to the Liver Meridian. This shows that the theory of meridian tropism comes mainly from clinical practice.

The theory of meridian tropism should be applied in consideration of the four natures, five flavors, as well as the action of lifting, lowering, floating and sinking. As drugs attributive to the same Meridian may have different functions due to the difference of nature, flavor or lifting, lowering, floating and sinking. e. g. Huang Qin (Radix Scutellariae), Gan Jiang (Rhizoma Zingiberis), Bai He (Bulbus Lilii) and Ting Li Zi (Semen Lepidii seu Descurainiae) are all attributive to the Lung Meridian. Yet Huang Qin (Radix Scutellariae) can clear away Lung-Heat, Gan Jiang (Rhizoma Zingiberis) can warm the Lung, Bai He (Bulbus Lilii) can treat Lung-Deficiency, while Ting Li Zi (Semen Lepidii seu Descurainiac) can purge Lung-Fire. Therefore, only by a comprehensive study and analysis of the drugs can a correct application of them be abtained. In addition, the physiological inter-relation between Zang-Fu and Channels and Collaterals and their influence on each other in pathology should be taken into consideration in treating an illness. For instance, when a pathological change occurs in a certain Meridian, apart from using drugs attributive to this meridian, drugs attributive to other meridians should also be selected for treatment. e. g. drugs for strengthening the Spleen are used for treating Lung diseases, drugs for tonifying the Kidney-Yin are used for treating hyperactivity of Liver-Yang.

4. Toxicity

In Chinese medical books, some drugs are labeled "toxic", "mildly toxic", "highly toxic" or "deadly toxic" etc. This means the dosage for treatment is close to the dosage of poisoning, or within the range of poisoning, above which, poisoning reaction or big side-effect may occur.

In order to ensure the safety of drug administration, drugs with toxicity or side-effect should be selected and administered in consideration of the degree of the toxicity, the constitution and age of the patient as well as the severity of illness. For the highly-poisonous drugs, overdose is forbidden. Besides, the toxicity may be lowered by processing of the drug or by being used together with other drugs or by refining treatment.

Certain toxic drugs manifest marked therapeutic function. According to the principle of "using poison as an antidote to poison," they can be applied to severe and intractable diseases on condition of safety.

Processing of Crude Drugs

The processing of crude drugs indicates that the crude drugs are treated to comform appropriate specifications through processing procedures so as to obtain the processed drugs fulfilling the requirements of therapeutic, dispersing or manufacturing usage, thus assuring the safety and efficacy of the drugs.

1. Objectives of Processing

The objectives of drug processing are as follows:

(1) To eliminate or lower the toxicity, intensity and side-effect of certain drugs. For instance, Chuan Wu (Radix Aconiti), Cao Wu (Radix Aconiti Kusnezoffii) and Gan Sui (Radix Euphorbiae Kansui) can be made less poisonous by processing; Ba Dou (Fructus Crotonis), a strong purgative, can become milder with oil and frost removed; while Chang Shan (Radix Dichroae), a strongly emetic drug, can be made milder after being stir-fried with wine.

(2) To strengthen the function. For instance, Yan Hu Suo (Rhizoma Corydalis) prepared with vinegar can strengthen its pain-relieving effect; honey-prepared Bai Bu (Radix Stemonae) and Kuan Dong Hua (Flos Farfarae) can enhance their function of moistening

the Lung and relieving cough.

(3) To change the character of the drug so as to meet the needs. e. g. Sheng Di Huang (Radix Rehmanniae) is cold in nature and used for cooling Blood; while the prepared one (Radix Rehmanniae Praeparata) is warm in nature and used for reinforcing Blood; Dai Huang (Radix et Rhizoma Rhei) is a strong purgative, yet the prepared one is milder in purgation while carbonized one has almost no purgative effect but with blood-arresting function.

(4) To fit for making decoction, refining treatment and storage. Herbs are cut to slices so that effective elements are easily soluble in decoction. Also sliced herbs can be conveniently made into powder or other forms of medicine. On the other hand, minerals and shells should be calcined until they are crisp and easily crushed. Some fresh drugs must be dried to avoid mildew or rot.

(5) To remove the foreign matters, such as dirt, skin (for some herbs), head and feet or wing (for some animals) or unpleasant smell (for some sea-food).

2. Methods of Processing

Generally, there are 5 methods of processing drugs.

(1) Sorting and cutting. First, sort out the specified part used and eliminate the foreign matters. Second, crush or powder the crude drugs for further processing or for application. Third, cut the crude drugs into sections, pieces, slices or slivers in accordance with different requirements so as to be fit for making decoctions and further processings, and to be convenient for drying, storage and dispensation.

(2) Processing with water. First, wash the crude drugs clean with water for the purpose of removing the dirt or foreign matters. Second, soften the drugs for cutting by sprinkling water or other liquid frequently on the drugs. Third, eliminate salty, stinky smell or toxic

drugs in clear or flowing water. Fourth, levigating. Add a quantity of water to the insoluble minerals (granulated first) and pulverize to fine powders, then add more water, stir, decant the supernatant suspension, repeat the operation on the precipitate for several times, remove the foreign matters and combine the suspensions. Allow to stand, seperate the precipitate, dry and pulverize to fine powder. The advantage of levigating is getting very fine powder with little loss of the drug.

(3) Processing with fire

This includes direct and indirect treatment with fire, such as stir-frying, stir-frying with liquid, calcining, stewing, etc.

A. Stir-frying: Stir continuously while frying the crude drug in a pot. It may be subdivided into stir-frying by itself and stir-frying mixed with excipient. ①Stir-fry the crude drugs without excipient to proper conditions, that is, to brown, chared or carbonized conditions. The first means to stir-fry the crude drug till the surface of the drug turns brown while there is no change inside; and the second means to stir-fry the drug till the surface of the drug turns deep brown and the cross section becomes brown, while the third means to carbonize the drug to the degree of half-burnt with the nature of the drug preserved. ②Stir-fry with excipient, such as Zao Xin Tu (Terra Flava Usta), bran, rice, talcum, powder of Ge Ke (Concha Meretricis seu Cyclinae).

B. Stir-frying with liquid: Stir-fry the crude drug with such liquid as honey, wine, vinegar, salt-water, ginger juice, etc, for the purpose of strengthening the therapeutic effect or changing the nature of the drug or decreasing the side-effect. For example, drugs stir-fried with honey will reinforce the function of tonifying the middle-jiao, promoting the circulation of Qi and nourishing the Lung to arrest cough, it can also make the nature of the drug milder and decrease the side-effect; drugs processed with vinegar are capable of strengthening the funcuion of calming the liver and alleviating pain; while drugs processed with salt-water can reinforce the function of tonifying the kidney and Yin to suppress Fire, and drugs stir-fried with vinegar juice will strengthen the function for stopping vomiting and the cold nature of the drug,and it also decreases the toxicity and side-effect.

C. Calcining: Put the drug directly on fire or indirectly in a refractory container, calcine the drug to red hot and dip it into vinegar or water to make it crisp and easily crushed , so that the effective elements can be decocted out, or the nature of the drug can be changed to strengthen the effect. Generally, minerals and shells are calcined directly, while Xue Yu Tan (Crinis Carbonisatus), Chen Zong Tan (Trachycarpi Carbonisatus),etc are calcined indirectly.

D. Roasting: Wrap the drug with flour paste or with wet paper, then roast it in fresh cinders till the paste or paper becomes black and burnt,so as to decrease the fat,spicy substances,the intensity or toxicity or side-effect of the drug.

(4) Processing with both fire and water. The purpose of this treatment is to strengthen the therapeutic effect of the drug, decrease the toxicity,change the nature of the drug and make it fit for storage. The methods include:

A. Steaming,a method to heat the drug by steaming.

B. Boiling, a method to heat the drug by boiling both the drug and water or other liquid.

C. Calcining, a method to make the drug crisp by dipping the red-hot drug into the cold water or other liquid.

D. Blanching in boiling water, a method to heat the drug by putting it in boiling water and taking it out instantly.

E. Others. Some drugs are processed according to particular requirements such as germination,fermination,frostation,etc.

Application of the Drugs

Clinical application of traditional Chinese drugs should be guided by the theory of traditional Chinese medicine (TCM) and consideration should be given to the particular condition of the patient, the properties of the drugs and the requirement of the treatment. Generally, four aspects are involved in the application: compatibility, contraindication, dosage and administration.

1. Compatibility

In treating an illness, sometimes a drug is used alone, sometimes several drugs are applied together. Compatibility means selecting more than two kinds of drugs and applying them together so as to bring the curative components into full play.

From long-term clinical practice, the ancient TCM practitioners summarized seven conditions under which a single drug is used alone or more than two drugs are used together. They are:

(1) Danxing——treating an illness with one drug alone;

(2) Xiangxu——two kinds of drugs with similar properties used in combination to reinforce each other's action;

(3) Xiangshi——two or more ingredients in a prescription used in

combination, one being the principal substance while the rest play a subsidiary role to reinforce the action of the former;

(4) Xiangwei——mutual restraining effect of different ingredients to weaken or neutralize each other's toxicity or side-effect;

(5) Xiangsha——the property of one drug or ingredient to neutralize the toxicity of another drug or ingredient;

(6) Xiangwu——the property of one drug or ingredient to weaken the action of another drug or ingredient;

(7) Xiangfan——incompatibility. Severe side-effect may result when two incompatible ingredients are used in combination.

To sum up, drugs (excluding the first type, Danxing) will have interaction when they are used in combination, some may interpromote the curative effect, others may interrestrain to decrease each other's toxicity or side-effect, still others may weaken the original action or even result in toxicity or side-effect. Therefore, correct choice of the drugs used in combination is necessary to ensure the therapeutic effect and decrease the side-effect. As Xiangxu and Xiangshi can interpromote the curative effect, they are most commonly used in making a prescription, while Xiangwu and Xiangfan should be avoided as they can either decrease the action or result in toxicity, on the other hand, Xiangwei and Xiangsha can be considered when a poisonous drug is to be used.

2. Contraindication

During drug administration, some other drugs or certain food should be forbidden or should be taken with precaution. Contraindication includes contraindicated symptoms, incompatible dispensary, medicines contraindicated during pregnancy and food taboo.

(1) Contraindicated symptoms. Each kind of drugs and each drug has its own indications, beyond which are contraindicated symptoms. For instance, Ma Huang (Herba Ephedrae), which is acrid in flavor and warm in nature and capable of promoting perspiration, dispers-

ing cold and relieving dyspnea, can be used to treat affection of Wind-Cold with superficial sthenia symptoms like anhidrosis, cough and dyspnea due to stagnation of the Lung-Qi, while superficial asthenia syndromes such as spontaneous sweating, cough and dyspnea due to Lung-Deficiency are contraindicated syndromes.

(2) Incompatible dispensary. This refers to the toxicity or side-effect produced by or enhanced by the combined use of certain drugs. The ancient medical literature classified the incompatible conditions into "Shi Ba Fan" and "Shi Ju Wei".

"Shi Ba Fan"—eighteen incompatible medicaments, which, if given in combination, are believed to give rise to serious side-effect. They are: Wu Tou (Radix Aconiti) incompatible with Ban Xia (Rhizoma Pinelliae), Gua Lou (Fructus Trichosanthis), Bei Mu (Bulbus Fritillariae), Bai Lian (Radix Ampelopsis) and Bai Ji (Rhizoma Bletilae); Gan Cao (Radix Glycyrrhizae) incompatible with Da Ji (Radix Euphorbiae Pekinensis), Gan Sui (Radix Euphorbiae Kansui), Yuan Hua (Flos Genkwa) and Hai Zao (Sargassum); While Li Lu (Radix Veratri) incompatible with Ren Shen (Radix Ginseng), Sha Shen (Radix Adenophorae Strictae), Dan Shen (Radix Salviae Miltiorrhizae), Xuan Shen (Radix Scrophulariae), Xi Xin (Herba Asari) and Shao Yao (Radix Paeoniae Alba).

"Shi Ju Wei"—nineteen medicaments of mutual antagonism, which, if used in combination, may restrain or neutralize each other's action. These include: Sulfur is antagonistic to crude mirabilite, mercury to arsenic, Lang Du (Radix Euphorbiae Ebracteolatae) to Mi Tuo Seng (Lithargyrum), Ba Dou (Fructus Crotonis) to Qian Niu (Semen Pharbitidis), Ding Xiang (Flos Caryophylli) to Yu Jin (Radix Curcumae) and Chuan Wu (Radix Aconiti), Cao Wu (Radix Aconiti Kusnezoffii) to Xi Jiao (Cornu Rhinoceri Asiatici), crystalized mirabilite to San Leng (Rhizoma Sparganii), Guan Gui (Cortex Cinnamomi) to Chi Shi Zhi (Halloysitum Rubrum), Ren Shen (Radix Ginseng) to Wu Ling Zhi (Faeces Trogopterorum).

However, combined application of some of the incompatible drugs listed above are precedented in ancient and modern times. Experimental studies have shown that some of them will produce greater toxicity if given in combination, while some do not produce any toxicity. So far, there is yet no identical view, and further research in this field is to be carried on. As to the combined use of these drugs, it is prudent to use them cautiously and under no circumstances should they be used together before sound experimental basis and clinical experience are obtained.

(3) Contraindication During Pregnancy. Because some drugs can impair the original Qi of the fetus and lead to threatened abortion or even miscarriage, they should be prohibited or given cautiously during pregnancy. Most of the prohibited drugs are highly toxic or drastic, such as Ba Dou (Fructus Crotonis), Ban Mao (Mylabris), Qian Niu (Semen Pharbitidis), Da Ji (Radix Euphorbiae Pekinensis), Gan Sui (Radix Euphorbiae Kansui), Yuan Hua (Flos Genkwa), Shang Lu (Radix Phytolaccae), She Xiang (Moschus), San Leng (Rhizoma Sparganii), E Zhu (Rhizoma Zedoariae), Shui Zhi (Hirudo), Meng Chong (Tabanus), etc. Drugs which should be used with caution include those which remove Blood stasis to restore menstrual flow, or relieve stagnation of Qi or those with acrid and hot properties, or with lowering and sinking actions, such as Tao Ren (Semen Persicae), Hong Hua (Flos Carthami), Dai Huang (Radix et Rhizoma Rhei), Zhi Shi (Fructus Aurantii Immaturus), Fu Zi (Radix Aconiti Praeparata), Gan Jiang (Rhizoma Zingiberis), Rou Gui (Cortex Cinnamomi), etc. Unless it is absolutely necessary, these two types of drugs should not be applied during pregnancy for fear that it should cause any adverse consequence.

(4) Food Taboo During Medication. In the course of treatment with drugs, food unfit for the disease or contraindicative to a certain drug should be avoided or limited. In general, uncooked, cold, greasy, fishy and stinking, indigestible and irritating food should be avoided or restrained. Also, according to the condition of the patient, some particular food may have to be avoided. For instance, for Cold syndromes, uncooked or cold food should be avoided; for Heat syndromes, hot, spicy and greasy food should be avoided; for indigestion due to Deficiency of the Spleen and Stomach, deep-fried, sticky and greasy food should be avoided; for

suppurative skin infections with pruritus, fish, shrimps, crabs and other seafood and irritating food should be avoided; for patient with dizziness, insomnia and impetuous temperament, pepper, hot pepper and garlic should be avoided. In addition, according to ancient literature, Chang Shan (Radix Dichroae) counteracts scallion; Di Huang (Radix Rehmanniae) and Shou Wu (Radix Polygoni Multiflori) counteract scallion, garlic and turnip; Bo He (Herba Menthae) counteracts turtle flesh; Gan Cao (Radix Glycyrrhizae) counteracts silver carp; Fu Ling (Poria) counteracts vinegar; Tu Fu Ling (Rhizoma Smilacis Glabrae) and Shi Jun Zi (Fructus Quisqualis) counteract tea; while honey counteracts raw scallion. These may serve as a reference in dispensing medicine.

3. Dosage

Dosage refers to the amount of drugs to be used. In Chinese medicine, it chiefly refers to the daily amount of each drug for an adult, and also to the relative amount of different drugs in a recipe. The amount or dosage of each drug in this book, unless otherwise indicated, refers to an adult's daily amount of dried drug in a decoction.

Because dosage is directly related to the curative effect and therefore should be properly determined. Since most of the traditional Chinese drugs are crude drugs with a wide range of safe dosage, the dosage of drugs is not as strict as that of chemicals. Some of them, however, are very drastic in nature or highly toxic, so the dosage of such drugs should be strictly controlled to prevent poisoning. Generally, the following aspects must be taken into consideration in determining the dosage.

(1) The property of the drug. Drugs with toxic and drastic property should be prescribed in small dosages at the beginning and gradually increased to larger dosages but within the range of safe dosage. As soon as the patient's condition improves, the dosage should be reduced or the application discontinued to avoid drug poi-

soning or side-effect. Drugs of great density such as minerals and animal shells should be given in large dosages whereas the light ones such as flowers, leaves, or volatile aromatic drugs can be given in small dosages. Those greasy and thick in tastes should be given in relatively large dosages.

(2) Compatibility and dosage form. As a rule, the same drug, when used alone, may be given in larger dosage than used in a compound recipe; larger in a decoction than in bolus or powder form, larger as a principal ingredient in the compound recipe than as a supplementary one.

(3) The condition of the disease, the age and constitution of the patient. Generally speaking, severe illnesses, emergency cases or intractable diseases need to be treated with larger dosages while the mild and chronic ones with smaller dosages; patients with strong constitution can be given larger dosages than the aged, the weak, postpartum patients and babies. As a rule, the dosage for a child over six years of age is half the dosage for an adult, under five, a quarter, and for an infant, even smaller.

4. Administration

This section covers the decoction of drugs and administration of the different dosage forms of drugs.

(1) Methods for making decoctions. Decoction is a very common form of Chinese pharmaceutical preparations. It is a liquid preparation made by boiling drugs with water or other liquids such as wine or vinegar. When preparing a decoction, drugs are put into a container which has relatively stable chemical properties, such as an earthenware, or an enamal, never an iron or copper pot. Then clean water is added into the container to the level of 2cm above the top of the drugs to soak the drugs for 30～60 minutes. Afterwards, boil the drugs first with a strong fire then with a soft fire for a certain period of time and decant the liquid decoction and add clean water again to the same level to be boiled for the second time. Generally,

two decoctions are got from the same drugs and they are mixed and taken in two times.

The amount of water used and the decocting duration should be decided in line with the properties of the drugs. Drugs for relieving superficies-syndromes and drugs for clearing away heat should be added with less water and decocted with a strong fire for a short time, that is, 5～10 minutes after it boils; while tonics should be added with more water and decocted with a soft fire for a long time that is, 30～40 minutes after it boils. Because of their particular characters, some drugs should be dealt with individually as in the following:

A. To be decocted prior to other drugs: Some minerals and animal shells should be crushed and decocted 20～30 minutes prior to other ingredients because their active compositions can not be extracted easily. These include Sheng Shi Gao (Gypsum Fibrosum), Mu Li (Concha Ostreae), Shi Jue Ming (Concha Haliotidis), Gui Ban (Plastrum Testudinis), Bie Jia (Carapax Trionycis), etc.

B. To be decocted later than other drugs: Some aromatic drugs should be put in after other drugs have been boiled for 10～15 minutes in order to avoid volatilization of their active compositions. These drugs include Bo He (Herba Menthae), Qing Hao (Herba Artemisiae Annuae), Mu Xiang (Radix Aucklandiae), Sha Ren (Fructus Amomi), etc.

C. To be wrapped for decocting: Some powder-like, sticky and villous drugs should be wrapped in a piece of gauze for decocting so that the decoction will not be turbid, irritating to the throat or burnt at the bottom of the pot. These drugs include Xuan Fu Hua (Flos Inulae), Che Qian Zi (Semen Plantaginis), Zao Xin Tu (Terra Flava Usta), etc.

D. To be decocted separately: Some precious drugs, such as Ren Shen (Radix Ginseng), Xi Yang Shen (Radix Panacis Quinquefolii), Ling Yang Jiao (Cornu Antelopis), etc. should be decocted separately so as to avoid any waste of these precious drugs. The decoction obtained can be taken separately or together with the decoction of other drugs after they are mixed.

E. To be infused in boiling water or in finished decoction: Some drugs unsuitable for decocting should be ground into fine powder and then infused with boiling water or in finished decoction for administraion, e. g. Hu Po (Succinum), San Qi (Radix Notoginseng), Zhu Sha (Cinnabaris), etc.

F. To be melted: Some gluey and very sticky drugs should be melted or dissolved in boiling water or finished decoction, e. g. E Jiao (Colla Corii Asini), malt sugar, etc.

(2) Methods of administration. This includes the time for administration and methods of drug application.

A. Time for administration: Usually one dose a day or two doses a day in acute diseases, taken in two or three times. For mild or chronic illness, twice a day in early morning and late evening; for severe and acute diseases, once every four hours. Tonics can be taken before meals; drugs irritating to the stomach and drugs for strengthening the stomach should be taken after meals; anthelmintics and purgatives should be taken with an empty stomach; anti-malaria drugs should be taken two hours prior to the attack; tranquilizers should be taken before bed-time. Drugs for chronic diseases should be taken at regular time; drugs for acute diseases should be taken instantly. Time for administration should always be 1～2 hours before or after meals so as to assure the therapeutic effect.

B. Methods of drug application: As a rule, decoction is taken while it is warm. Cold-natured drugs for treating Heat syndromes may be taken cold, while hot-natured drugs for treating Cold syndromes may be taken hot. In case of Cold syndrome with pseudo-Heat symptoms, it is better to take the medicine of hot nature when it is cold, and on the other hand, Heat syndrome with pseudo-Cold syndromes, hot decoction of drugs of cold nature can be taken. For unconscious or lockjaw patients, the decoction can be given by nasal feeding. For vomiting, the decoction can be concentrated and given frequently in small amount. Pills, boluses and powder should be taken with warm boiled water unless otherwise stated.

CLASSIFIED INTRODUCTION

Superficies-syndrome Relieving Drugs

Drugs whose principal action is dispersing the pathogenic factors from the superficies of the body and relieving superficies-syndromes are included in this category.

Superficies-syndrome relieving drugs are ususlly acrid in flavor, volatile in property, and are indicated for chilliness, fever, headache, general pain with or without sweat, floating pulse, etc. caused by affection of exopathogenic factors. In addition, drugs of this category can also promote the dispersing function of the Lung, relieve asthma, promote diuresis and skin eruptions, and therefore they are also indicated for asthmatic cough, edema and incomplete skin eruptions.

According to differences of their properties, superficies-syndrome relieving drugs can be divided into two groups: superficies-syndrome relieving drugs with acrid flavor and warm nature, and superficies-syndrome relieving drugs with acrid flavor and cool nature. They should be chosen in accordance with different syndromes and used in combination with drugs of other categories to promote Qi circulation, strengthen Yang or tonify Yin.

As these drugs are acrid, aromatic and diaphoretic in property, care should be taken to avoid excessive sweating, lest it consume the Qi and Body-Fluid. So they are contraindicated in profuse sweating, impairment of Body-Fluid by febrile diseases, fever due to Yin Deficiency as well as suppurative skin infections, stranguria and bleedings. In addition, these drugs should not be decocted for very long for fear of decreasing their efficacy.

1. Superficies-syndrome Relieving Drugs with Acrid Flavor and Warm Nature

Drugs of this group are also referred to as drugs for dispersing Wind-Cold, as they are mainly capable of dispersing pathogenic Wind-Cold. These drugs are indicated in chilliness, anhidrosis, headache and general aching, floating and tense pulse, etc. caused by affection of Wind-Cold, or in another word, common cold. Some of them can also be used for Wind-Cold with Dampness, the onset of rheumatic pain, edema and other superficies-syndromes characterized by Wind-Cold.

As these drugs are potent in inducing perspiration, they should not be applied to syndromes not appropriate for diaphoretics.

1.1. Ma Huang (Herba Ephedrae)

Description The herbaceous stem of Ephedra sinica stapf, Ephedra equisetina Bge. Family Ephedraceae.

Characteristics Acrid and slightly bitter in flavor, warm in nature, and attributive to the Lung and Urinary Bladder Channels.

Action Inducing sweat to expel the exogenous pathogens from the body surface, promoting the function of Lung to relieve asthma, and promoting diuresis to reduce edema.

Indications

(1) Superficial sthenia-syndromes caused by affection of exogenous evils manifested by chilliness, fever, pain all over the body, blocked nose, thin and white tongue-coat, floating and taut pulse, and anhidrosis. Usually it is used with Gui Zhi (Ramulus Cinnamo-

mi), e. g. Mahuang Tang (Herba Ephedrae Decoction).

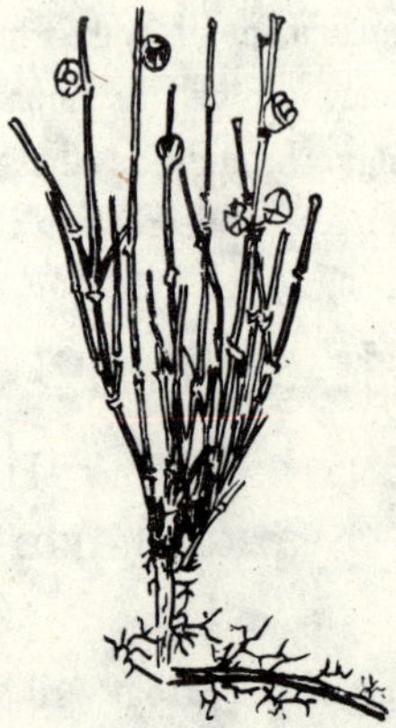

(2) Cough and dyspnea due to Wind-Cold and stagnation of the Lung-Qi. Usually used with Xing Ren (Semen Armeniacae Amarum) and Gan Cao (Radix Glycyrrhizae), e. g. Sanao Tang (Decoction of Three Crude Drugs). In the case of dyspnea and cough due to invasion by pathogenic Heat into the Lung, Shi Gao (Gypsum Fibrosum) and Xing Ren (Semen Armeniacae Amarum) can be used together with Ma Huang (Herba Ephedrae), e. g. Ma Xing Shi Gan Tang (Decoction of Herba Ephedrae, Semen Armeniacae Amarum, Gypsum Fibrosum and Radix Glycyrrhizae); in the case of attack of superficies by Wind-Cold and retention of Phlegm in the Lung, it is used with Xi Xin (Herba Asari), Gan Jiang (Rhizoma Zingiberis), Ban Xia (Rhizoma Pinelliae), Wu Wei Zi (Fructus Schisandrae), etc., as in Xiao Qinglong Tang (Minor Decoction of Green Dragon).

(3) Edema complicated with superficies-syndrome. Usually used together with Sheng Jiang (Rhizoma Zingiberis Recens), Bai Zhu (Rhizoma Atractylodis Macrocephalae), etc. e. g. Yuebi Jiazhu Tang (Decoction for Relieving Edema plus Rhizoma Atractylodis Macrocephalae).

(4) Rheumatism, arthralgia-syndromes, carbuncles and subcutaneous nodules or itching from urticaria. To treat rheumatism and arthralgia, Gui Zhi (Ramulus Cinnamomi), Bai Zhu (Rhizoma Atractylodis Macrocephalae) can be used together with Ma Huang (Herba Ephedrae), e. g. Mahuang Jia Zhu Tang (Decoction of Herba Ephedrae with Rhizoma Atractylodis Macrocephalae); for carbuncles and subcutaneous nodules, Shu Di (Radix Rehmanniae Praeparata), Bai Jie Zi (Semen Sinapis Albae), etc. may be used together with Ma Huang (Herba Ephedrae), e. g. Yanghe Tang (Yang-activating

Decoction); for itching from urticaria, Jing Jie (Herba Schizonepetae), Fang Feng (Radix Ledebouriellae) and Chan Tui (Periostracum Cicadae) can be used together with Ma Huang (Herba Ephedrae).

Administration 1.5~9g for making a decoction. Unprepared for superficies-syndromes, prepared for relieving asthma.

Precautions Not administered to patients with spontaneous sweating due to Deficiency of superficies or with night sweat due to Yin Deficiency, or with asthma and cough resulting from failure of the Kidney-Qi to aid the Lung in regulating inspiration.

1.2. Gui Zhi (Ramulus Cinnamomi)

Description The tender branch of Cinnamomum cassia Presl. Family Lauraceae.

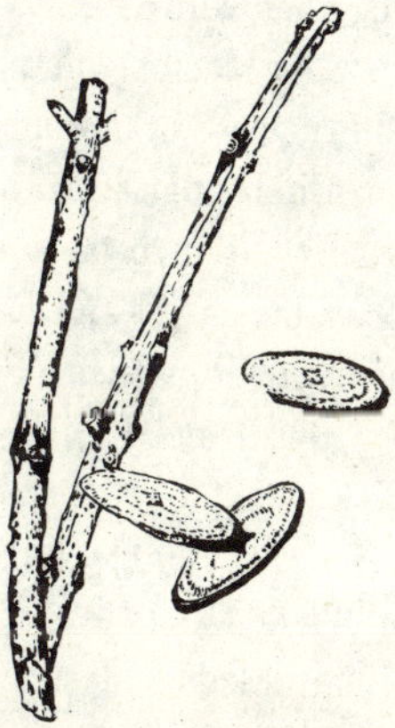

Characteristics Acrid and sweat in flavor, warm in nature, and acting on the Heart, Lung, Spleen and Urinary Bladder Channels.

Action Inducing perspiration to expel the pathogenic evils from the body surface, warming the meridians and reinforcing Yang.

Indications

(1) Superficies-syndromes caused by Wind-Cold with or without sweat. In the case of absence of sweat, Ma Huang (Herba Ephedrae) can be used together, e.g. Mahuang Tang (Herba Ephedrae Decoction); in the case of presence of sweat, Bai Shao (Radix Paeoniae Alba) can be used together, e.g. Guizhi Tang (Ramulus Cinnamomi Decoction).

(2) Arthralgia due to Wind-Cold-Dampness, pain in the shoulder joints. Usually used together with Fu Zi (Radix Aconiti Praeparata) and Sheng Jiang (Rhizoma Zingiberis Recens), e.g. Guizhi Fuzi

Tang (Decoction of Ramulus Cinnamomi and Radix Aconiti Praeparata); it can also be used together with Qiang Huo (Rhizome seu Radix Noto-pterygii), Xi Xin (Herba Asari) and Fang Feng (Radix Ledebouriellae). In the case of Deficiency in Ying and Wei, arthralgia due to stagnation of Blood, Huang Qi (Radix Astragali seu Hedysari) and ShaoYao (Radix Paeoniae Alba) can be used together with Gui Zhi (Ramulus Cinnamomi), e. g. Huang Qi Guizhi Wuwu Tang (Decoction of Five Drugs Including Radix Astragali seu Hedysari and Ramulus Cinnamomi).

(3) Deficiency of Heart-Yang, chest pain radiating to the back, back pain radiating to the heart, or tight chest, palpitation, precordial pain and irregular, slow and intermittent pulse. For the former, used together with Gua Lou (Fructus Trichosanthis) and Xie Bai (Bulbus Allii Macrostemi), as in Zhishi Xiebai Guizhi Tang (Decoction of Fructus Aurantii Immaturus, Bulbus Allii Macrostemi and Ramulus Cinnamomi); for the latter, usually used together with Gan Cao (Radix Glycyrrhizae), e. g. Guizhi Gancao Tang (Decoction of Ramulus Cinnamomi and Radix Glycyrrhizae); it can also be used together with Ren Shen (Radix Ginseng), Mai Men Dong (Radix Ophiopogonis) and E Jiao (Colla Corii Asini), e. g. Zhi Gancao Tang (Decoction of Prepared Radix Glycyrrhizae).

(4) Deficiency of Heart-Yang and Spleen-Yang resulting in retention of Water-Dampness, Phlegm retention and Water retention in the Urinary Bladder, dysuria and edema. For Phlegm retention, usually used with Bai Zhu (Rhizoma Atractylodis Macrocephalae) and Fu Ling (Poria), e. g. Ling Gui Zhu Gan Tang (Decoction of Poria, Ramulus Cinnamomi, Atractylodis Macrocephalae and Glycyrrhizae); for hypofunction of Urinary Bladder, usually used with Fu Ling (Poria), Ze Xie (Rhizoma Alismatis), e. g. Wu Ling San (Powder of Five Drugs Including Poria).

(5) Stagnation of Blood-Cold leading to amenorrhea and menorrhalgia. Usually used together with Dang Gui (Angelicae Sinensis), Chuan Xiong (Rhizoma Ligustici Chuanxiong) and Wu Zhu Yu (Fructus Euodiae), e. g. Wenjing Tang (Decoction for Warming the Channels). In the case of amenorrhea complicated

with a mass in the lower abdomen, used with Mu Dan Pi (Cortex Moutan Radicis), Shao Yao (Radix Paeoniae Alba), Tao Ren (Semen Persicae) and Fu Ling (Poria), e. g. Guizhi Fuling Wan (Bolus of Ramulus Cinnamomi and Poria).

(6) Stagnation of Yin-Cold, adverse rising of the vital energy of the Chong Channel leading to gas rushing up, or gangrene of the finger or toe, and chilblain. For the former, usually used with Gan Cao (Radix Glycyrrhizae) and Sheng Jiang (Rhizoma Zingiberis Recens); for the latter, usually used with Xi Xin (Herba Asari), Dang Gui (Radix Angelicae Sinensis), Tong Cao (Medulla Tetrapanacis), e. g. Danggui Sini Tang (Decoction of Radix Angelicae Sinensis for Restoring Yang).

Administration 3～10g for making a decoction.

Precautions Administered with caution to patients with internal Heat due to Yin Deficiency or patients with Heat Excess. Not applied to pregnant women or women with hypermenorrhea.

1. 3. Jing Jie (Herba Schizonepetae)

Description The branch and leaf with inflorescence of Schizonepeta tenuifolia (Benth). Briq. and S. multifida (L.) Briq.. Family Labiatae.

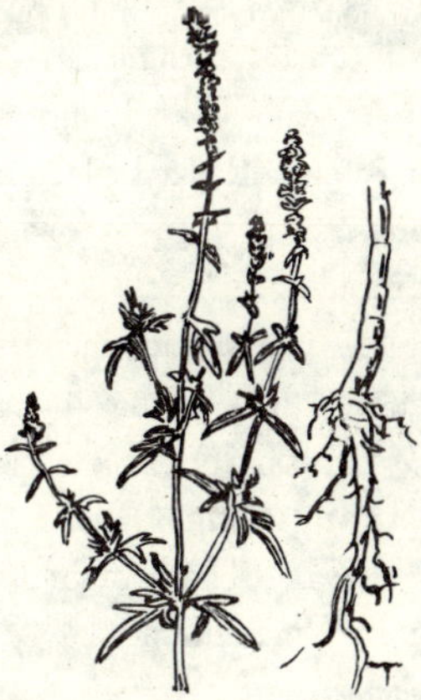

Characteristics Acrid in flavor, slightly warm in nature, and acting on the Lung and Liver Channels.

Action Expelling pathogenic Wind, inducing diaphoresis, promoting eruptions and arresting bleeding.

Indications

(1) Affection of pathogenic Wind, fever, anhidrosis, headache and general aching of the body. In the case of affection of Wind-Cold, usually used together with Fang Feng (Radix Ledebouriellae)

and Qiang Huo (Rhizoma seu Radix Noto-pterygii), e. g. Jing Fang Baidu San (Schizonepeta and Ledebouriella Powder for Expelling Wind); in the case of Wind-Heat manifested as sore throat and red eyes, often used together with Bo He (Herba Menthae), Niu Bang Zi (Fructus Arctii) and Jin Yin Hua (Flos Lonicerae), e. g. Yin Qiao San (Powder of Flos Lonicerae and Fructus Forsythiae)); in the case of severe sore throat and hoarseness, used with Jie Geng (Radix Platycodi) and Gan Cao (Radix Glycyrrhizae), e. g. Jing Jie Tang (Decoction of Herba Schizonepetae and Radix Platycodi).

(2) Incomplete eruption of measles and itching from urticaria. In the case of Wind-Cold, used with Fang Feng (Radix Ledebouriellae) and Ma Huang (Herba Ephedrae); in the case of Wind-Heat, used with Bo He (Herba Menthae), Chan Tui (Periostracum Cicadae) and Niu Bang Zi (Fructus Arctii).

(3) Epistaxis, hemafecia and metrorrhagia. Usually carbonized and used with Ce Bai Ye (Cacumen Biotae), stir-fried Huai Hua (Flos Sophorae), Di Yu Tan (Radix Sanguisorbae Carbonisatus), etc.

(4) Early-stage skin inflammation with superficies-syndromes such as furuncles, carbuncles, scrofula and anal fistula. Usually used with Jin Yin Hua (Flos Lonicerae), Lian Qiao (Fructus Forsythiae) and Fang Feng (Radix Ledebouriellae).

Administration 3～6g for making a decoction. Carbonized for arresting bleeding.

Precautions Not administered to patients with spontaneous perspiration due to Deficiency of the superficies, or with Yin Deficiency and Fire Excess. Not decocted for too long.

1. 4. Fang Feng (Radix Ledebouriellae)

Description The root of Ledebouriella divaricata (Turcz.) Hiroe. Family Umbelliferae.

Characteristics Acrid and sweet in flavor, slightly warm in nature and acting on the Lung, Liver, Spleen and Urinary Bladder Channels.

Action Expelling Wind and inducing diaphoresis to relieve superficies-syndromes, dispersing Cold and Dampness, relieving spasm and pain.

Indications

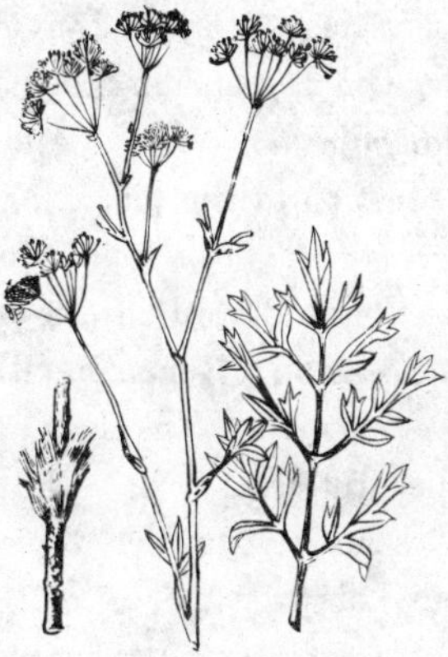

(1) Headache, general aching, fever and chilliness caused by affection of pathogenic evils. In the case of Wind-Cold invasion, usually used together with Zi Su (Folium Perillae), Jing Jie (Herba Schizonepetae), etc.; for Wind-Heat type, used with Jing Jie (Herba Schizonepetae), Lian Qiao (Fructus Forsythiae), Bo He (Herba Menthae), etc.; in the case of measles, urticaria or itching, used with Jing Jie (Herba Schizonepetae, Bai Ji Li (Fructus Tribuli), etc.

(2) Affection of pathogenic Wind-Dampness or pain from arthralgia. Usually used together with Qiang Huo (Rhizome seu Radix Noto-pterygii), Du Huo (Radix Angelicae Pubescentis), Chuan Xiong (Rhizoma Ligustici Chuanxiong), etc., e. g. Qianghuo Shengshi Tang (Decoction of Rhizoma seu Radix Noto-pterygii for Dispersing Dampness).

(3) Opisthotonos and lockjaw caused by tetanus, deviation of mouth and eye caused by invasion of Wind-evil. For the former, usually used with Qiang Huo (Rhizoma seu Radix Noto-pterygii), Tian Nan Xing (Rhizoma Arisaematis) and Tian Ma (Rhizoma Gastrodiae), etc., e. g., Yu Zhen San (Powder with Marvellous Effect); for the latter, usually used with Qiang Huo (Rhizoma seu Radix Noto-pterygii), Jiang Can (Bombyx Batryticatus), Quan Xie (Scorpio), etc.

(4) Abdominal distension or pain, diarrhea due to stagnation of the iver-Qi and Deficiency of the Spleen. Usually used with Chen Pi (Pericarpium Citri Reticulatae), Bai Zhu (Rhizoma Atractylodys Macrocephalae) and Bai Shao (Radix Paeoniae Alba), e. g. Tong Xie Yao Fang (Prescription of Importance for Diarrhea with Pain).

(5) Carbonized to treat fresh bloody stools, metrorrhagia and

metrostaxis. Usually used with Jing Jie Tan (Herba Schizonepetae Carbonisatus), Di Yu Tan (Radix Sanguisorbae Carbonisatus), Huang Qin Tan (Radix Scutellariae Carbonisatus), etc.

Administration 3～10g for making a decoction. It can also be made into powder or pills.

Precautions Not applied to Yin Deficiency and Fire Excess, or spasm due to Blood Deficiency.

1. 5. Zi Su (Herba Perillae)

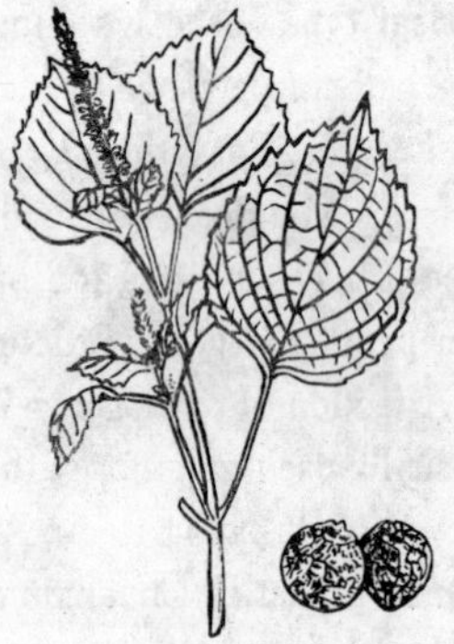

Description The herb of Perilla frutescens (L.) Britt. var. acuta (Thunb.) Kudo. Family Labiatae.

Characteristics Acrid in flavor, warm in nature, and acting on the Lung and Spleen Channels.

Action Inducing perspiration to expel the exogenous Cold from the body surface, promoting the circulation of Qi to soothe the Middle-jiao, detoxicating fish and crab poison.

Indications

(1) Common cold of Wind-Cold type manifested as chilliness, anhidrosis, in some cases accompanied with cough and stuffiness sensation in the chest. For inducing diaphoresis, usually it is used together with Jing Jie (Herba Schizonepetae) and Fang Feng (Radix Ledebouriellae), and in the case of accompanying cough, usually used with Qian Hu (Radix Peucedani) and Xing Ren (Semen Armeniacae Amarum), e. g. Xing Su San (Powder of Semen Armeniacae Amarum and Herba Perillae); in the case of tight chest, usually used together with Chen Pi (Pericarpium Citri Reticulatae) and Xiang Fu (Rhizoma Cyperi), e. g. Xiang Su San (Powder of Rhizoma Cyperi and Herba Perillae).

(2) Tight chest, vomiting, etc. caused by stagnation of Spleen-Qi

and Stomach-Qi. In the case of excessive Cold, used with Huo Xiang (Herba Agastachis); in the case of excessive Heat, used with Huang Lian (Rhizome Coptidis); in the case of Phlegm retention and Qi stagnation, used with Hou Po (Cortex Magnoliae Officialis) and Ban Xia (Rhizome Pinelliae); while in the case of morning sickness complicated by stuffy sensation in the chest and abdomen, and threatened abortion, usually used with Sha Ren (Fructus Amomi) and Chen Pi (Pericarpium Citri Reticulatae).

(3) Abdominal pain, vomiting and diarrhea caused by eating fish or crab. Used either alone or together with fresh ginger and garlic for making a decoction, the compound recipe being more effective.

Administration 3～10g for making a decoction.

Precautions Not used for Yin Deficiency, internal Heat or Heat-Excess syndromes.

1. 6. Xiang Ru (Herba Elsholtziae seu Moslae)

Description Herb of Elsholtzia splendens Nakai ex F. Maekawa and Mosla chinensis Maxim., Family Labiatae.

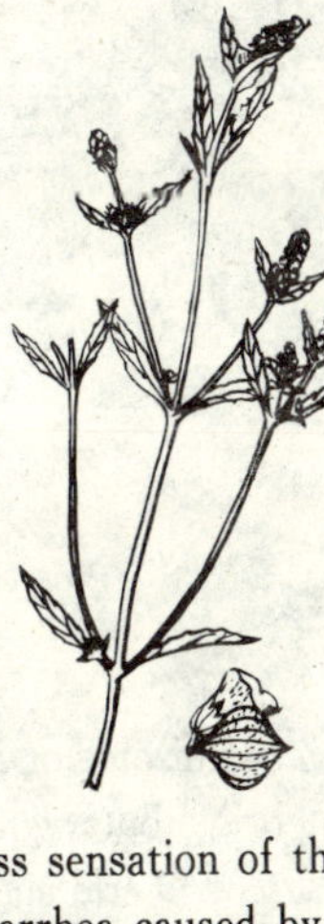

Characteristics Acrid in flavor, slightly warm in nature, and acting on the Lung and Stomach Channels.

Action Inducing diaphoresis, dispersing Dampness and regulating the Middle-jiao, promoting diuresis to relieve edema.

Indications

(1) Chilliness, anhidrosis, heaviness sensation of the head with headache, tight chest, vomiting and diarrhea caused by affection of both exogenous Cold and internal Dampness during summer and autumn time. For treatment, usually used together with Bian Dou (Semen Dolichoris Album) and Hou Po (Cortex Magnoliae Officinalis), e. g. Xiangru Yin (Herba Elsholtziae seu Moslae Drink).

(2) Edema and dysuria caused by retention of Water-Dampness. Usually used alone or together with Bai Zhu (Rhizome Atractylodis Macrocephalae), e. g. Xiangru Wan (Herba Elsholtziae seu Moslae Bolus). For treating edema due to Spleen Deficiency, it is used with Bai Zhu (Rhizome Atractylodis Macrocephalae), Fu Ling (Poria) and Yi Yi Ren (Semen Coicis).

Administration 3～10g for making a decoction. It can also be made into boluses or powder. Decocted a short time for treating superficies-syndromes, a long time for edema.

Precautions Not administered for superficies Deficiency with much perspiration.

1.7. Qiang Huo (Rhizome seu Radix Notopterygii)

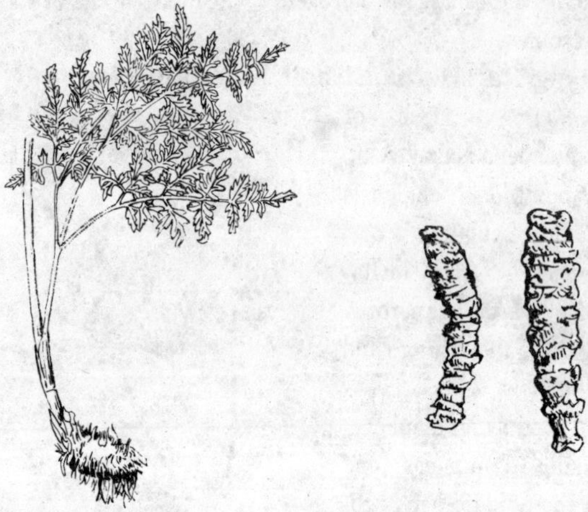

Description Rhizome or root of Notopterygium incisum Ting ex H. T. Chang or Notopterygium forbesii Boiss. Family Umbelliferae.

Characteristics Acrid and bitter in flavor, warm in nature, and acting on the Urinary Bladder and Kidney Channels.

Action Expelling Cold, inducing diaphoresis, removing Wind and Dampness, relieving pain and rheumatism.

Indications

(1) Chilliness, fever, headache, general pain, etc. caused by com-

mon cold of Wind-Cold type. Usually used together with Fang Feng (Radix Ledebouriellae), Xi Xin (Herba Asari) and Bai Zhi (Radix Angelica Dahuricae), e. g. Jiuwei Qianghuo Tang (Notopterygii Decoction of Nine Ingredients). In the case of severe headache and blocked nose due to affection of Wind-Cold, Chuan Wu (Radix Aconiti) and Xi Xin (Herba Asari) may be applied with Qiang Huo (Rhizome seu Radix Notopterygii), e. g. Jiawei Qiang Wu San (Augmented Powder of Notopterygii and Aconiti).

(2) Pain and soreness of the limbs, joints, shoulders and back, especially pain of the upper body caused by pathogenic Wind-Cold and Dampness. Usually used with Fang Feng (Radix Ledebouriellae), Jiang Huang (Rhizome Curcumae Longae), Dang Gui (Radix Angelicae Sinensis), e. g. Juan Bi Tang (Decoction for Removing Pain and Soreness).

(3) Lockjaw, stiffness of nape and opisthotonos caused by tetanus. Usually used with Fang Feng (Radix Ledebouriellae), Bai Zhi (Radix Angelicae Dahuricae), Bai Fu Zi (Rhizome Typhonii), e. g. Yuzhen San (Powder with Marvellous Effect).

Administration 3~10g for making a decoction.

Precautions Not applied to Blood Dryness due to Yin Deficiency.

1. 8. Bai Zhi (Radix Angelicae Dahuricae)

Description Root of Angelica dahurica (Fisch. ex Hoffm.) Benth. et Hook. f. var formosana (Boiss.) Shan et Yuan. Family Umbelliferae.

Characteristics Acrid in flavor, warm in nature, and acting on the Lung and Stomach Channels.

Action Expelling pathogenic Cold by inducing diaphoresis, removing pathogenic Wind and Dampness, regulating meridians to relieve pain, subduing swelling and promoting pus discharge.

Indications

(1) Headache, blocked nose or sinusitis leading to headache caused by affection of exopathogenic Wind-Cold. In the case of headache and blocked nose, used either alone or together with Qiang Huo (Rhizome seu Radix Notopterygii) and Fang Feng (Radix Lede-

bouriellae), e. g. Jiuwei Qiang Huo Tang (Notopterygii Decoction of Nine Ingredients); in the case of sinusitis leading to headache, used with Cang Er Zi (Fructus Xanthii), Xin Yi (Flos Magnoliae), etc.

(2) Pain of ossa frontale, recurrent headache and toothache caused by pathogenic Wind, used with Chuan Xiong (Rhizome Ligustici Chuanxiong), Fang Feng (Radix Ledebouriellae), e. g. Chuanxiong Cha Tiao San (Chuanxiong Mixture); in the case of toothache induced by Wind-Cold, used with Xi Xin (Herba Asari); while in the case of toothache induced by Wind-Heat, usually used together with Shi Gao (Gypsum Fibrosum), Huang Qin (Radix Scutellariae), Jing Jie (Herba Schizonepetae), etc. e. g. Qing Yang San Huo Tang (Decoction for Clearing Yang and Dispersing Fire).

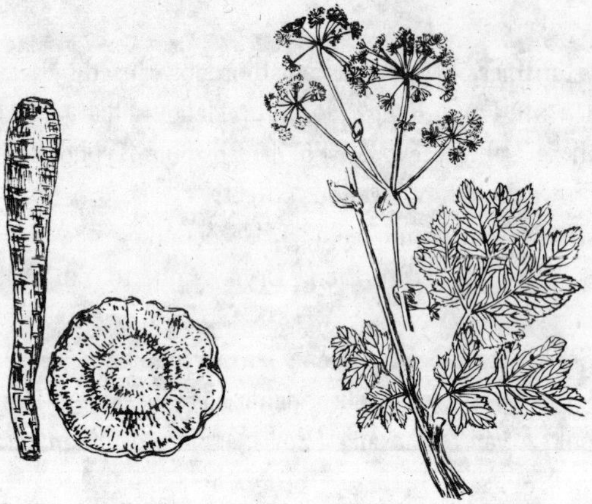

(3) Swelling and pain of carbuncle. In the initial stage of carbuncle, usually used with Gua Lou (Fructus Trichosanthis), Zhe Bei Mu (Bulbus Fritillariae Thunbergii), Pu Gong Ying (Herba Taraxaci), etc.; while in the case of pus formation, used with Dang Gui (Radix Angelicae Sinensis), Zao Jiao Ci (Spina Gleditsiae), Chuan Shan Jia (Squama Mantis), etc.

(4) Pruritus of skin and leukorrhea due to Cold-Dampness. For pruritus, used with Bai Xian Pi (Cortex Dictamni Radicis), Chan Tui (Periostracum Cicadae), etc., for the latter, usually used with Fu

Ling (Poria), Bai Zhu (Rhizoma Atractylodis Macrocephalae), Hai Piao Xiao (Os Sepiae), etc.

Administration 3～10g for making a decoction.

Precautions Not administered to patients with Yin Deficiency and Fire Excess, or Deficiency of both Liver-Yin and Kidney-Yin, or asthenia of Liver-Yang.

1.9. Xin Yi (Flos Magnoliae)

Description The flower bud of Magnolia biondii Pamp., Magnolia denudata Desr. or Magnolia sprengeri Pamp. Family Magnoliaceae.

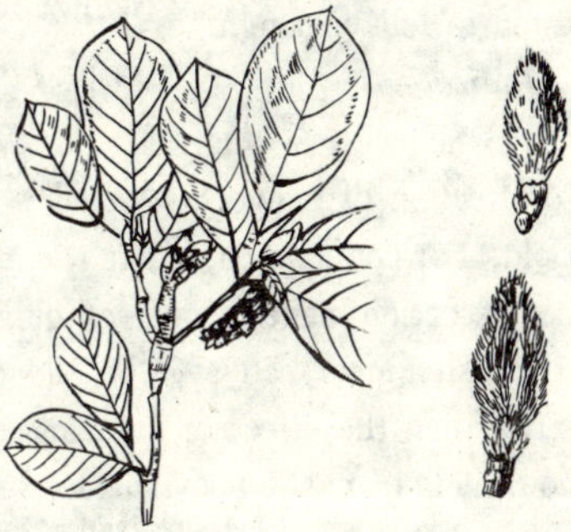

Characteristics Acrid in flavor, warm in nature, and acting on the Lung and Stomach Channels.

Action Expelling Wind and Cold, and clearing the nasal passage.

Indications

Headache, blocked nose and sinusitis caused by affection of exogenous Wind-Cold. For treating headache and blocked nose, used with Fang Feng (Radix Ledebouriellae), Bai Zhi (Radix Angelicae Dahuricae) and Chuan Xiong (Rhizoma Ligustici Chuanxiong); for treating sinusitis manifested by blocked nose, headache, loss of sense of smell, and frequent and turbid nasal discharge, used together with Bai Zhi (Radix Angelicae Dahuricae), Xi Xin (Herba Asari), etc. for Wind-Cold type, and used with Bo He (Herba Menthae), Huang Qin (Radix Scutellariae), etc. for Wind-Heat type.

Administration 3～10g for making a decoction (usually wrapped in cloth).

Precautions Not used for Yin Deficiency and Fire Excess, or asthenia of Liver-Yang.

1.10. Sheng Jiang (Rhizoma Zingiberi Recens)

Description Rhizome of Zingiber officinale (Wild.) Rosc. Family Zingiberaceae.

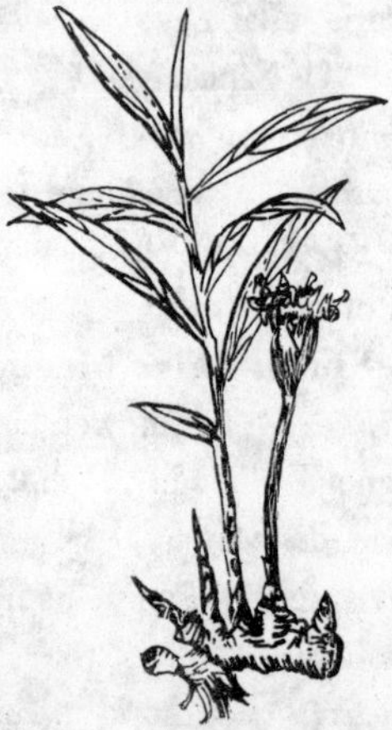

Characteristics Acrid in flavor, slightly warm in nature, and acting on the Lung and Spleen Channels.

Action Inducing diaphoresis, warming the Middle-jiao to arrest vomiting, warming the Lung to relieve cough.

Indications

(1) Superficies-syndromes due to affection of exogenous Wind-Cold. For common cold, take the hot decoction made from fresh ginger after adding brown sugar into it. Fresh ginger can also be added into some other decoctions to strengthen the effect of inducing perspiration and expelling exogenous evils from the body surface, e. g. Guizhi Tang (Ramulus Cinnamomi Decoction).

(2) Vomiting, pain and mass in the abdomen caused by retention of fluid. For treating vomiting due to Stomach-Cold, usually used with Ban Xia (Rhizoma Pinelliae), e. g. Xiao Banxia Tang (Minor Decoction of Rhizoma Pinelliae); for treating vomiting due to Stomach-Heat, usually used with Zhu Ru (Caulis Bambusae in Taeniam) and Huang Lian (Rhizoma Coptidis). In the case of pain and mass in the abdomen caused by retention of fluid, usually used with Ban Xia (Rhizoma Pinelliae), Huang Lian (Rhizoma Coptidis), Dang Shen (Radix Codonopsis Pilosulae), etc., e. g. Shengjiang Xiexin Tang (Ginger Decoction for Clearing Stomach-Heat).

(3) Cough, profuse phlegm and tight chest due to Phlegm retention from Wind-Cold. Usually used with Ma Huang (Herba Ephedrae) and Xing Ren (Semen Armeniacae Amarum).

(4) Detoxication for Ban Xia (Rhizoma Pinelliae), Nan Xing (Rhizoma Arisaematis), fish and crab. For poison of Ban Xia (Rhizoma Pinelliae) or Nan Xing (Rhizoma Arisaematis), fresh ginger can be pounded into a paste and taken after being infused with boiling wa-

ter or after being made into a decoction; for poison of fish and crab, usually used together with Zi Su (Folium Perillae).

Administration 3～10g for making a decoction or infusion after being pounded into a paste.

Precautions Not used for Fire-Heat syndromes like internal Heat due to Yin Deficiency or preponderance of Heat.

2. Superficies-syndrome Relieving Drugs with Acrid Flavor and Cool Nature

Also called medicines for dispersing Wind-Heat. Mainly indicated for fever, mild chilliness, dry throat and thirst, thin yellowish tongue coat, floating and rapid pulse, etc. caused by affection of exogenous Wind-Heat or early stage seasonal febrile diseases. Some drugs in this group are also capable of treating headache, redness of the eyelids, sore throat, and some are capable of opening the inhibited Lung-Qi to relieve cough, and dispersing Wind to promote skin eruption. Usually they are used together with Heat-clearing and anti-toxic drugs.

2.1. Bo He (Herba Menthae)

Description The branch and leaf of Mentha haplocalyx Briq. Family Labiatae.

Characteristics Acrid in flavor, cool in nature, acting on the Liver and Lung Channels.

Action Dispersing Wind-Heat, clearing away Heat from head and eyes, and promoting skin eruptions.

Indications

(1) Fever, mild chilliness, headache, anhidrosis, etc. induced by common cold of Wind-Heat type, and early stage seasonal febrile diseases. Usually used together with Jin Yin Hua (Flos Lonicerae), Lian Qiao (Fructus Forsythiae), Niu Bang Zi (Fructus Arctii), etc. e.g. Yin Qiao San (Powder of Flos Lonicerae and Fructus Forsythi-

ae).

(2) Headache, dizziness, red eyelids, or sore throat caused by attack of pathogenic Wind-Heat. For headache and red eyelids, Bo He (Herba Menthae) is used together with Sang Ye (Folium Mori), Ju Hua (Flos Chrysanthemi), Huang Qin (Radix Scutellariae), etc.; for sore and swelling of the throat, used together with Jie Geng (Radix Platycodi), Jiang Can (Bombyx Batryticatus) and Jing Jie (Herba Schizonepetae). e. g. Liu Wei Tang (Decoction of Six Ingredients).

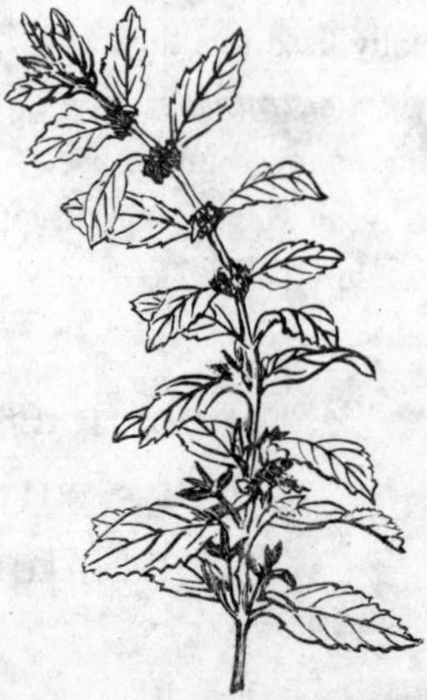

(3) Early stage eruptive diseases and urticaria, itching, etc. Usually used with Chan Tui (Periostracum Cicadae), Jing Jie (Herba Schizonepetae), Niu Bang Zi (Fructus Arctii) and Lian Qiao (Fructus Forsythiae), e. g. Jiajian Gegen Tang (Modified Radix Puerariae Decoction).

(4) Tight chest and distending pain in the costal region caused by stagnation of Qi and depression of Liver-Qi. Usually used in combination with Chai Hu (Radix Bupleuri), Chen Pi (Pericarpium Citri Reticulatae), Bai Shao (Radix Paeoniae Alba), e. g. Xiao Yao San (Ease Powder).

(5) Abdominal pain, vomiting and diarrhea caused by attack of Summer-Heat. Usually used with Huo Xiang (Herba Agastachis) and Xiang Fu (Rhizoma Cyperi).

Administration 2～10g for making a decoction. Not to be decocted too long.

Precautions Not applied to patients with weak constitution and with much perspiration.

2. 2. Sang Ye (Folium Mori)

Description Leaf of Morus alba L., Family Moraceae.

Characteristics Bitter and sweet in flavor, cold in nature, and acting on the Lung and Liver Channels.

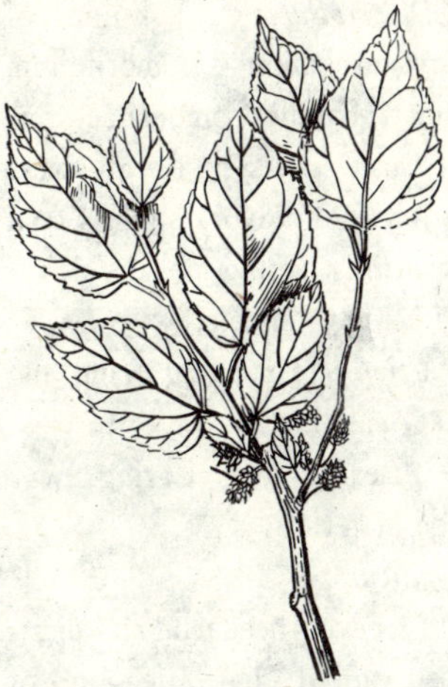

Action Dispersing Wind and Heat, clearing away Liver-Fire to treat eye diseases.

Indications

(1) Fever, dizziness, headache, cough and sore throat caused by affection of Wind-Heat. Usually used together with Ju Hua (Flos Chrysanthemi), Lian Qiao (Fructus Forsythiae), Jie Geng (Radix Platycodi), etc., e. g. Sang Ju Yin (Drink of Folium Mori and Flos Chrysanthemi).

(2) Cough with thick and scanty phlegm, dry nose and dry throat due to impairment of the Lung by the pathogenic Dryness. Usually used with Xing Ren (Semen Armeniacae Amarum), Mai Dong (Radix Ophiopogonis), etc. e. g. Sang Xing Tang (Decoction of Folium Mori and Semen Armeniacae Amarum).

(3) Redness, swelling, pain and profuse tear of the eye due to upward attack of the Wind-Heat or sthenic-Heat of the Liver Meridian. Usually used in combination with Ju Hua (Flos Chrysanthemi) and Jue Ming Zi (Semen Cassiae) to make a decoction. Sang Ye (Folium Mori) can also be decocted alone for a wash. In the case of Yin Deficiency of the Liver and Kidney leading to blurring of vision, usually made into pills with Hei Zhi Ma (Semen Sesami Nigrum) and prepared honey, e. g. Sang Ma Wan (Pill of Folium Mori and Semen Sesami Nigrum).

Administration 5～10g for making a decoction. it can also be made into pills or powder.

Precautions Applied with caution to patients with poor appetite or with diarrhea.

2. 3. Ju Hua (Flos Chrysanthemi)

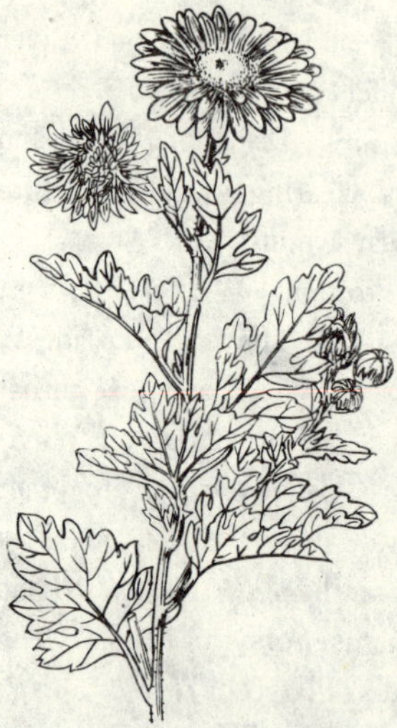

Description Capitulum of Chrysanthemum morifolium Ramat. Family Compositae.

Characteristics Acrid, sweet and bitter in flavor, slightly cold in nature, acting on the Liver and Lung Channels.

Action Expelling Wind and Heat, calming the Liver to treat eye diseases, and clearing away toxic materials.

Indications

(1) Fever, headache and dizziness caused by affection of Wind-Heat or early stage febrile diseases. Usually used together with Sang Ye (Folium Mori) and Bo He (Herba Menthae), e. g. Sang Ju Yin (Drink of Folium Mori and Flos Chrysanthemi). In the case of high fever, usually used together with Huang Qin (Radix Scutellariae) and Lu Gen (Rhizoma Phragmitis).

(2) Redness, swelling and pain of the eye caused by Wind-Heat in the Lung Meridian or upward attack of Liver-Fire, blurring of vision due to Yin Deficiency of the Liver and Kidney, for the former, usually used with Sang Ye (Folium Mori), Xia Ku Cao (Spica Prunellae), Chan Tui (Periostracum Cicadae), etc.; for the latter, usually used with Gou Qi Zi (Fructus Lycii) and Shu Di Huang (Radix Rehmanniae Praeparata), e. g. Qi Ju Dihuang Wan (Bolus of Rehmannia with Wolfberry and Chrysanthemum).

(3) Headache and dizziness due to hypoactivity of Liver-Yang. Usually used in combination with Shi Jue Ming (Concha Haliotidis), Bai Shao (Radix Paeoniae Alba), Gou Teng (Ramulus Uncariae cum Uncis), etc, e. g. Lingyang Gouteng Tang (Decoction of Cornu Antilopis and Ramulus Uncariae cum Uncis).

(4) Swelling and redness from carbuncles. Usually used with Jin

Yin Hua (Flos Lonicerae), Gan Cao (Radix Glycyrrhizea), etc.

Administration 10～15g for making a decoction. It can also be made into boluses or powder.

Precautions Decreased dosage for weak constitution and poor appetite.

2. 4. Niu Bang Zi (Fructus Arctii)

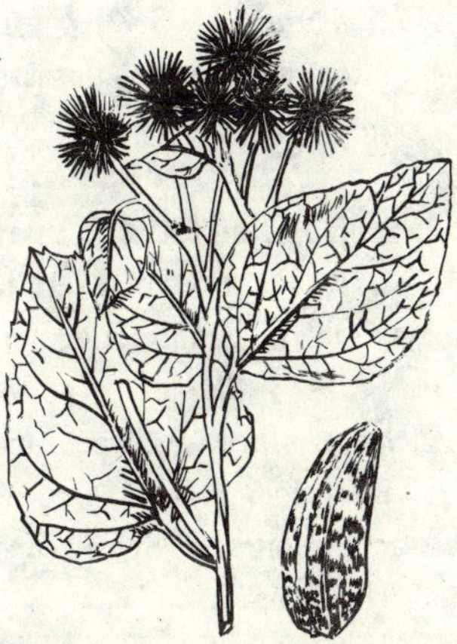

Description Fruit of Arctium lappa L. Family Compositae.

Characteristics Acrid and bitter in flavor, cold in nature, acting on the Lung and Stomach Channels.

Action Expelling Wind and Heat, detoxicating, promoting skin eruptions, and easing throat inflammation.

Indications

(1) Common cold of Wind-Heat type manifested as fever, slight chilliness, headache and sore throat, cough with Phlegm retention, etc. Usually used in combination with Bo He (Herba Menthae), Jie Geng (Radix Platycodi), Jing Jie (Herba Schizonepetae), etc., e. g. Niubang Tang (Fructus Arctii Decoction); in the case of intensive Heat, Ban Lan Gen (Radix Isatidis) and Huang Qin (Radix Scutellariae) may be used with Niu Bang Zi (Fructus Arctii).

(2) Onset or incomplete eruption of measles or rashes due to Wind-Heat, etc. In the mild cases, usually used in combination with Chan Tui (Periostracum Cicadae), Bo He (Herba Menthae), Ge Gen (Radix Puerariae), etc; in the case of Heat Excess, usually used together with Da Qing Ye (Folium Isatidis), Zi Cao (Radix Arnebiae seu Lithospermi), Chi Shao (Radix Paeoniae Rubra), etc.

(3) Pyogenic infection and ulcerous disease of skin as well as mump. Usually used together with Ban Lan Gen (Radix Isatidis),

Lian Qiao (Fructus Forsythiae), Ye Ju Hua (Flos Chrysanthemi Indici), etc. Niu Bang Zi (Fructus Arctii) can also be used to treat epidemic disease characterized by swelling and redness of face due to upward attack of Wind-Heat, usually with Huang Qin (Radix Scutellariae) and Ban Lan Gen (Radix Isatidis), e. g. Pu Ji Xiaodu Yin (Universal Relief Decoction for Disinfection).

Administration 3～10g for making a decoction. It can also be made into a powder or boluses.

Precautions Not applied to patients with Qi Deficiency or loose stools.

2. 5. Ge Gen (Radix Puerariae)

Description Root of Pueraria lobata Ohwi. Family Leguminosae.

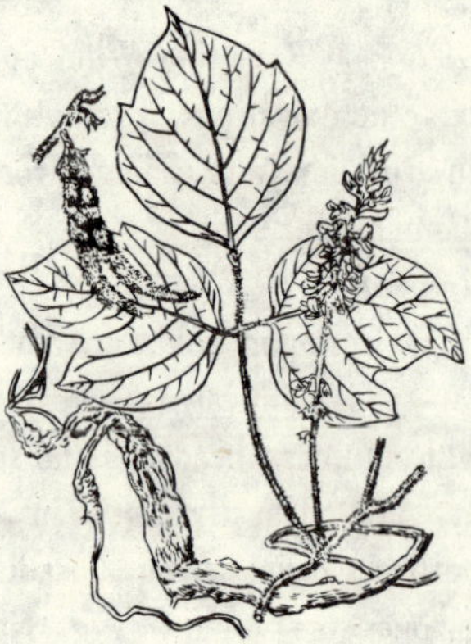

Characteristics Sweet and acrid in flavor, cool in nature, and acting on the Spleen and Stomach Channels.

Action Expelling the pathogenic factors from superficies and muscles, promoting the production of body fluid to quench thirst, promoting the eruption of measles and lifting the lucid Yang.

Indications

(1) Common cold with fever, headache, anhidrosis, stiffness and pain of nape and back. In the case of affection of Wind-Heat with headache, usually used with Chai Hu (Radix Bupleuri), Huang Qin (Radix Scutellariae), etc.; in the case of affection of Wind-Cold with chilliness and anhidrosis, stiffness and pain of nape and back, usually used with Ma Huang (Herba Ephedrae) and Gui Zhi (Ramulus Cinnamomi), e. g. Ge Gen Tang (Radix Puerariae Decoction).

(2) Febrile diseases with thirst or diabetes. Usually used alone or together with Mai Men Dong (Radix Ophiopogonis), Tian Hua Fen

(Radix Trichosanthis),etc.

(3) Diarrhea and dysentery due to Damp-Heat or loose stools due to Spleen Deficiency. For the former, used together with Huang Lian (Rhizoma Coptidis) and Huang Qin (Radix Scutellariae), e.g. Gegen Qin Lian Tang (Decoction of Puerariae, Scutellariae and Coptidis); for the latter, usually used with Dang Shen (Radix Codonopsis Pilosulae), Bai Zhu (Radix Atractylodis Macrocephalae), etc., e.g. Qiwei Baizhu San (Atractylodis Macrocephalae Powder of Seven Ingredients).

(4) Onset or incomplete eruption of measles. Usually used together with Sheng Ma (Rhizoma Cimicifugae) and Chi Shao (Radix Paeoniae Rubra), e.g. Shengma Gegen Tang (Decoction of Rhizoma Cimicifugae and Radix Puerariae); Niu Bang Zi (Fructus Arctii), Jing Jie (Herba Schizonepetae), Chan Tui (Periostracum Cicadae), etc. can also be used in combination for the same purpose.

Administration 10～20g for making a decoction. It can also be made into boluses or powder.

Precautions Applied with caution to Stomach-Yin Deficiency, for the ancients stated "Ge Gen (Radix Puerariae) consumes Stomach-fluid".

2. 6. Chai Hu (Radix Bupleuri)

Description Root of Bupleurum chinense DC. and the root and herb of B. scorzonerifolium Willd. Family Umbelliferae.

Characteristics Bitter and acrid in flavor, slightly cold in nature, and acting on the Pericardium, Liver, Triple-jiao and Gallbladder Channels.

Action Regulating related organs to clear away Heat, dispersing the stagnated Liver-Qi, lifting up the depressed Yang.

Indications

(1) Common cold with fever or affection of pathogenic Cold from ShaoYang Channel, alternate chills and fever. For common cold with fever, usually used with Gan Cao (Radix Glycyrrhizae), e.g. Chaihu Tang (Radix Bupleuri Decoction); or used together with Ge Gen (Radix Puerariae), etc., e.g. Chai Ge Jieji Tang (Bupleurum and Pueraria Decoction for Dispelling Pathogenic Factors from Superfi-

cial Muscles). For affection of Cold from ShaoYang Channel manifested by alternate chills and fever, stuffiness sensation in the chest and hypochondrium, bitterness of the mouth, dry throat, dizziness, etc., usually used together with Huang Qin (Radix Scutellariae), Ban Xia (Rhizoma Pinelliae), etc., e.g. Xiao Chaihu Tang (Minor Bupleuri Decoction). In the case of alternate chills and fever due to malaria, used with Qing Hao (Herba Artemisiae Chinghao) and Huang Qin (Radix Scutellariae).

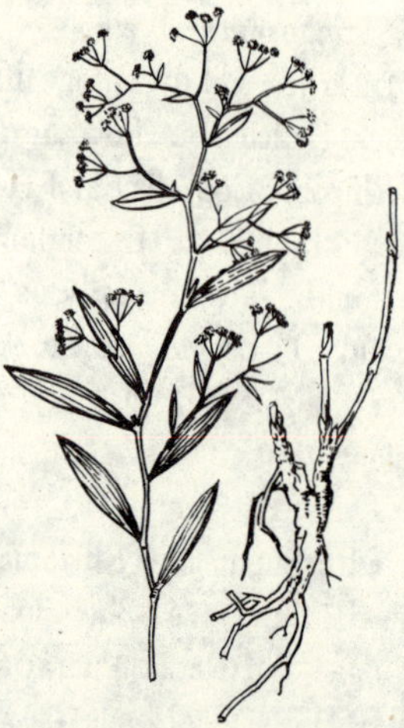

(2) Disorders of chest, hypochondrium and abdomen, or irregular or painful menstruation, amenorrhea, etc., caused by stagnation of Liver-Qi. For treating various disorders of chest, hypochondrium and abdomen, usually used together with Xiang Fu (Rhizoma Cyperi), Chuan Xiong (Rhizoma Ligustici Chuanxiong), Zhi Ke (Fructus Aurantii), etc., e.g. Chaihu Shugan San (Bupleurum Powder for Relieving Liver-Qi). For treating menstrual disorders, usually used together with Bai Shao (Radix Paeoniae Alba), Dang Gui (Radix Angelicae Sinensis), etc., e.g. Xiao Yao San (Ease Powder). In the case of hypochondriac pain caused by Damp-Heat of Liver and Gallbladder, usually used with Yin Chen Hao (Herba Artemisiae Scopariae), Zhi Zi (Fructus Gardeniae), etc.

(3) Prolapse of anus due to prolonged diarrhea, visceroptosis as well as shortness of breath, fatigue, etc. Usually used in combination with Sheng Ma (Rhizoma Cimicifugae), Ren Shen (Radix Ginseng) and Huang Qi (Radix Astragali seu Hedysari), e.g. Buzhong YiQi Tang (Decoction for Reinforcing Middle-jiao and Replenishing Qi).

Administration 3～10g for making a decoction. Stir-fried with vinegar for removing stagnation of Liver-Qi.

Precautions Not applied to such cases as those with Yin Deficiency and Fire Excess or hyperactivity of Liver Yang.

2.7. Sheng Ma (Rhizoma Cimicifugae)

Description Rhizome of Cimicifuga heracleifolia Kom., C. dahurica (Turcz.) Maxim. and C. foetida L. Family Ranunculaceae.

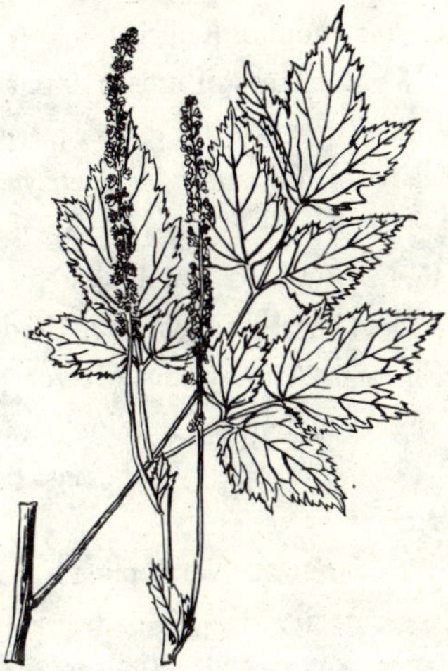

Characteristics Acrid and sweet in flavor, slightly cold in nature, and acting on the Lung, Spleen, Large Intestine and Stomach Channels.

Action Promoting diaphoresis and skin eruption, clearing away Heat and toxin, lifting up the depressed Yang.

Indications

(1) Common cold of Wind-Heat type with headache, onset or incomplete eruption of measles. For the former, usually used with Ge Gen (Radix Puerariae), e. g. Shengma Gegen Tang (Decoction of Cimicifugae and Puerariae); for the latter, usually used with Ge Gen (Radix Puerariae), Niu Bang Zi (Fructus Arctii), Huang Qi (Fructus Scutellariae), Bo He (Herba Menthae), etc., e. g. Shengma Tang (Rhizoma Cimicifugae Decoction). In the case of intensive Heat in measles, Zi Cao (Radix Arnebiae seu Lithospermi) and Niu Bang Zi (Fructus Arctii) may be used in combination.

(2) Toothache due to stomach Heat, aphthae, sore throat, swelling and pain from carbuncles, skin eruption due to Heat pathogen, etc. For toothache due to stomach Heat and aphthae, usually used in combination with Sheng Di (Radix Rehmannia) and Huang Lian (Rhizoma Coptidis), e. g. Qingwei San (Powder for Clearing Stomach-Heat). For sore throat, usually used with Xuan Shen (Radix Scrophulariae) and Jie Geng (Radix Platycodi), e. g.

Niubangzi Tang (Fructus Arctii Decoction), while for swelling and pain from carbuncles, skin eruption due to Heat pathogen, usually used with Da Qing Ye (Folium Isatidis), Lian Qiao (Fructus Forsythiae), Chi Shao (Radix Paeoniae Rubra) and Mu Dan Pi (Cortex Moutan Radicis).

(3) Shortness of breath, fatigue, prolonged diarrhea with prolapse of anus, prolapse of uterus caused by either collapse of Middle-jiao or collapse of Qi due to Deficiency of vital energy, or metrorrhagia due to Deficiency of Qi. Usually used in combination with Chai Hu (Radix Bupleuri) and Qi-replenishing drugs such as Ren Shen (Radix Ginseng), Huang Qi (Radix Astragali seu Hedysari), Bai Zhu (Rhizoma Atractylodis Macrocephalae), etc., e. g. Buzhong YiQi Tang (Decoction for Reinforcing Middle-jiao and Replenishing Qi).

Administration 3 ~ 10g. Processed for raising the collapsed Yang.

Precautions Not applied to patients with Yin Deficiency and Fire Excess or dyspnea with adverse flow of Qi.

2. 8. Chan Tui (Periostracum Cicadae)

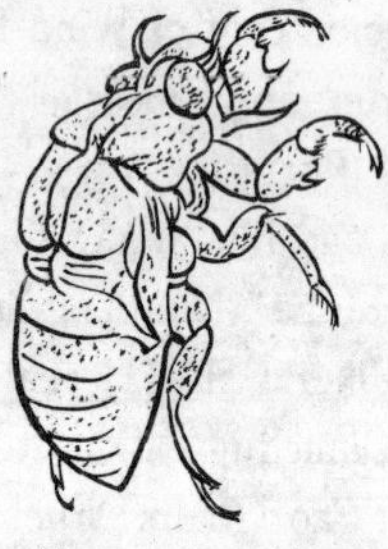

Description The exuviae of nymph during emergence of Cryptotympana pustulata Fabricius. Family Cicadidae.

Characteristics Sweet in flavor, cold in nature, and acting on the Lung and Liver Channels.

Action Expelling Wind and Heat, promoting skin eruption and alleviating itching, improving eyesight and removing nebula, eliminating Wind to relieve spasm.

Indications

(1) Affection of Wind-Heat or onset of febrile diseases with fever, headache, sorethroat, etc. Usually used with Lian Qiao (Fructus Forsythiae), Ju Hua (Flos Chrysanthemi), Bo He (Herba Menthae), etc.

(2) Wind-Heat accumulation in the Lung with sorethroat, hoarse-

ness and other symptoms. Usually used together with Pang Da Hai (Semen Sterculiae Scaphigerae), Niu Bang Zi (Fructus Arctii) and Jie Geng (Radix Platycodi).

(3) Onset or incomplete eruption of measles. Usually used in combination with Ge Gen (Radix Puerariae) and Niu Bang Zi (Radix Platycodi). For treating German measles, it is equally effective when used together with Jing Jie (Herba Schizonepetae), Bai Ji Li (Fructus Tribuli), etc.

(4) Wind-Heat in the Liver Meridian with redness of eyes, nebula, profuse tears, etc. Usually used with Ju Hua (Flos Chrysanthemi), Gu Jing Cao (Flos Eriocauli)., e.g. Chan Hua San (Powder of Cicadae and Chrysanthemi).

(5) Morbid crying and nocturnal fretfulness in infants as well as tetanus. Used alone or with Quan Xie (Scorpio), Jiang Can (Bombyx Batryticatus) and Gou Teng (Ramulus Uncariae cum Uncis).

Administration 3～10g for making a decoction. It can also be made into boluses or powder.

2.9. Dan Dou Chi (Semen Sojae Praeparatum)

Description The fermented seeds of Glycine max (L.) Merr. Family Leguminosae.

Characteristics Acrid, sweet and slightly bitter in taste, cold in nature, and acting on the Lung and Stomach Channels.

Action Expelling the exogenous pathogens from the body surface, clearing Heat to remove vexation.

Indications

(1) Fever, chilliness, headache, etc., caused by affection of exogenous pathogens from the body surface. In the Wind-Cold case, used together with Cong Bai (Bulbus Allii Fistulosi), e.g. Cong Chi Tang (Decoction of Sojae Praeparatum and Allii Fistulosi); in the case of Wind-Heat, usually used with Bo He (Herba Menthae), Jing Jie (Herba Schizonepetae) and Niu Bang Zi (Fructus Arctii), as in Yin Qiao San (Powder of Flos Lonicerae and Fructus Forsythiae).

(2) Febrile disease with chest upset, vexation and insomnia. Usually used with Zhi Zi (Fructus Gardeniae), e.g. Zhizi Chi Tang (Decoction of Gardeniae and Sojae Praeparatum). In the case of relapse

of disease due to overstrain with fever accompanied by restlessness, tight chest and loss of appetite, usually used together with Zhi Shi (Fructus Aurantii Immaturus) and Zhi Zi (Fructus Gardeniae), e.g. Zhishi Zhizi Chi Tang (Decoction of Aurantii Immaturus, Gardeniae and Sojae Praeparatum).

Administration 10～15g for making a decoction.

Heat-clearing Drugs

Drugs with clearing internal Heat as their main function are called Heat-clearing drugs

Heat-clearing drugs are cold or cool in nature and are characterized by purging Heat and Fire, cooling Blood, detoxicating, clearing away asthenic Heat, etc., and they are mainly applied to febrile diseases with high fever, Heat-type disentery, carbuncles as well as Yin Deficiency with internal Heat and other Heat-type symptoms.

According to their main actions, Heat-clearing drugs are classified into five categories: Heat-clearing and Fire-purging drugs, Heat-clearing and Dampness-eliminating drugs, Heat-clearing and Blood-cooling drugs, Heat-clearing and toxin-removing drugs as well as drugs for lowering asthenic fever. Clinical application should be in accordance with variation of cases, e. g. in the case of interior Heat accompanied with superficies syndromes, the latter should be treated first or together with the former; in the case of asthenic Heat in the Qi system complicated by Heat invasion of the Blood system, it is approperiate to clear away Heat in both systems.

As Heat-clearing drugs are cool or cold in nature, they are likely to damage Yang and Stomach and therefore they should be used with caution for asthenic Cold of the Spleen and Stomach. In the case of Yang being kept externally by the excessive Yin inside the body which manifests as pseudo-Heat-syndromes in appearance but real Cold-syndromes in nature, it is extremely important to make a correct diagnosis in order to avoid the wrong application of the drugs. Also, Heat-clearing drugs should be suspensed as soon as the disease is cured so as to protect the Vital Qi from being impaired.

1. Heat-clearing and Fire-purging Drugs

1.1 Shi Gao (Gypsum Fibrosum)

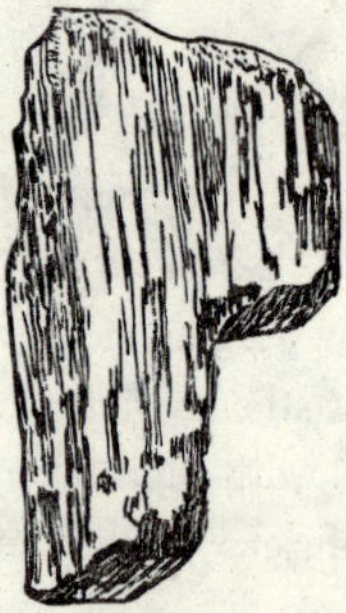

Description The monoclinic system of gypsum ore, containing hydrous calcium sulfate.

Characteristics Sweet and acrid in flavor, extremely cold in nature, and acting on the Lung and Stomach Channels.

Action Clearing away Heat, purging Fire, quenching thirst, arresting bleeding and tightening up the skin.

Indications

(1) Sthenic Heat in the Qi system marked by fever, excessive thirst, full and rapid pulse, etc. Usually used together with Zhi Mu (Rhizoma Anemarrhenae), e. g. Baihu Tang (White Tiger Decoction). For excessive Heat in both Qi and Blood due to deep invasion of pathogenic Heat manifested by high fever and skin eruptions, usually used together with Mu Dan Pi (Cortex Moutan Radicis), Xuan Shen (Radix Scrophulariae), Sheng Di (Radix Rehmannia), etc., e. g. Huaban Tang (Decoction for Relieving Feverish Rash).

(2) Lung-Heat syndrome with dyspnea, cough and turbid phlegm. Uaually used with Ma Huang (Herba Ephedrae), Xing Ren (Semen

Armeniacae Amarum),etc. ,e.g. Ma Xing Shi Gan Tang (Decoction of Ephedrae, Apricot Kernel,Gypsum and Licorice).

(3) Headache, swelling and pain of gum due to hyperactivity of Stomach-Fire. Usually used with Zhi Mu (Rhizoma Anemarrhenae), Niu Xi (Radix Achyranthis Bidentatae), etc., e.g. Yunü Jian (Decoction of Gypsum Fibrosum).

(4) Calcined Shi Gao (Gypsum Fibrosum) for external application to unhealing ruptured lesions, eczema, scalds and burns, bleeding from trauma, etc. Usually used alone or with Qing Dai (Indigo Naturalis) and Huang Bo (Cortex Phellodendri).

Administration 15~60g for making a decoction. Unprepared for internal use; calcined for external use; crushed and decocted earlier than other ingredients.

Precautions Not administered to asthenic Cold of the Spleen and Stomach, or Yin Deficiency with internal Heat.

1.2. Zhi Mu (Rhizoma Anemarrhenae)

Description Rhizoma of Anemarrhena asphodeloides Bunge. Family Liliaceae.

Characteristics Bitter and sweet in flavor, cold in nature, acting on the Lung, Stomach and Kidney Channels.

Action Clearing away Heat and Fire, nourishing Yin, moisturizing Dryness, and promoting the production of Body-Fluid to quench thirst.

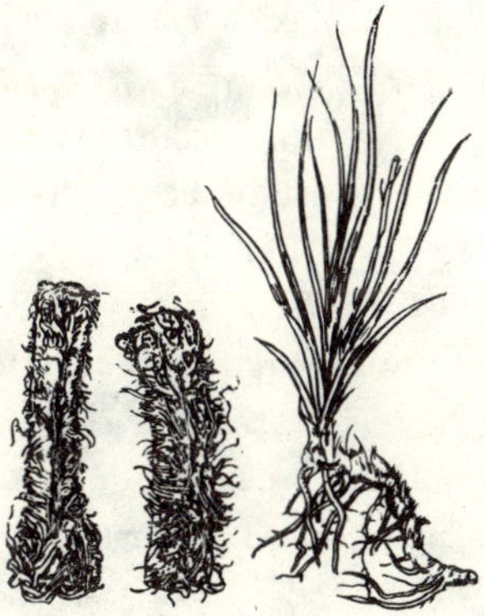

Indications

(1) Seasonal febrile diseases with high fever, excessive thirst, full and rapid pulse, etc. Usually used with Shi Gao (Gypsum Fibrosum), Gan Cao (Radix Glycyrrhizae), etc., e.g. Baihu Tang (White Tiger Decoction).

(2) Cough of Lung-Heat type, dry cough of Yin-Deficiency type

or cough with turbid sputum. Usually used together with Bei Mu (Bulbus Fritillariae Thunbergii),e.g. Ermu Wan (Bolus of Anemarrhenae and Fritillariae Thunbergii).

(3) Yin-Deficiency and Fire-Excess with hectic fever and night sweat, nocturnal emission, etc. Usually used together with Huang Bo (Cortex Phellodendri), Sheng Di (Radix Rehmanniae), etc., e.g. Zhi Bo Dihuang Wan (Bolus of Anemarrhena, Phellodendri and Rehmannia).

(4) Diabetes with thirst and profuse urine. Usually used together with Tian Hua Fen (Radix Trichosanthis), Mai Men Dong (Radix Ophiopogonis), Wu Wei Zi (Fructus Schisandrae), etc., e.g. Yuye Tang (Decoction for Promoting the Production of Body-Fluid).

Administration 5～12g for making a decoction.

Precautions Not used for Spleen Deficiency with diarrhea.

1.3. Zhi Zi (Fructus Gardeniae)

Description Fruit of Gardenia jasminoides Ellis var. radicans (Thunb.) Makino. Family Rubiaceae.

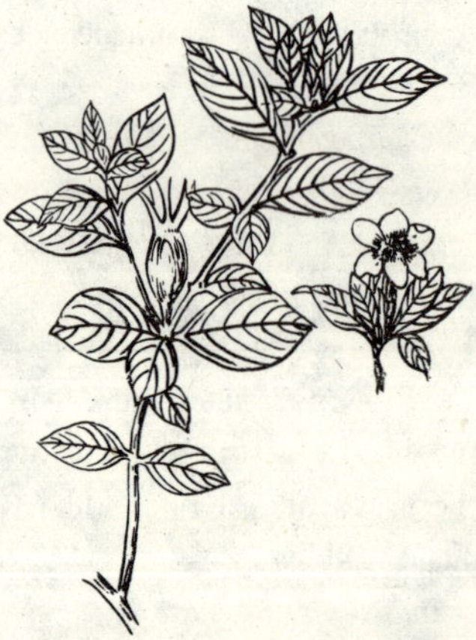

Characteristics Bitter in flavor, cold in nature, acting on the Heart, Liver, Lung, Stomach and Triple-jiao Channels.

Action Purging sthenic Fire to relieve vexation, clearing away Heat, promoting diuresis, cooling the Blood, removing toxins, eliminating Blood stasis and stopping bleeding.

Indications

(1) Febrile diseases with irritability, melancholia and restlessness. Usually used together with Dan Dou Chi (Semen Sojae Praeparatum), e.g. Zhizi Chi Tang (Decoction of Gardeniae and Sojae Praeparatum). In the case of high fever, restlessness and deliri-

um, Huang Lian (Rhizoma Coptidis) and Lian Qiao (Fructus Forsythiae) may be added, e. g. Huanglian Jiedu Tang (Coptidis Decoction for Detoxication).

(2) Jaundice, fever and stranguria of Dampness-Heat type. Usually used together with Yin Chen Hao (Herba Artemisiae Scopariae), e. g. Yinchenhao Tang (Decoction of Artemisiae Scopariae and Artemisiae Annuae).

(3) Heat in the Blood marked by epistaxis, hematemesis, hematuria, etc. Usually used together with Sheng Di (Radix Rehmanniae), Huang Qin (Radix Scutellariae) and Bai Mao Gen (Rhizoma Imperatae).

(4) Trauma with local swelling and pain. Usually powdered and used alone for external application.

Administration 3～9g for making a decoction; q. s. for external use.

Precautions Administered with caution for asthenic Cold of the Spleen and Stomach, or for poor appetite with diarrhea.

1. 4. Xia Ku Cao (Spica Prunellae)

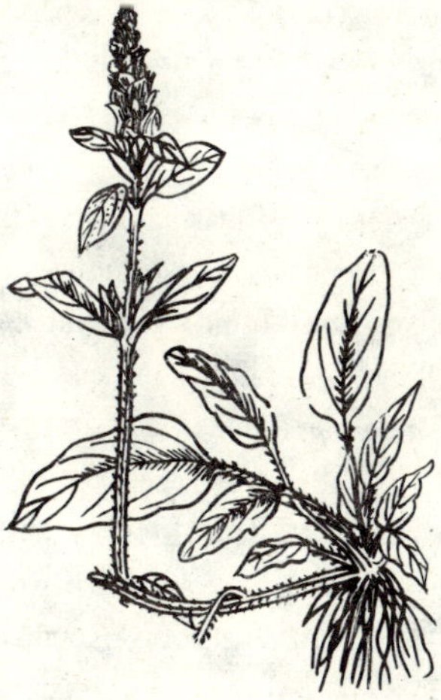

Description The whole plant or spike of Prunella vulgaris L. Family Labiatae.

Characteristics Bitter and acrid in flavor, cold in nature, and acting on the Liver and Gallbladder Channels.

Action Clearing away Liver-Fire and dispersing stagnation.

Indications

(1) Hyperactivity of Liver-Fire with conjunctivitis, photophobia, lacrimation, headache and dizziness. Usually used with Ju Hua (Flos Chrysanthemi), Pu Gong Ying (Herba Taraxaci), etc. In the case of pain of the eyeball more intense in the night, Dang Gui

(Radix Angelicae Sinensis), Bai Shao (Radix Paeoniae Alba), etc. may be used in combination

(2) Stagnation of Phlegm-Fire with scrofula, goiter, etc. Usually used alone by taking the decoction of it or by taking the semi-fluid extract made from it, or by applying the extract on the affected area. It can also be used together with Kun Bu (Thallus Laminariae seu Eckloniae), Hai Zao (Sargassum), etc.

(3) Hyperactivity of Liver-Yang or adverse ascending of Liver-Fire with vertigo, headache, etc. Used alone in large quantity for treating hypertension of Liver-Heat and Yang-Excess type or together with Shi Jue Ming (Concha Haliotidis), Huang Qin (Radix Scutellariae), Bai Shao (Radix Paeonia Alba), etc.

Administration 10～15g for making a decoction or semi-fluid extract.

1.5. Tian Hua Fen (Radix Trichosanthis)

Description Root of Trichosanthes kirilowii Maxim. Family Cucurbitaceae.

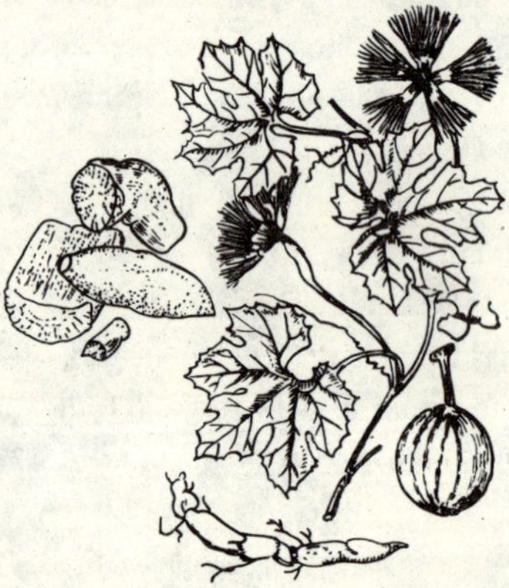

Characteristics Bitter and slightly sweet in flavor, cold in nature, acting on the Lung and Stomach Channels.

Action Clearing away Heat, promoting the production of Body-Fluid, relieving swelling and draining the pus.

Indications

(1) Febrile diseases with impairment of Body-Fluid, vexation and thirst or dry cough due to Lung-Heat. For the former, used with Mai Dong (Radix Ophiopogonis), Zhi Mu (Rhizoma Anemarrhenae), etc.; for the latter, used with Tian Dong (Radix Asparagi), Mai Dong (Radix Ophiopogonis), Sha Shen (Radix Adenophorae Strictae), etc.

(2) Diabetes. Usually used together with Sheng Di (Radix

Rehmanniae), Mai Dong (Radix Ophiopogonis), Ge Gen (Radix Puerariae) and Wu Wei Zi (Fructus Schisandrae). In the case of extreme thirst with excessive drinking and impairment of both Qi and fluid, used with Ren Shen (Radix Ginseng), Huang Qi (Radix Astragali seu Hedysari), etc.

(3) Pyogenic infections due to Heat pathogens with redness, swelling and burning pain. Usually used with Jin Yin Hua (Flos Lonicerae), Bai Zhi (Radix Angelicae Dahuricae), Chi Shao (Radix Paeoniae Rubra), etc., as in Xianfang Huoming Yin (Fairy Decoction for Saving Life).

(4) Mass in the abdomen with pain or extra-uterine pregnancy.

Administration 10~15g for making a decoction. It can also be prepared into powder or boluses.

Precautions Contraindicated for Spleen Deficiency with lingering diarrhea, Stomach Deficiency with Damp-Phlegm or pathogenic factors attacking the superficies.

2. Heat-clearing and Dampness-eliminating Drugs

Drugs of this type are indicated for stagnated Damp-Heat in the body or transmision of Heat from pathogenic Dampness. Clinical manifestations are fever, recessive fever, scanty urine and greasy tongue coat due to retention of Damp-Heat in the body; and diarrhea, dysentery as well as hemorrhoids and fistula due to accumulation of Damp-Heat in the Stomach and Intestines; distending pain of the ribs and jaundice with reddish urine, otitis media with pus discharge due to Damp-Heat steaming the Liver and Gallbladder; leucorrhagia with discharge of pus and blood, stranguria of Heat type with pain, swollen and painful joints due to descending of Damp-Heat; or eczema, exudative skin damage caused by invasion of Damp-Heat.

In order to avoid impairment of Yin and Stomach, drugs of this type should be used in combination with drugs for replenishing Stomach and tonifying Yin.

2. 1. Huang Qin (Radix Scutellariae)

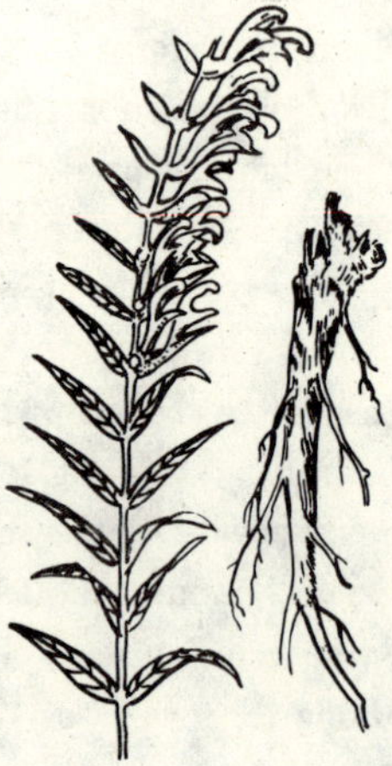

Description Root of Scutellaria baicalensis Georgi. Family Labiatae.

Characteristics Bitter in favor, cold in nature, acting on the Lung, Gallbladder and Large Intestine Channels.

Action Clearing away Heat, eliminating Dampness, purging Fire, detoxicating, stopping bleeding and preventing miscarriage.

Indications

(1) Diarrhea, dysentery, jaundice, Damp-Heat syndromes, stranguria of Heat type and pyogenic infection. For diarrhea and dysentery with abdominal pain, used together with Shao Yao (Radix Paeoniae Alba) and Gan Cao (Radix Glycyrrhizae), as in Huangqin Tang (Radix Scutellariae Decoction); for jaundice due to Damp-Heat, usually used with Yin Chen (Herba Artemisiae Scopariae), Zhi Zi (Fructus Gardeniae), etc.; for Damp-Heat syndromes marked by fever, stuffiness sensation in the chest and abdomen with greasy tongue coat, usually used with Hua Shi (Talcum) and Tong Cao (Medulla Tetrapanacis)); for stranguria of Heat type, used with Sheng Di (Radix Rehmanniae) and Mu Tong (Caulis Akebiae), as in Huofu Dan (Pill for Removing Excessive Heat from the Heart); for pyogenic infection, used with Tian Hua Fen (Radix Trichosanthis), Bai Zhi (Radix Angelicae Dahuricae) and Lian Qiao (Fructus Forsythiae).

(2) Febrile diseases with high fever, excessive thirst, yellowish tongue coat and rapid and forceful pulse. Usually used with Huang Lian (Rhizoma Coptidis) and Shi Gao (Gypsum Fibrosum); for al-

ternate chills and fever, used with Chai Hu (Radix Bupleuri), as in Xiao Chaihu Tang (Minor Decoction of Radix Bupleuri).

(3) Cough due to Lung-Heat. Used alone or with Sang Bai Pi (Cortex Mori Radicis), Zhi Mu (Rhizoma Anemarrhenae) and Bei Mu (Bulbus Fritillariae Cirrhosae), as in Qingyan Ningfei Tang (Decoction for Easing the Throat and Calming the Lung).

(4) Hematemesis due to invasion of Blood by excessive Heat. For treatment, it can be carbonized and made into a decoction by itself, or used in combination with Sheng Di (Radix Rehmanniae), San Qi (Radix Notoginseng), Bai Mao Gen (Rhizoma Imperatae), etc.

(5) Threatened abortion. Usually used together with Bai Zhu (Rhizoma Atractylodis Macrocephalae), Dang Gui (Radix Angelicae Sinensis), etc., as in Danggui San (Powder of Radix Angelicae Sinensis).

Administration 3～10g for making a decoction; it can also be made into powder and pills.

Precautions Contraindicated for poor appetite due to asthenic Cold of the Spleen and Stomach, or loose stools.

2. 2. Huang Lian (Rhizoma Coptidis)

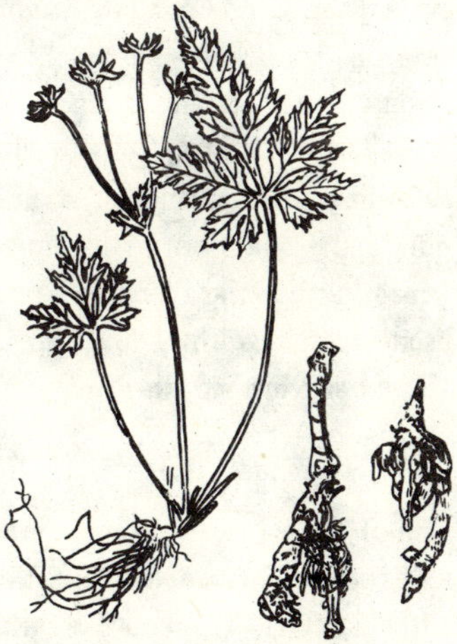

Description Rhizoma of Coptis chinensis Franch, or Coptis deltoidea Cheng et Hsiao, or Coptis teetoides Cheng. Family Ranunculaceae.

Characteristics Bitter in flavor, cold in nature, acting on the Heart, Liver, Stomach and Large Intestine Channels.

Action Clearing away Heat, eliminating Dampness, purging Fire and detoxicating.

Indications

(1) Damp-Heat syndromes of various kinds, especially marked by dysentery and vomiting. In the

mild case, Huang Lian (Rhizoma Coptidis) is used alone; in the case of accompanying tenesmus, used together with Mu Xiang (Radix Aucklandiae), as in Xiang Lian Wan (Pill of Radix Aucklandiae and Rhizoma Coptidis); in the case of accompanying superficies-syndromes with fever, usually used with Ge Gen (Radix Puerariae) and Huang Qin (Radix Scutellariae), as in Gegen Qin Lian Tang (Decoction of Radix Puerariae, Radix Scutellariae and Rhizoma Coptidis) in the case of prolonged dysentery with red and white stools and decreased Damp-Heat syndrome, used together with Wu Mei (Fructus Mume). For treating vomiting induced by Stomach-Heat or Liver-Fire, used with Wu Zhu Yu (Fructus Euodiae), named Zuojin Wan (Pill for Purging Liver-Fire and Regulating the Stomach); or with Ban Xia (Rhizoma Pinelliae) and Zhu Ru (Caulis Bambusae in Taeniam), as in Huanglian Zhuru Banxia Tang (Decoction of Rhizoma Coptidis, Caulis Bambusae in Taeniam and Rhizoma Pinelliae).

(2) Febrile diseases marked by high fever, restlessness, unconsciousness, delirium and other manifestations induced by excessive Heart-Fire. For treatment, used together with Huang Qin (Radix Scutellariae), Zhi Zi (Fructus Gardeniae), etc., as in Huanglian Jiedu Tang (Decoction of Rhizoma Coptidis for Detoxication). In the case of insufficiency of Yin Blood and Body-Fluid, excessive Fire, vexation and insomnia, used together with Huang Qin (Radix Scutellariae), E Jiao (Colla Corii Asini) and Bai Shao (Radix Paeoniae Alba), as in Huanglian Ejiao Tang (Decoction of Rhizoma Coptidis and Colla Corii Asini); in the case of excessive Heart-Fire which invades the Blood and results in hematemesis and epistaxis, used together with Huang Qin (Radix Scutellariae) and Dai Huang (Radix et Rhizoma Rhei), as in Xiexin Tang (Decoction for Purging Heart-Fire).

(3) Suppurative infection on the body surface such as swelling and pain of the ears, canker sores in the mouth, swelling of the gum and foul breath. For pyogenic infection induced by Heat pathogens, used with Lian Qiao (Fructus Forsythiae), Jin Yin Hua (Flos Lonicerae), Ye Ju Hua (Flos Chrysanthemi Indici), etc.; for swelling and pain of the ear and eyes, usually used with Zhi Zi (Fructus Gardeniae), Chi

Shao (Radix Paeoniae Rubra), Xia Ku Cao (Spica Prunellae), etc.; for swelling of the gum and foul breath, used with Sheng Ma (Rhizoma Cimicifugae), Shi Gao (Gypsum Fibrosum) and Sheng Di (Radix Rehmanniae).

(4) Diabetes due to excessive Stomach-Fire. Usually used together with Tian Hua Fen (Radix Trichosanthis), Sheng Di (Radix Rehmanniae), Ge Gen (Radix Puerariae), etc.

Administration 2～10g for making a decoction. It can also be made into powder or pills.

Precautions Contraindicated for Deficiency-Cold of the Spleen and Stomach.

2. 3. Huang Bo (Cortex Phellodendri)

Description Bark of Phellodendron chinensis Schneid. or P. amurense Rupr. Family Rutaceae.

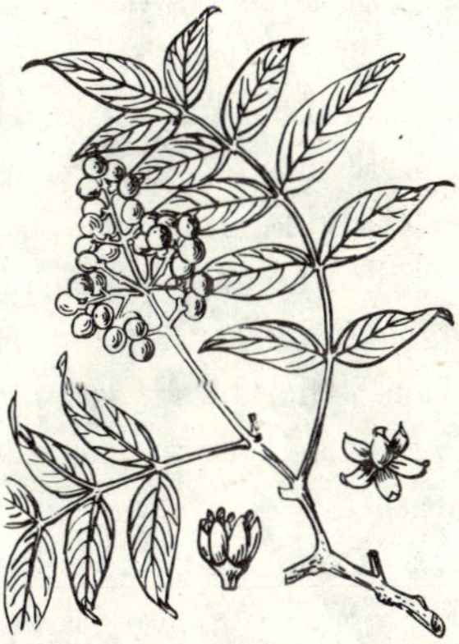

Characteristics Bitter in flavor and cold in nature, acting on the Kidney, Urinary Bladder and Large Intestine Channels.

Action Clearing away Heat and Dampness, purging Fire, detoxicating and reducing asthenia Heat.

Indications

(1) Various Damp-Heat syndromes such as diarrhea, dysentery, jaundice, leukorrhagia, flaccidity of the lower limbs as well as stranguria of Heat type. For diarrhea and dysentery, usually used together with Huang Lian (Rhizoma Coptidis) and Bai Tou Weng (Radix Pulsatillae), as in Baitouweng Tang (Decoction of Radix Pulsatillae); for jaundice, usually used together with Zhi Zi (Fructus Gardeniae), Yin Chen (Herba Artemisiae Scopariae), Che Qian Zi (Semen Plantaginis), etc.; for leukorrhagia with yellowish and foul vaginal discharge, usually used in combination with Bai Guo (Semen

Ginkgo) and Che Qian Zi (Semen Plantaginis), as in Yihuang Tang (Decoction for Removing Yellow Leukorrhagia); for flaccidity of the lower limbs or swelling and pain of the joints, usually used with Cang Zhu (Rhizoma Atractylodis) and Niu Xi (Radix Achyranthis Bidentatae), as in San Miao Wan (Bolus of Three Wonderful Drugs); for stranguria of Heat-type, used with Zhu Ye (bamboo leaves) and Mu Tong (Caulis Akebiae).

(2) Pyogenic infection on the body surface or eczema induced by Heat pathogen. For skin infection due to Heat pathogen, used internally together with Huang Lian (Rhizoma Coptidis) and Zhi Zi (Fructus Gardeniae), externally by mixing the powder of it with pig's bile or with eggwhite; for eczema, used together with Ku Shen (Radix Sophorae Flavescentis), Jing Jie (Herba Schizonepetae), etc.

(3) Asthenic fever due to Yin Deficiency, hectic fever with night sweat, nocturnal emission, etc. Usually used with Zhi Mu (Rhizoma Anemarrhenae), Shu Di (Rhizoma Rehmanniae Praeparatae), etc., as in Zhi Bo Dihuang Wan (Bolus of Rhizoma Anemarrhenae, Cortex Phellodendri and Rhizoma Rehmanniae).

Administration 3～10g for making a decoction. It can also be made into bolus or powder. q.s. for external application.

Precautions Contraindicated for asthenic Cold of the Spleen and Stomach.

2.4. Long Dan Cao (Radix Gentianae)

Description The root and rhizome of Gentiana manshurica Kitag., or Gentiana scabra Bge., or Gentiana triflora Pall., or Gentiana rigescens Franch. Family Gentianaceae.

Characteristics Bitter in flavor and cold in nature, acting on the Liver, Gallbladder and Stomach Channels.

Action Clearing away Heat, eliminating Dampness and purging Fire in the Liver.

Indications

(1) Jaundice due to Damp-Heat, swelling and pruritus of vulva, leukorrhagia, eczema, etc. For jaundice, used with Yin Chen (Herba Artemisiae Scopariae), Zhi Zi (Fructus Gardeniae), Yu Jin (Radix Curcumae), etc.; for perineal pruritus and swelling with yellowish

and foul vaginal discharge or eczema, usually used with Huang Bo (Cortex Phellodendri), Ku Shen (Radix Sophorae Flavescentis), Che Qian Zi (Semen Plantaginis), etc.

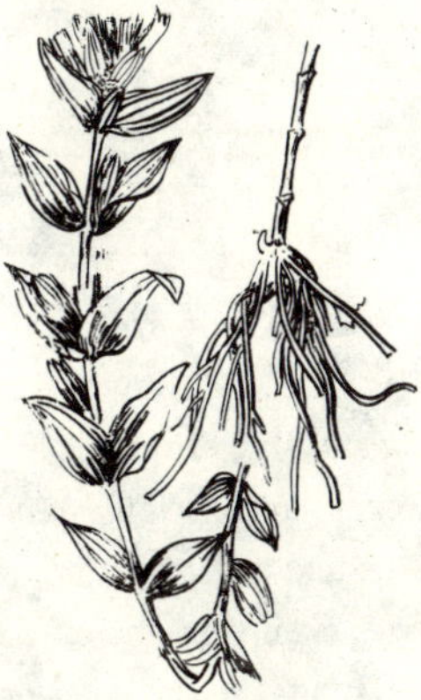

(2) Flaring-up of sthenic Fire in the Liver and Gallbladder manifested by headache, bitter taste in the mouth, red eyes, deafness, hypochondriac pain, etc. Usually used together with Chai Hu (Radix Bupleuri), Huang Qin (Radix Scutellariae), Zhi Zi (Fructus Gardeniae), Sheng Di (Radix Rehmanniae) and Che Qian Zi (Semen Plantaginis), as in Longdan Xiegan Tang (Decoction of Radix Gentianae for Purging Liver-Fire).

(3) Excessive Heat in the Liver Meridian inducing Wind-syndromes marked by sthenic fever and convulsion. Usually used with Gou Teng (Ramulus Uncaria cum Uncis), Niu Huang (Calculus Bovis), Huang Lian (Rhizoma Coptidis), Qing Dai (Indigo Naturalis), etc., as in Liangjing Wan (Pill for Removing Heat from the Liver and Relieving Convulsion).

(4) Impairment of Yin by Stomach-Heat leading to dry mouth, poor appetite, abdominal distension from meals, glossy tongue without coat, etc. Usually used with Shi Hu (Herba Dendrobii), Sha Shen (Radix Adenophorae Strictae), Mai Dong (Radix Ophiopogonis), etc.

Administration 3～6g for making a decoction.

Precautions Contraindicated for asthenic Cold of the Spleen and Stomach.

3. Heat-clearing and Blood-cooling Drugs

Drugs of this type are capable of removing pathogenic Heat from the Ying and Blood systems and they are indicated for hematemesis and epistaxis, skin eruptions and all sorts of bleedings as well as nocturnal fever, unconsciousness and delirium, deep red tongue with prickly fur and other symptoms.

Because of impairment of Yin and Body-Fluid when Heat invades Ying and Blood, a combined use of drugs for tonifying Yin and increasing fluid is necessary. In the case of excessive Heat without invasion of the Ying and Blood, drugs of this type are not recommended.

3.1. Sheng Di Huang (Radix Rehmanniae)

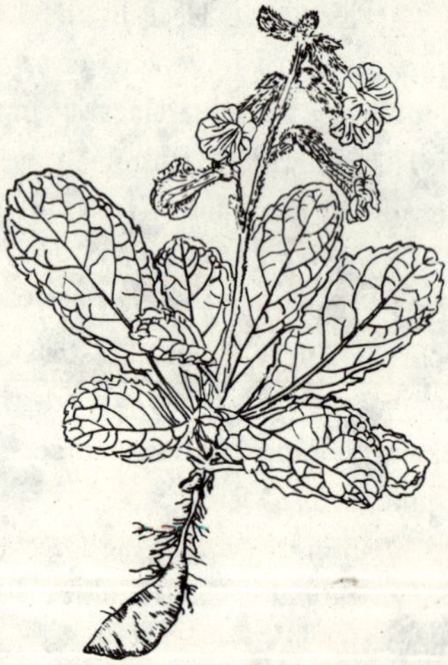

Description Root of Rehmannia glutinosa Libosch. Family Scrophulariaceae.

Characteristics Sweet and bitter in flavor, cold in nature, acting on the Heart, Liver and Kidney Channels

Action Clearing away Heat from the Blood, tonifying Yin to promote the production of Body-Fluid.

Indications

(1) Epidemic febrile diseases with Heat invasion into the Yin and Blood manifested by fever, thirst, deep red tongue, etc. Usually used with Xuan Shen (Radix Scrophulariae) and Mai Dong (Radix Ophiopogonis), as in Qingying Tang (Decoction for Clearing Away Heat in the Ying System).

(2) Lingering low fever at the late stage of febrile disease when Heat-evil is retreating, or Yin Deficiency and Heat in the interior due to a chronic disease, or diabetes. For lingering low fever, usually used with Qing Hao (Herba Artemisiae Annuae), Bie Jia (Carapax Trionycis), Zhi Mu (Rhizoma Anemarrhenae), etc., as in Qinghao Biejia Tang (Decoction of Herba Artemisiae Annuae and Carapax Trionycis); for febrile diseases with thirst due to impairment of Body-Fluid, used together with Mai Dong (Radix Ophiopogonis), Sha Shen (Radix Adenophorae Strictae), Yu Zhu (Rhizoma Polygonati Odorati), etc., as in Yiwei Tang (Decoction for Strengthening the Stomach); for diabetes, used with Tian Hua Fen (Radix Trichosanthis), Mai Dong (Radix Ophiopogonis), Wu Wei Zi (Fructus Schisandrae), etc., as in Tianhua San (Radix Trichosanthis Powder).

(3) Bleeding due to invasion of Blood by pathogenic Heat, or skin eruptions. For the former such as hematemesis, epistaxis, hematuria, bloody stools, metrorrhagia and metrostaxis, usually used together with Ce Bo Ye (Cacumen Biotae), Sheng Ai Ye (Folium Artemisiae Argyi), Sheng He Ye (Folium Nelumbinis), etc., as in Si Sheng Wan (Bolus of Four Fresh Drugs); for the latter, used with Chi Shao (Radix Paeoniae Rubra), Mu Dan Pi (Cortex Moutan Radicis), etc.

(4) Urticaria and skin tinea of Blood-Heat type. Usually used with Fang Feng (Radix Ledebouriellae), Chan Tui (Periostracum Cicadae), Bai Ji Li (Fructus Tribuli), etc.

Administration 10~30g for making a decoction. Unprepared for clearing away Heat and promoting the production of Body-Fluid; carbonized for arresting bleeding.

Precautions Contraindicated for Deficiency of the Spleen with Damp pathogen marked by abdominal distension and loose stools.

3. 2. Xuan Shen (Radix Scrophulariae)

Description Root of Scrophularia ningpoensis Hemsl. Family Scrophulariaceae.

Characteristics Bitter, sweet and salty in flavor, cold in nature, acting on the Lung, Stomach and Kidney Channels.

Action Clearing away Heat from the Blood, removing toxins to disperse mass, tonifying Ying and purging Fire.

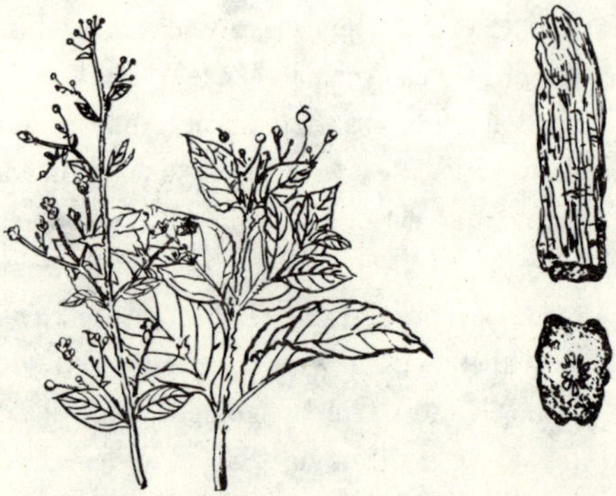

Indications

(1) Epidemic febrile diseases with Heat pathogen invading the Ying system and the Heart marked by fever accompanied with restlessness, thirst, insomnia, unconsciousness, delirium, etc. Usually used together with Sheng Di Huang (Radix Rehmanniae), Huang Lian (Rhizoma Coptidis), Jin Yin Hua (Flos Lonicerae), Lian Qiao (Fructus Forsythiae), etc., as in Qingying Tang (Decoction for Clearing Away Heat in the Ying System).

(2) Epidemic diseases with excessive Blood-Heat marked by maculas and eruptions. Usually used with Zhi Mu (Rhizoma Anemarrhenae), Shi Gao (Gypsum Fibrosum), etc., as in Huaban Tang (Decoction for Relieving Feverish Rash).

(3) Sore throat, scrofula, subcutaneous nodules, gangrene of finger or toe, etc. For sore throat due to affection of exopathogens, usually used with Niu Bang Zi (Fructus Arctii), Bo He (Herba Menthae); for flaring up of asthenic Fire, used with Sheng Di Huang (Radix Rehmanniae), Mai Dong (Radix Ophiopogonis), Sheng Gan Cao (Radix Glycyrrhizae), etc.; for scrofula and subcutaneous nodules, usually used with Bei Mu (Bulbus Fritillariae Cirrhosae), Mu Li (Concha Ostreae), etc.; for gangrene of finger or toe, used with Jin Yin Hua (Flos Lonicerae), Dang Gui (Radix Angelicae Sinensis)

and Gan Cao (Radix Glycyrrhizae), as in Simiao Yongan Tang (Decoction of Four Wonderful Drugs for Quick Restoration of Health).

(4) Febrile diseases at the late stage when exhaustion of Body-Fluid and impairment of Yin result in constipation. Usually used in combination with Sheng Di Huang (Radix Rehmanniae), Mai Men Dong (Radix Ophiopogonis), etc., as in Zengye Tang (Decoction for Increasing Body-Fluid).

Administration 10~15g for making a decoction.

Precautions Contraindicated for asthenic Cold of the Spleen and Stomach. Antagonistic to Li Lu (Radix Veratri).

3. 3. Mu Dan Pi (Cortex Moutan Radicis)

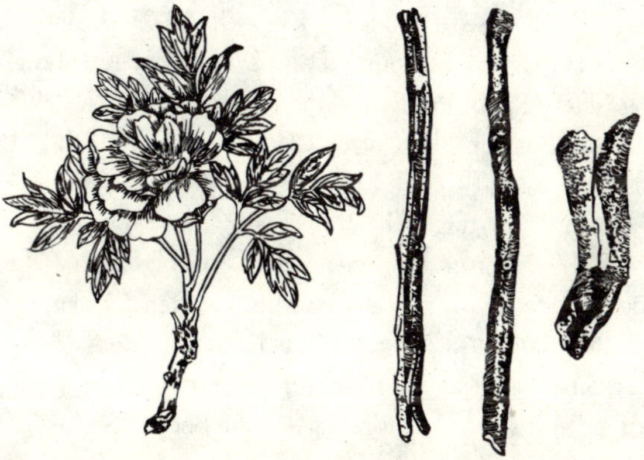

Description Cortex of Paeonia suffruticosa Andr. Family Ranunculaceae.

Characteristics Bitter and acrid in flavor, slightly cold in nature, acting on the Heart, Liver and Kidney Channels.

Action Clearing away Heat from the Blood, activating Blood circulation to disperse Blood stasis.

Indications

(1) Epidemic febrile diseases with Heat invading the Blood system manifested as maculas, hematemesis, epistaxis, etc. Usually used with Sheng Di Huang (Radix Rehmanniae) and Chi Shao (Radix Paeoniae Rubra), in the severe cases, Shui Niu Jiao (Cornu Bubali)

can be added; in the case of obvious macule purplish dark in color, Da Qing Ye (Folium Isatidis) and Ban Lan Gen (Radix Isatidis) can be added.

(2) Febrile diseases at the late stage when Heat invades the Yin system manifested by nocturnal fever or Yin Deficiency and Heat in the interior. Usually used together with Qing Hao (Herba Artemisiae Annuae), Bie Jia (Carapax Trionycis), Sheng Di Huang (Radix Rehmanniae), etc., as in Qinghao Biejia Tang (Decoction of Herba Artemisiae Annuae and Carapax Trionycis).

(3) Liver stagnation and Fire excess marked by fever, vertigo, headache, red eyes and cheeks as well as irregular menstruation, distension of the breasts during menstruation and fever prior to menstruation. Usually used in combination with Zhi Zi (Fructus Gardeniae), Chai Hu (Radix Bupleuri), Dang Gui (Radix Angelicae Sinensis), Bai Shao (Radix Paeoniae Alba), etc., as in Dan Zhi Xiaoyao San (Ease Powder of Cortex Moutan Radicis and Fructus Gardeniae).

(4) Amenorrhea, menorrhalgia, mass in the abdomen, trauma or pain due to Blood-stasis. For amenorrhea, menorrhalgia and mass in the abdomen, usually used together with Tao Ren (Semen Persicae) and Gui Zhi (Ramulus Cinnamomi), as in Guizhi Fuling Wan (Pill of Ramulus Cinnamomi and Poria); for trauma, used with Chi Shao (Radix Paeoniae Rubra), Ru Xiang (Resina Boswelliae Carterii), Mo Yao (Myrrha), etc.

(5) Suppurative infection on the body surface or appendicitis resulting from stagnation of excessive Blood-Heat. For the former, used with Jin Yin Hua (Flos Lonicerae), Lian Qiao (Fructus Forsythiae) and Bai Zhi (Radix Angelicae Dahuricae); for the latter, used together with Chi Shao (Radix Paeoniae Rubra), Da Huang (Radix et Rhizoma Rhei), Tao Ren (Semen Persicae), Dong Gua Ren (Semen Benincasae), etc., as in Dahuang Mudanpi Tang (Decoction of Radix et Rhizoma Rhei and Cortex Moutan Radicis).

Administration 6～12g for making a decoction.

Precautions Applied with caution to pregnant women or in cases of menorrhagia.

3.4. Chi Shao (Radix Paeoniae Rubra)

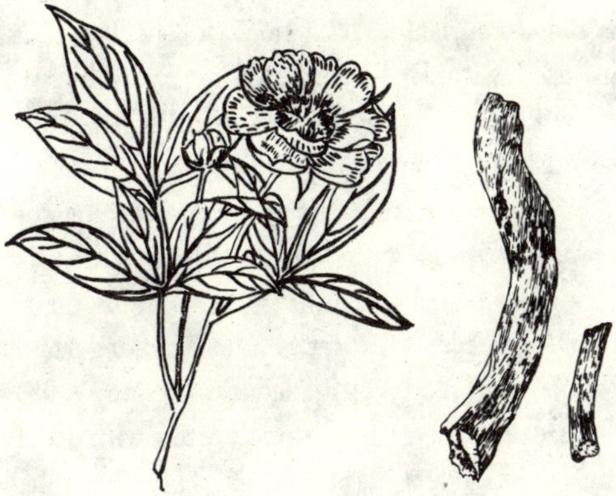

Description Root of Paeonia lactiflora Pall., or Paeonia veitchii Lynch. Family Ranunculaceae.

Characteristics Bitter in flavor, slighly cold in nature, acting on the Liver Channel.

Action Clearing away Heat from the Blood, eliminating Blood-stasis to relieve pain.

Indications

(1) Epidemic febrile diseases with Heat pathogen invading the Blood system marked by fever, maculae or eruptions, hematemesis and epistaxis. Usually used together with Mu Dan Pi (Cortex Moutan Radicis), Sheng Di Huang (Radix Rehmanniae), Chan Tui (Periostracum Cicadae), etc.

(2) Impairment of Blood collaterals by Heat leading to stranguria complicated by hemoturia, or dysentery of Heat type. For the former, usually used with Xiao Ji (Herba Cephalanoploris), Qu Mai (Herba Dianthi), etc; for the latter, used together with Dai Huang (Radix et Rhizoma Rhei), Bing Lang (Semen Arecae), Mu Xiang (Radix Aucklandiae), etc., as in Shao Yao San (Radix Paeoniae Rubra Powder).

(3) Amenorrhea, menorrhalgia due to Blood-stasis, or swelling due to trauma, etc. For regulating menstruation, used together with

Chuan Xiong (Rhizoma Ligustici Chuanxiong), Dang Gui (Radix Angelicae Sinensis), Dan Pi (Cortex Moutan Radicis), etc., as in Zixue Tang (Blood-nourishing Decoction); for swelling due to traumatic injury, used with Ru Xiang (Resina Boswelliae Carterii), Hong Hua (Flos Carthami), Tao Ren (Semen Persicae), etc.

(4) Suppurative infection on the body surface, pain of the eyes due to Liver-Fire, or hemiplegia. For suppurative infections on the body surface, usually used with Bei Mu (Bulbus Fritillariae Cirrhosae), Zao Ci (Spina Gleditsiae), Jin Yin Hua (Flos Lonicerae) and Bai Zhi (Radix Angelicae Dahuricae), as in Xianfang Huoming Yin (Fairy Decoction for Treating Cutaneous Infection); for swelling pain of the eyes due to Liver-Fire, usually used with Ju Hua (Flos Chrysanthemi) and Bo He (Herba Menthae); for hemiplegia, used with Huang Qi (Radix Astragali seu Hedysari), Dang Gui (Radix Angelicae Sinensis), Chuan Xiong (Rhizoma Ligustici Chuanxiong), etc., as in Buyang Huanwu Tang (Decoction for Strengthening Yang and for Recuperation).

Administration 3～15g for making a decoction.

Precautions Used with caution for Blood Deficiency without Blood-stasis, or for ulcerated pyogenic infection. Antagonistic to Li Lu (Radix Veratri).

4. Heat-clearing and Toxin-removing Drugs

Drugs of this category are mainly indicated for various syndromes caused by pathogenic Fire or Heat, such as epidemic febrile diseases, sore throat due to excessive Fire, diarrhea and dysentery due to Heat, carbuncles and furuncles, snake bite or insect sting or malignant tumour, etc.

As noxious Heat syndromes cover a wide range of diseases, clinical application of these drugs should vary in accordance with differences of cases and they should be used in combination with other compatible drugs so as to achieve a satisfactory result.

4.1. Jin Yin Hua (Flos Lonicerae)

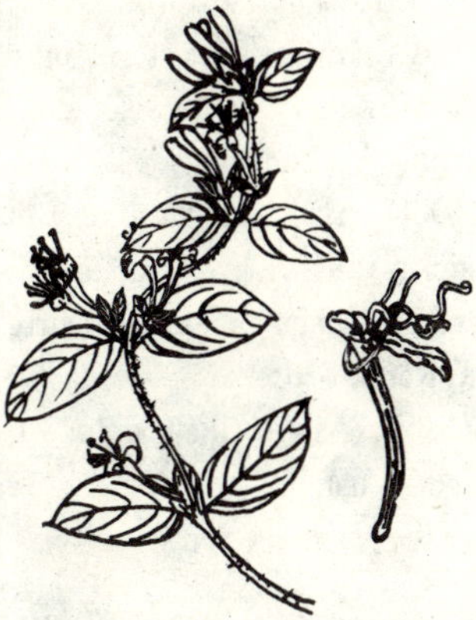

Description The flower bud of Lonicera japonica Thunb., L. hypoglauca Miq. and L. confusa DC. Family Caprifoliaceae.

Characteristics Sweet in flavor, cold in nature, acting on the Lung, Stomach and Large Intestine Channels.

Action Clearing away Heat and detoxicating, dispersing pathogenic Wind-Heat, cooling Blood and arresting dysentery.

Indications

(1) Affection of Wind-Heat or epidemic febrile diseases at the early stage, marked by fever and slight chilliness. Usually used in combination with Lian Qiao (Fructus Forsythiae), Jing Jie (Herba Schizonepetae), Bo He (Herba Menthae), etc., e.g. Yin Qiao San (Powder of Flos Lonicerae and Fructus Forsythiae). In the case of invasion of the Qi system by Heat marked by high fever, excessive thirst, full and large pulse, usually used with Shi Gao (Gypsum Fibrosum) and Zhi Mu (Rhizoma Anemarrhenae); in the case of invasion of Blood system by Heat manifested by appearance of skin eruption, restlessness, coma, purple tongue with thready and rapid pulse, usually used together with Mu Dan Pi (Cortex Moutan Radicis), Sheng Di Huang (Radix Rehmanniae), etc., e.g. Qing Ying Tang (Decoction for Clearing Heat in the Ying System).

(2) Sores, carbuncles, furuncles and swellings due to noxious Heat. Used either alone or with Ye Ju Hua (Flos Chrysanthemi Indici), Zi Hua Di Ding (Herba Violae), Pu Gong Ying (Herba Taraxaci), etc., e.g. Wu Wei Xiao Du Yin (Antiphlogistic Decoction of Five Drugs). Jin Yin Hua (Flos Lonicerae) can also be used to treat mastitis at the early stage with red, swelling, feverish and

painful breast, and it is usually used together with Gua Lou (Fructus Trichosanthis), Zao Ci (Spina Gleditsiae), Qing Pi (Pericarpium Citri Reticulatae Viride),etc. For appendicitis, it is used with Yi Yi Ren (Semen Coicis), Huang Qin (Radix Scutellariae),Dang Gui (Radix Angelicae Sinensis),etc. ,e. g. Qing Chang Yin (Drink for Treating Appendicitis).

(3) Diarrhea and dysentery due to Heat pathogen,sore throat, tonsillitis,pharyngitis,etc. For diarrhea and dysentery,it can be decocted alone and taken frequently,or decocted together with Huang Qin (Radix Scutellariae),Huang Lian (Rhizoma Coptidis),Bai Shao (Radix Paeoniae Alba) and Ge Gen (Radix Puerariae); for throat ailments, usually used together with Ban Lan Gen (Radix Isatidis), Xuan Shen (Radix Scrophulariae) and Ma Bo (Lasiosphaera seu Calvatia).

Administration 10～30g for making a decoction; q. s. for external application.

Precautions Applied with caution to pyogenic skin infections with Qi defficiency.

4. 2. Lian Qiao (Fructus Forsythiae)

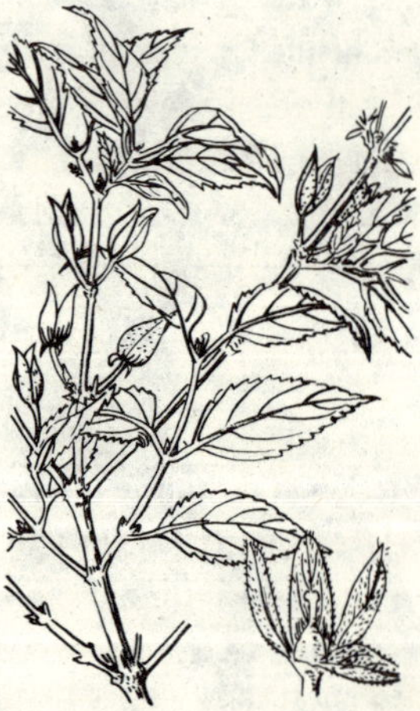

Description Fruit of Forsythia suspensa (Thunb.) Vahl. Family Oleaceae.

Characteristics Bitter in flavor,slightly cold in nature, acting on the Lung,Heart and Gallbladder Channels.

Action Clearing away Heat and detoxicating, expelling Wind-Heat, dispersing lumps and stagnation.

Indications

(1) Fever due to either epidemic febrile diseases or affection of pathogenic factors. Usually used together with Jin Yin Hua

(Flos Lonicerae), for the onset of epidemic febrile diseases or affection of pathogenic factors, Yin Qiao San (Powder of Flos Lonicerae and Fructus Forsythiae) is usually applied, while for the late stage, Qing Ying Tang (Decoction for Removing Heat from the Ying System) is used.

(2) Various kinds of suppurative infections on the body surface, or scrofula and tuberculous adenitis. For the former, usually used with Jin Yin Hua (Flos Lonicerae), Pu Gong Ying (Herba Taraxaci), Chi Shao (Radix Paeoniae Rubra), etc; for the latter, usually used with Xia Ku Cao (Spica Prunellae), Zhe Bei Mu (Bulbus Fritillariae Thunbergii), Xuan Shen (Radix Scrophulariae), etc. It can also be used for mastitis with swelling and pain, usually together with Gua Lou (Fructus Trichosanthis), Jin Yin Hua (Flos Lonicerae), Chuan Shan Jia (Squama Manitis), etc., e. g. Xiao Ru Tang (Decoction for Relieving Mastitis).

(3) Frequent and painful urination with scanty urine caused by downward flow of Heat-Fire. Usually used with Bai Mao Gen (Rhizoma Imperatae), Sheng Di (Radix Rehmannia), Dan Zhu Ye (Herba Lophatheri) and Gan Cao (Radix Glycyrrhizae) (fine roots only).

Administration 6～15g for making a decoction.

Precautions Applied with caution to asthenic Cold of the Spleen and Stomach or to chilblain.

4. 3. Niu Huang (Calculus Bovis)

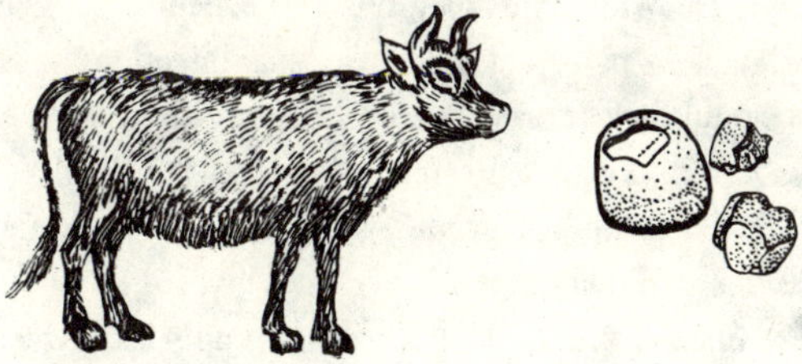

Description The stones in the gallbladder or biliary ducts of Bos taurus domesticus Gmelin. Family Bovidae.

Characteristics Bitter in flavor, cool in nature, acting on the Liver and Heart Channels.

Action Clearing away Heat and toxins, checking the Wind pathogen to relieve convulsion, resolving Phlegm to induce resuscitation.

Indications

(1) Excessive Heat pathogen, up-stirring of the Liver-Wind marked by spasm and convulsion. Usually used with Gou Teng (Ramulus Uncariae cum Uncis), Quan Xie (Scorpio), etc., e. g. Niuhuang San (Powder of Calculus Bovis).

(2) Invasion of intense Heat into the pericardium in epidemic febrile diseases, or apoplexy, epilepsy due to retention of Phlegm-Heat in the interior marked by high fever, coma, delirium, lockjaw, etc. Applied alone after being powdered and infused with the decoction of Dan Zhu Li (Herba Lophatheri), or with She Xiang (Moschus), Bing Pian (Borneolum Syntheticum), Yu Jin (Radix Curcumae), Zhu Sha (Cinnabaris), etc., e. g. An Gong Niuhuang Wan (Calculus Bovis Bolus for Resurrection).

(3) Sore throat, canker sores in the mouth or on the tongue caused by intense Heat flowing adversely upward. For treatment, blow the powdered Niu Huang (Calculus Bovis) alone onto the affected parts, or the mixed powder of Bing Pian (Borneolum Syntheticum), Zhen Zhu (Margarita) and Niu Huang (Calculus Bovis) onto the affected parts. It can also be taken internally with Huang Lian (Rhizoma Coptidis), Xiong Huang (Realgar), etc., as in Niuhuang Jie Du Wan (Antitoxic Bolus of Calculus Bovis).

(4) Carbuncles, boils and other pyogenic infection, scrofula, subcutaneous nodule and breast cancer. Usually used with She Xiang (Moschus), Ru Xiang (Resina Boswelliae Carterii), Mo Yao (Myrrha), etc., as in Xi Huang Wan (Pill of Cornu Rhinoceri Asiatici and Calculus Bovis).

Administration 0.15～0.5g for making pills or powder.

Precautions Not to be used for non-sthenic Heat syndromes; used with caution for pregnant women.

4.4. Da Qing Ye (Folium Isatidis)

Description Leaf of Isatis tinctoria L. Family Cruciferae or Baphicacanthus cusia (Nees) Brem. Family Acanthaceae.

Characteristics Bitter in flavor, very cold in nature, acting on the Heart, Lung and Stomach Channels.

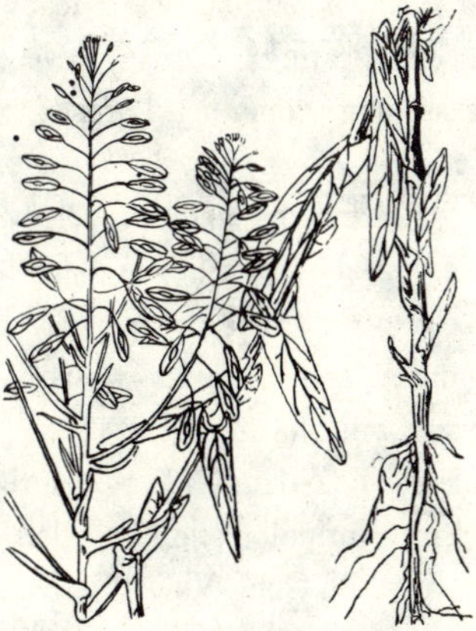

Action Clearing away Heat and detoxicating, cooling Blood and eliminating skin eruptions.

Indications

(1) Epidemic febrile diseases with excessive Heat syndromes such as high fever, restlessness and thirst. In the case of no invasion of Heat into the Blood system, usually used together with Jin Yin Hua (Flos Lonicerae), Lian Qiao (Fructus Forsythiae), Shi Gao (Gypsum Fibrosum), Zhi Mu (Rhizoma Anemarrhenae), etc.; in the case of invasion of Heat into the Blood system, marked by coma and skin eruptions, usually used in combination with Zhi Zi (Fructus Gardeniae).

(2) Sorethroat, mumps, aphthae, etc. Usually used with Niu Bang Zi (Fructus Arctii), Jie Geng (Radix Platycodi), Lian Qiao (Fructus Forsythiae) and Sheng Ma (Rhizoma Cimicifugae).

(3) Carbuncles, furuncles, boils, erysipelas and rubella induced by Heat. For treatment, fresh herb of Da Qing Ye (Folium Isatidis) may be smashed into juice which is then taken by mouth, dry herb may be used in combination with Pu Gong Ying (Herba Taraxaci), Jin Yin Hua (Flos Lonicerae), Xuan Shen (Radix Scrophulariae), etc.

Administration 9～15g for making a decoction.

Precautions An overdose will lead to malaise in Stomach and Intestines.

4. 5. Pu Gong Ying (Herba Taraxaci)

Description Herb of Taraxacum mongolicum Hand. -Mszz. or other species in the same genus. Family Compositae.

Characteristics Bitter and sweet in flavor, cold in nature, acting on the Liver and Stomach Channels.

Action Clearing away Heat and detoxicating, treating eye diseases and promoting diuresis.

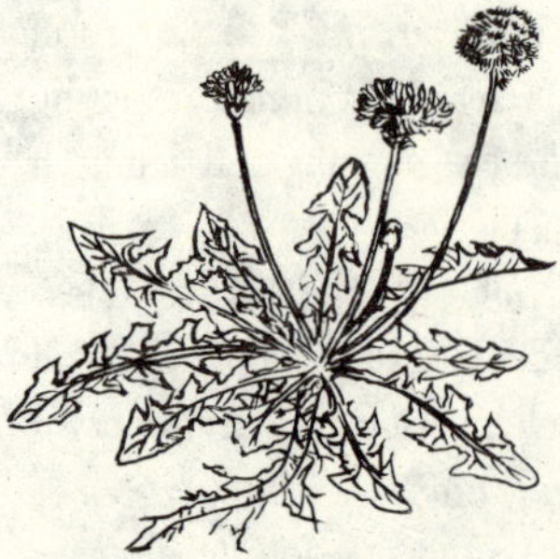

Indications

(1) Carbuncles and furuncles caused by Heat pathogen, and abscess of internal organs. For carbuncles and furuncles, usually used with Jin Yin Hua (Flos Lonicerae), Zi Hua Di Ding (Herba Violae), etc., as in Wu Wei Xiao Du Yin (Antiphlogistic Decoction of Five Drugs). For treating mastitis, fresh Pu Gong Ying (Herba Taraxaci) may be applied alone internally or smashed for external application, it can also be smashed with Ren Dong Teng (Caulis Lonicerae) to squeeze out juice for oral application. For pulmonary abscess with cough, spitting of foul and thick phlegm, usually used in combination with Yu Xing Cao (Herba Houttuyniae), Lu Gen (Rhizoma Phragmitis), Tao Ren (Semen Persicae), etc. For appendicitis with intense Heat, usually used with Chi Shao (Radix Paeoniae Rubra), Mu Dan Pi (Cortex Moutan Radicis), DaiHuang (Radix et Rhizoma Rhei), etc.

(2) Redness, pain and swelling of the eye. Usually used together with Xia Ku Cao (Spica Prunellae), Chi Shao (Radix Paeoniae Rubra), etc.

(3) Stranguria of Heat type, jaundice of Damp-Heat type. For the former, used together with Shi Wei (Folium Pyrrosiae), Che Qian Cao (Herba Plantaginis), etc.; for the latter, used together with Yin Chen (Herba Artemisiae Scopariae), Ban Lan Gen (Radix Isatidis), Jin Qian Cao (Herba Lysimachiae), etc.

Administration 10～30g for making a decoction.

Precautions Overdosage may result in chronic diarrhea.

4. 6. Yu Xing Cao (Herba Houttuyniae)

Description Herba of Houttuynia cordata Thunb. Family Saururaceae.

Characteristics Acrid in flavor, slightly cold in nature, acting on the Lung, Kidney and Urinary Bladder Channels.

Action Clearing away Heat and toxins, relieving carbuncles, draining the pus and promoting diuresis.

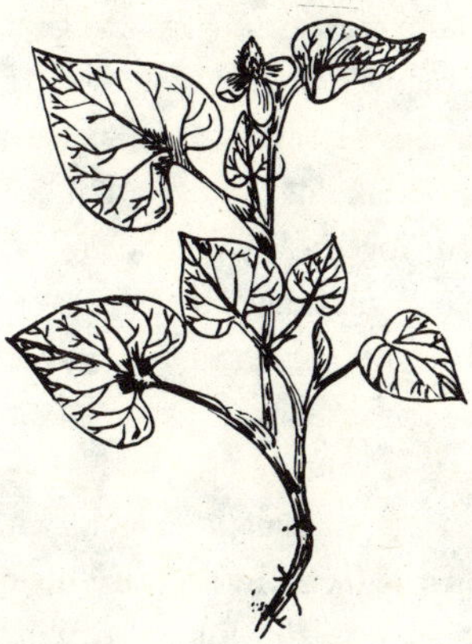

Indications

(1) Abscess of Lung with pus-and-blood-mixed sputum of foul odor, or Lung-Heat with thick yellow phlegm. In the case of pulmonary abscess without pus formation, usually used with Jin Yin Hua (Flos Lonicerae), Lu Gen (Rhizoma Phragmitis), Yi Yi Ren (Semen Coicis), etc., as in Qianjin Wei Jing Tang (Decoction for Eliminating Pulmonary Abscess); in the case of pus formation, usually used with Jie Geng (Radix Platycodi). For cough due to Heat pathogen, usually used with Ye Ju Hua (Flos Chrysanthemi Indici), Pu Gong Ying (Herba Taraxaci), etc.

(2) Stranguria of Heat type. Usually used with Che Qian Zi (Semen Plantaginis), Bai Mao Gen (Rhizoma Imperatae), Chuan Niu Xi (Radix Cyathulae), etc.

Administration 15～30g for making a decoction, q. s. for external application.

Precautions As it contains volatile oil, long boiling is not recommended.

4.7. She Gan (Rhizoma Belamcandae)

Description Rhizome of Belamcanda chinensis (L.) DC. Family Iridaceae.

Characteristics Bitter in flavor, cold in nature, acting on the Lung Channel.

Action Clearing away Heat and toxins, eliminating sputum and easing the throat.

Indications

(1) Sore throat with profuse phlegm of Heat type. Usually used together with Xuan Shen (Radix Scrophulariae), Jing Jie (Herba

Schizonepetae), Niu Bang Zi (Fructus Arctii), etc., as in Shegan Xiaodu Yin (Belamcandae Drink for Detoxication); or used together with Sheng Ma (Rhizoma Cimicifugae), Ma Bo (Lasiosphaera seu Calvatia), etc., as in Shegan Tang (Belamcandae Decoction).

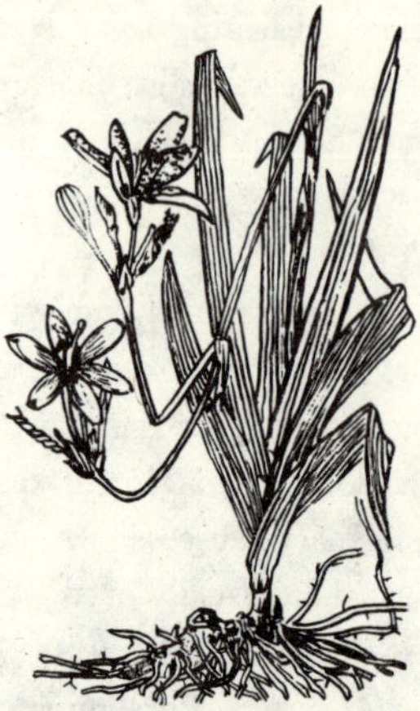

(2) Asthmatic cough with much phlegm. In the case of invasion into the Lung by Wind-Heat marked by profuse phlegm, cough and sore throat, usually used with Jie Geng (Radix Platycodi), Qian Hu (Radix Peucedani) and Bei Mu (Bulbus Fritillariae Cirrhosae); in the case of dyspnea due to attack of Wind-Cold, usually used with Ma Huang (Herba Ephedrae), Xi Xin (Herba Asari), Ban Xia (Rhizoma Pinelliae), Zi Wan (Radix Asteris), etc., as in Shegan Mahuang Tang (Decoction of Rhizoma Belamcandae and Herba Ephedrae); while in the case of Lung-Heat with thick and sticky sputum, usually used in combination with Sang Bai Pi (Cortex Mori Radicis), Ma Dou Ling (Fructus Aristolochiae), etc., as in Shegan Douling Tang (Decoction of Rhizoma Belamcandae and Fructus Aristolochiae).

(3) Redness, swelling and pain of the breast due to stagnation of Heat pathogen. Usually used with Xuan Cao (Radix Hemerocallis) and Pu Gong Ying (Herba Taraxaci).

Administration 6～12g for making a decoction.

Precautions Contraindicated for pregnant women.

4.8. Ma Bo (Lasiosphaera seu Calvatia)

Description The sporophore of Lasiosphaera fenzlii Reich, Calvatia gigantea (Batsch. ex Pers.) Lloyd and C. lilacina (Mont. et Berk.) Lloyd. Family Lycoperdaceae.

Characteristics Acrid in flavor, mild in nature, acting on the Lung Channel.

Action Clearing away Lung-Heat, easing the throat and arresting bleeding.

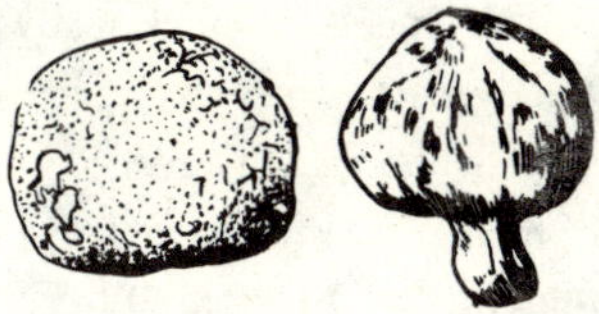

Indications

(1) Cough, sorethroat and aphonia due to Lung-Heat. For treatment, hold the powdered Ma Bo (Lasiosphaera seu Calvatia) in the mouth or the mixed powder with Xuan Shen (Radix Scrophularia) and Ban Lan Gen (Radix Isatidis) in the mouth and melt it slowly. In the case of rotten throat with difficult swollowing, used together with Ban Lan Gen (Radix Isatidis) and Jin Yin Hua (Flos Lonicerae), as in Qing Yan Xiaodu Yin (Drink for Easing the Throat and Detoxication).

(2) Hematemesis and epistaxis due to Blood-Heat or bleeding from trauma. For the former, used alone or together with other hemostat; for the latter, apply the powdered Ma Bo (Lasiosphaera seu Calvatia) to the cut to stop bleeding.

Administration 3～6g for making a decoction; it can also be made into pills or powder.

Precautions Wrapped for making a decoction.

4. 9. Bai Tou Weng (Radix Pulsatillae)

Description Root of Pulsatilla chinensis (Bunge) Regel. Family Ranunculaceae.

Characteristics Bitter in flavor, cold in nature, acting on the Large Intestine and Liver Channels.

Action Clearing away Heat and toxins, cooling Blood, arresting dysentery, treating trichomoniasis and pruritus.

Indications

(1) Dysentery of Heat or Damp type with pus and blood, tenesmus, fever and abdominal pain. Usually used with Huang Lian (Rhizoma Coptidis), Huang Bo (Cortex Polygonati), Qin Pi (Cortex Fraxini), etc., as in Baitouweng Tang (Radix Pulsatillae Decoction). Recently, generally used for acute bacillary or amebic dysentery with remarkable effect.

(2) Descending of Damp-Heat in the Lung Meridian resulting in

morbid leukorrhea and pruritus of female pudendum. Usually used together with Ku Shen (Radix Sophorae Flavescentis), She Chuang Zi (Fructus Cnidii), Bai Bu (Radix Stemonae), etc. for fumigation and wash; also a decoction can be made for internal application with Sheng Di Huang (Radix Rehmanniae), Long Dan Cao (Radix Gentianae), Tu Fu Ling (Rhizoma Smilacis Glabrae), Huang Bo (Cortex Phellodendri), etc.

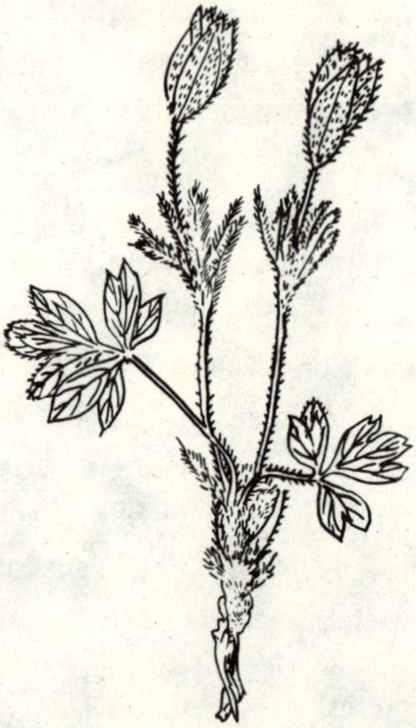

(3) Malaria of warm type. Usually used together with Chai Hu (Radix Bupleuri), Huang Qin (Radix Scutellariae) and Bing Lang (Semen Arecae).

Administration 6~15g for making a decoction; q. s. for external use.

4. 10. Tu Fu Ling (Rhizoma Smilacis Glabrae)

Description Rhizome of Smilax globra Roxb. Family Liliaceae.

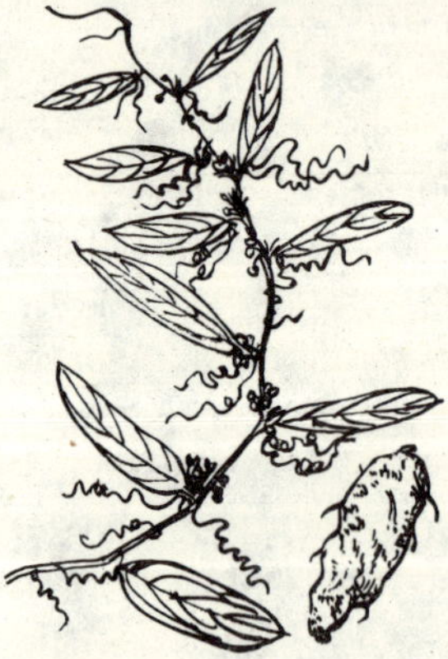

Characteristics Sweet and insipid in flavor, mild in nature, acting on the Liver and Stomach Channels.

Action Clearing away Heat and toxins, eliminating Dampness and easing the joint.

Indications

(1) Syphilis and mercurialism. Used either alone in large dosage or with Jin Yin Hua (Flos Lonicerae), Bai Xian Pi (Cortex

Dictamni Radicis), Gan Cao (Radix Glycyrrhizae), etc., as in Fufang Tufuling Tang (Composite Smilacis Glabrae Decoction).

(2) Rheumatism with red, swelling and painful joints and high fever. Usually used together with Ren Dong Teng (Caulis Lonicerae), Shi Gao (Gypsum Fibrosum), Zhi Mu (Rhizoma Anemarrhenae), Niu Xi (Radix Achyranthis Bidentatae), etc.

(3) Carbuncles and furuncles as well as stranguria of Heat type. For carbuncles and furuncles, usually used together with Jin Yin Hua (Flos Lonicerae), Lian Qiao (Fructus Forsythiae), Pu Gong Ying (Herba Taraxaci), etc.; for stranguria, usually used with Mu Tong (Caulis Akebiae) and Bian Xu (Herba Polygoni Avicularis).

Administration 15～60g for making a decoction.

Precautions Used with caution for Yin deficiency of the Liver and Kidney. Food taboo: tea.

5. Drugs for Lowering Asthenic Fever

Drugs in this group are capable of clearing away asthenic Heat from the Blood and they are indicated for hectic or tidal fever due to Yin deficiency, lingering low fever, burning sensation of five centres, insomnia due to vexation, dryness sensation in the mouth and throat, night sweat and nocturnal emission, red tongue with scanty coat, thready and rapid pulse. They can also be used for the late stage epidemic febrile diseases marked by lingering fever, impairment of Yin and consumption of Body-Fluid, nocturnal fever and listlessness.

Drugs for lowering asthenic fever are usually used in combination with Yin tonics so as to treat both the principal and the secondary aspects of the disease at the same time.

5.1. Qing Hao (Herba Artemisiae Annuae)

Description Herb of Artemisia annua L. Family Compositae.

Characteristics Bitter and acrid in flavor, cold in nature, acting on the Liver, Gallbladder and Kidney Channels.

Action Lowering asthenic fever, clearing away Summer-Heat, preventing the recurrence of malaria, cooling the Blood and arresting bleeding.

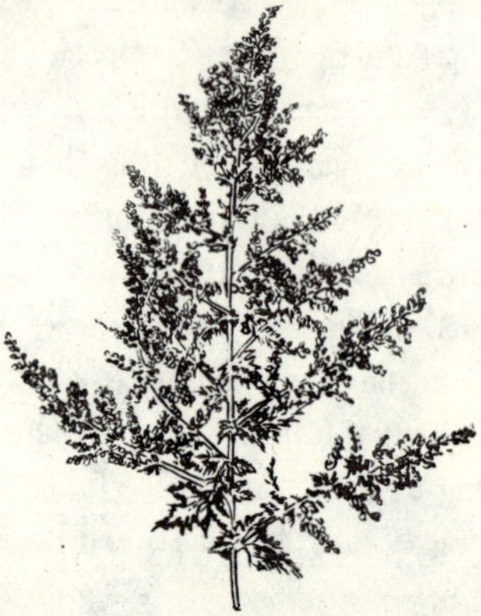

Indications

(1) Fever of Yin deficiency type, hectic or tidal fever, or late stage epidemic febrile diseases when Heat enters the Ying system marked by nocturnal fever and defervescence without sweating. For fever of Yin Deficiency type, usually used with Qin Jiao (Radix Gentianae), Bie Jia (Carapax Trionycis), Zhi Mu (Rhizoma Anemarrhenae), Di Gu Pi (Cortex Lycii Radicis), etc., as in Qing Gu San (Powder for Bone Heat); for late stage epidemic febrile diseases with lingering low fever, usually used together with Sheng Di (Radix Rehmanniae), Dan Pi (Cortex Moutan Radicis), Bie Jia (Carapax Trionycis), etc., as in Qinghao Biejia Tang (Decoction of Artemisia Annuae and Carapax Trionycis).

(2) Affection of Summer-Heat, fever without sweat, or epidemic febrile diseases with alternate spells of high fever and mild chills. For the former, fresh Qing Hao (Herba Artemisiae Annuae) is used in combination with Jin Yin Hua (Flos Lonicerae), mung beans, Dan Zhu Ye (Herba Lophatheri), flower of Dolichos lablab, etc.; for the latter, used together with Chai Hu (Radix Bupleuri), Huang Qin (Radix Scutellariae), etc.

(3) Malaria with fever and chills. For treatment, take the juice from large quantity of the fresh herb of Qing Hao (Herba Artemisiae Annue). In the case of accompanying vexation, stuffiness sensation in the chest and rich tongue coat, usually used with Huang Qin (Radix Scutellariae), Ban Xia (Rhizoma Pinelliae) and Fu Ling (Poria), as in Hao Qin Qingdan Tang (Decoction for Clearing Away Damp-Heat in the Gallbladder).

(4) Epistaxis, skin eruptions, inflammatory diseases with redness

of skin, fireburn or scald, etc. For epistaxis, take the juice from the fresh herb; for skin eruptions due to Blood-Heat, used together with Sheng Di (Radix Rehmanniae), Chi Shao (Radix Paeoniae Rubra), Da Qing Ye (Folium Isatidis), etc.; for inflammatory diseases with redness of skin, fireburn or scald, apply the juice made from the fresh herb to the affected area.

Administration 9~15g, or 30g in a large dose, for making a decoction; fresh herb is made into juice.

Precautions Used with caution for Spleen Deficiency with loose stools. Not to be decocted for too long.

5.2. Di Gu Pi (Cortex Lycii Radicis)

Description The root cortex of Lycium chinensis Mill. and L. barbarum L. Family Solanaceae.

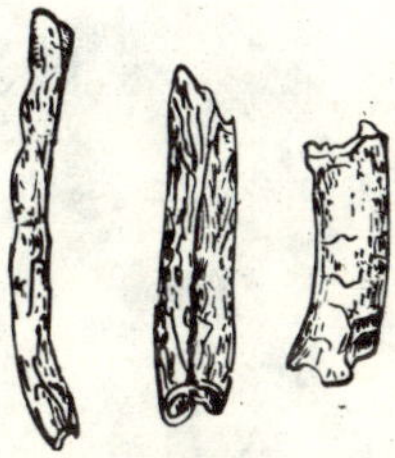

Characteristics Sweet and insipid in flavor, cold in nature, acting on the Lung, Liver and Kidney Channels.

Action Clearing away asthenic fever, purging Lung-Heat, and cooling Blood to treat hectic fever.

Indications

(1) Tidal fever due to Yin Deficiency and interior Heat, night sweat, as well as mulnutrition in children with fever. Usually used with Zhi Mu (Rhizoma Anemarrhenae), Bie Jia (Carapax Trionycis), etc., as in Digupi Tang (Decoction of Cortex Lycii Radicis).

(2) Dyspnea and cough due to Lung-Heat. Usually used together with Sang Bai Pi (Cortex Mori Radicis), Gan Cao (Radix Glycyrrhizae), etc., as in Xie Bai San (Powder for Expelling Lung-Fire).

(3) Adverse flow of Blood due to Heat marked by hematemesis, epistaxis and bloody urination. Usually used with Bai Mao Gen (Rhizoma Imperatae) and Ce Bai Ye (Cacumen Biotae).

(4) Diabetes. Usually used with Sheng Di Huang (Radix Rehman-

nia), Tian Hua Fen (Radix Trichosanthis), Sha Shen (Radix Adenophorae Strictae),etc.

Administration 6～12g for making a decoction.

Precautions Contraindicated for fever due to affection of Wind-Cold and asthenic Cold of the Spleen and Stomach.

5. 3. Bai Wei (Radix Cynanchi Atrati)

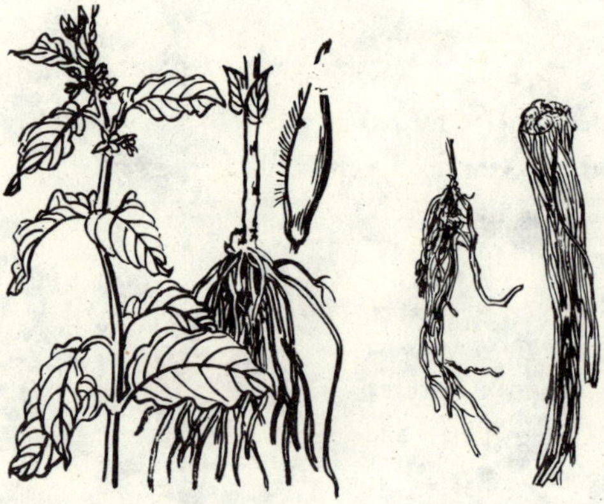

Description The root and rhizome of Cynanchum atratum Bunge or C. versicolor Bunge. Family Asclepiadaceae.

Characteristics Bitter and salty in flavor, cold in nature, acting on the Stomach, Liver and Kidney Channels.

Action Clearing away the Heat from the Blood, promoting diuresis to relieve stranguria, removing toxins to treat skin infections.

Indications

(1) Fever of various causes. It can clear away both asthenic and sthenic Heat. For fever due to affection of exopathogens, usually used with Jin Yin Hua (Flos Lonicerae), Lian Qiao (Fructus Forsythiae), etc.; For epidemic febrile diseases with Heat invasion into the Blood system and persistent fever, usually used with Sheng Di Huang (Radix Rehmanniae), Zhi Mu (Rhizoma Anemarrhenae), etc.; for hectic fever and night sweat due to Yin Deficiency and interior Heat, usually used with Di Gu Pi (Cortex Lycii Radicis), Qing Hao (Herba Artemisiae Annuae), etc.; for postpartum Blood Defi-

ciency with fever and coma, usually used with Dang Gui (Radix Angelicae Sinensis), Ren Shen (Radix Ginseng) and Gan Cao (Radix Glycyrrhizae), as in Bai Wei Tang (Cynanchi Atrati Decoction); while for cough due to Lung-Heat, usually used in combination with Bei Mu (Bulbus Fritillariae Cirrhosae), Hai Ge Ke (Concha Meretricis seu Cyclinae), etc.

(2) Stranguria of Heat type and stranguria complicated by hematuria. Usually used with Sheng Di Huang (Radix Rehmanniae), Mu Tong (Caulis Akebiae), Che Qian Zi (Semen Plantaginis), etc.

(3) Carbuncles, furuncles and other skin infections, sore throat, snake bite, etc. Used with Lian Qiao (Fructus Forsythiae), She Gan (Rhizoma Belamcandae), etc.; or applied alone to the affected part externally.

Administration 3～12g for making a decoction. q. s. for external use.

Precautions Used with caution for asthenic Cold of the Spleen and Stomach.

Purgatives

Drugs capable of inducing diarrhea or promoting laxation of the bowels are defined as purgatives.

Purgatives have heavy smells and flavors, lowering and sinking action, and they are characterized by relaxing the bowels and Stomach, expelling stagnation and retention of fluid, dispelling sthenic Heat and relieving edema. They are mainly indicated for constipation, food retention, accumulation of sthenic Heat in the interior, or other sthenic syndromes such as Cold stagnation and retention of water.

According to the medicinal properties and their characteristics, purgatives are divided into three types--drugs for clearing away Heat and relieving the bowels, drugs for moisturizing the intestines and drugs for purging Heat and retained fluid. Clinical application of purgatives varies accordingly with consideration to severity of the case, duration of stagnation, constitution of the patient and other aspects, also, compatible drugs are usually used in combination.

In spite of their quickness in taking effect, purgatives are liable to impair the vital Qi and therefore they should be discontinued as soon as the symptoms are relieved. Attention should be paid to avoiding overdosage or long-time application. For the old and the weak as well as pregnant women, purgatives should be avoided or used with precautions.

1. Drugs for Clearing Away Heat and Relieving the Bowels

Drugs of this type are mostly bitter in flavor, cold in nature and have lowering and sinking action. Being strongly purgative, they are mainly indicated for stagnation of Heat type with constipation and hard stools. When used in combination with drugs capable of warming the interior, some drugs of this type also have the function of treating constipation resulting from accumulation of Cold. As they can clear away Heat and Fire, they can also be used to treat high fever with coma, delirium and mania due to affection of exopathogenic Heat; headache, red eyes, sorethroat and gingival pain, epistaxis, etc. due to flaring up of Fire; or epidemic diseases, digestive syndromes in summer as well as food poisoning.

1.1. DaiHuang (Radix et Rhizoma Rhei)

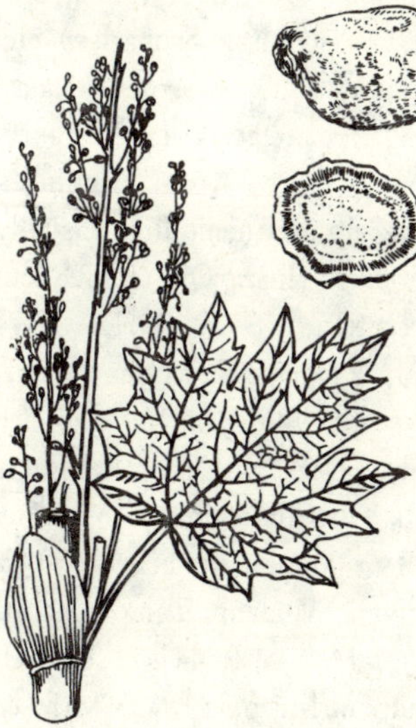

Description The root and rhizome of Rheum palmatum L., or Rheum tanguticum Maxim. ex Balf., or Rheum officinale Baill. Family Polygonaceae.

Characteristics Bitter in flavor, cold in nature, acting on the Spleen, Stomach, Large Intestine, Liver and Heart Channels.

Action Loosening the bowels, removing Heat and fire, clearing away toxins, promoting the circulation of Blood to dispel stasis.

Indications

(1) Constipation with abdomi-

nal pain, or even high fever, coma, delirium and mania due to accumulation of sthenic Heat in the Stomach and Intestines. For constipation resulting from Heat accumulation, usually used together with Mang Xiao (Natrii Sulfas), Zhi Shi (Fructus Aurantii Immaturus), Hou Po (Cortex Magnoliae Officinalis), etc., as in Da Cheng Qi Tang (Major Decoction for Purging Down Digestive Qi); for constipation due to accumulation of Cold, usually used with Fu Zi (Radix Aconiti Praeparata), Gan Jiang (Rhizoma Zingiberis), etc.

(2) Dysentery due to Damp-Heat, food retention and jaundice due to accumulation of Heat pathogen. For dysentery, used with Huang Lian (Rhizoma Coptidis), Mu Xiang (Radix Aucklandiae), Shao Yao (Radix Paeoniae Alba), etc., as in Shaoyao San (Radix Paeoniae Alba Powder); for food retention, usually used together with Shen Qu (Massa Fermentata Medicinalis), Zhi Shi (Fructus Aurantii Immaturus), Bai Zhu (Rhizoma Atractylodis Macrocephalae), Huang Lian (Rhizoma Coptidis), etc., as in Sanhuang Zhi Zhu Wan (Three Yellow Ingredients for Treating Indigestion); for jaundice due to accumulation of Heat-evil, used in combination with Zhi Zi (Fructus Gardeniae), Huang Bo (Cortex Phellodendri), Yin Chen (Herba Artemisiae Scopariae), etc., as in Zhizi Daihuang Tang (Decoction of Fructus Gardeniae and Radix et Rhizoma Rhei).

(3) Hematemesis and epistaxis due to invasion of Blood by Heat, red eyes, sore throat, swelling and pain of the gum, etc. due to flaring up of sthenic fire. Usually used with Huang Lian (Rhizoma Coptidis), Huang Qin (Radix Scutellariae), etc., as in Xie Xin Tang (Decoction for Purging Heart-Fire).

(4) Pyogenic infections due to Heat pathogen, and fireburn. For onset of cellulitis on the back accompanied by constipation, usually used together with Bai Zhi (Radix Angelicae Dahuricae); for appendicitis with abdominal pain and fever, usually used with Mu Dan Pi (Cortex Moutan Radicis), Tao Ren (Semen Persicae), etc., as in Daihuang Mudanpi Tang (Decoction of Radix et Rhizoma Rhei and Cortex Moutan Radicis); for fireburn, mix the powder of Dai Huang (Radix et Rhizoma Rhei) with sesame oil and apply the paste to the affected area.

(5) Amenorrhea due to Blood stasis, retention of lochia after delievery, mass in the abdomen or trauma. For postpartum Blood stasis with abdominal pain, usually used together with Zhe Chong (Eupolyphaga seu Steleophaga), Tao Ren (Semen Persicae), etc., as in Xia Yuxue Tang (Decoction for Discharging Blood Clots); for amenorrhea due to Blood stasis, usually used with Hong Hua (Flos Carthami), Chi Shao (Radix Paeoniae Rubra) and Dang Gui (Radix Angelicae Sinensis), as in Wu Ji Wan (Bolus for Regulating Menstruation By Dispelling Blood Stasis); for mass in the abdomen, usually used with Tao Ren (Semen Persicae), Meng Chong (Tabanus), etc., as in Daihuang Zhechong Wan (Pill of Radix et Rhizoma Rhei and Eupolyphaga seu Steleophaga); for traumatic injury with Blood stasis inside and tenderness all over the abdomen, usually used with Chuan Shan Jia (Squama Manitis), Hong Hua (Flos Carthami) and Tao Ren (Semen Persicae), as in Fuyuan Huoxue Tang (Decoction for Recovery and Activating Blood Circulation).

Administration 3～12g for making a decoction or a powder or pills; q. s. for external application. Processed with vinegar for treating Blood stasis; unprepared and added late for decocting when used for purgation.

Precautions Prohibited or used with caution for women during pregnancy, menstruation or breast feeding period.

1.2. Mang Xiao (Natrii Sulphas)

Prescription Monoclinic system of mirabilite, natrii sulfas as its chief component.

Characteristics Salty and bitter in flavor, cold in nature, acting on the Stomach and Large Intestine Channels.

Action Clearing away Heat, relaxing the bowels, moistening the Dryness and softening the hard mass.

Indications

(1) Constipation due to accumulation and retention of Heat. Usually used with Dai Huang (Radix et Rhizoma Rhei), as in Tiaowei Cheng Qi Tang (Purgative Decoction for Coordinating the Function of the Stomach).

(2) Accumulation of sthenic Heat in the chest with epigastic pain

and a very hard abdomen. Usually used with Dai Huang (Radix et Rhizoma Rhei), Gan Sui (Radix Euphorbiae Kansui), etc.

(3) Sore throat, canker sores, red eyes and pyogenic infection. Used alone externally or in combination with Peng Sha (Borax), Zhu Sha (Cinnabaris), Bing Pian (Borneolum Syntheticum), etc., as in Bing Peng San (Borneolum and Borax Powder). In addition, it can be used externally for abscess and swelling of breast, and also as lactifuge with desirable effect.

Administration 10～15g, infused in the decoction of other drugs or in hot boiled water for oral intake; q. s. for external application.

Precautions Contraindicated for pregnant women.

1. 3. Fan Xie Ye (Folium Sennae)

Description The leaflet of Cassia Angustifolia Vahl and C acutifolia Delile. Family Leguminosae.

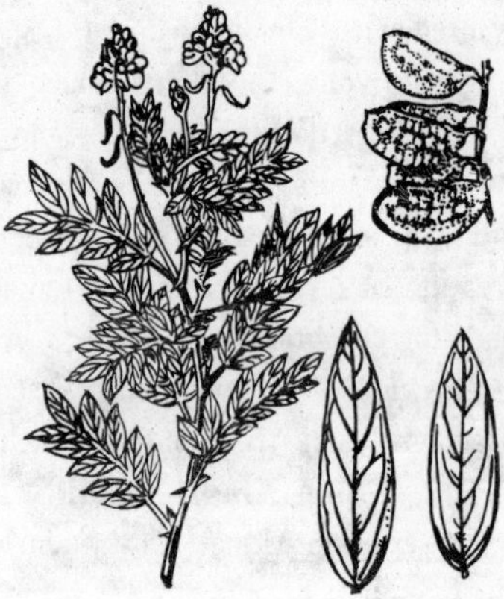

Characteristics Sweet and bitter in flavor, cold in nature, acting on the Large Intestine Channel.

Action Relaxing the bowels by purgation, expelling the Heat pathogen by leading it downward.

Indications Constipation, especially of Heat accumulation type. Used either alone or with Zhi Shi (Fructus Aurantii Immaturus), Hou Po (Cortex Magnoliae Officinalis), etc.

Administration 1. 5～3g for moistening the bowels; 5～10g for purgation. Soaked in boiling water and drunk like tea or decocted later than other ingredients.

Precautions Not to be applied to women drunk the period of menstruation, breast feeding or pregnancy. Overdosage will result in nausea, vomiting, abdominal pain and other side-effect.

2. Drugs for Moisturizing the Intestines

Drugs of this type are mostly seeds or kernels that are rich in oil and therefore they are capable of moisturizing the intestines. These drugs are used to treat constipation resulting from Yin deficiency, fluid exhaustion or Blood deficiency in patients who are old, weak, suffering from protracted illness or after childbirth. In clinical application of these drugs, the patient's particular conditions should be taken into consideration and these drugs should be used in combination with drugs for tonifying Yin, drugs for replenishing Qi, drugs for nourishing Blood or drugs for promoting the Qi circulation.

2.1. Huo Ma Ren (Fructus Cannabis)

Description The ripe seed of Cannabis sativa L. Family Moraceae.

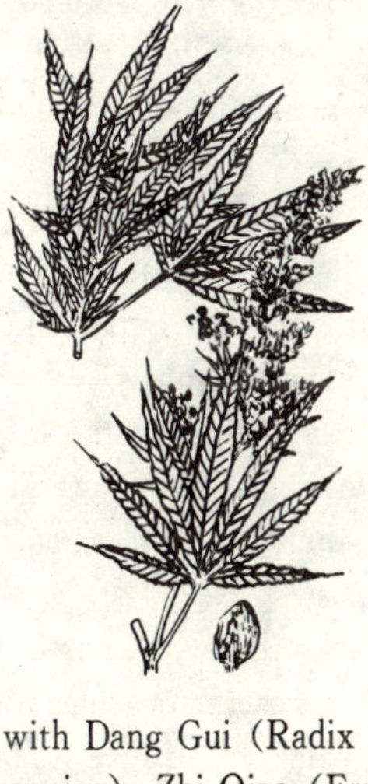

Characteristics Sweet in flavor, neutral in nature, acting on the Spleen and Large Intestine Channels.

Action Moisturizing the bowels to relieve constipation, tonifying the body to replenish Qi.

Indications Dry intestines and constipation. For constipation due to Deficiency of Yin-Blood, usually used together with Dang Gui (Radix Angelicae Sinensis), Sheng Di (Radix Rehmanniae), Zhi Qiao (Fructus Aurantii), etc., as in Yun Chang Wan (Pill for Moistening the Bowels); for constipation due to Dryness of Lung which prevents the pure Lung-Qi from descending, usually used with Xuan Shen (Radix Scrophulariae), Sheng Di (Radix Rehmanniae) and cow milk; for constipation due to Qi stagnation, used with Su Zi (Fructus Perillae) to make a gruel, as in Maren Sizi Zhou (Gruel of Fructus Cannabis and Fructus Perillae); for constipation due to Qi Deficiency, used with Huang Qi (Radix Astragali seu Hedysari), Chen Pi (Pericarpium Citri Reticulatae) and honey, as in Huangqi Tang (Decoction of Radix Astragali seu Hedysari); while for constipation due to Dry-Heat of the Stomach and Intestines, used with Xing Ren (Semen pruni Armeniacae), Bai Shao (Radix Paeoniae Alba), Dai Huang (Radix et Rhizoma Rhei), Zhi Shi (Fructus Aurantii Immaturus), etc., as in Maziren Wan (Fructus Cannabis Pill).

Administration 10 ~ 30g for making a decoction, powder or pills.

Precautions Overdosage is forbidden, an oral intake of above 60 ~ 120g once will be toxicated.

2. 2. Yu Li Ren (Semen Pruni)

Description The seed of Prunus humilis Bunge or P. japonica Thunb. Family Rosaceae.

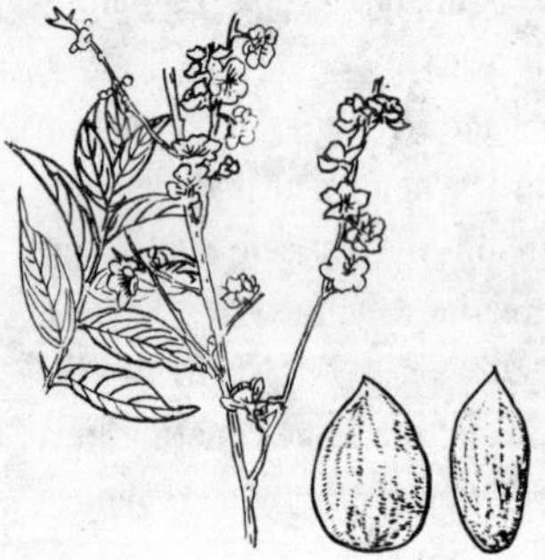

Characteristics Sweet and bitter in flavor, neutral in nature, acting on the Large and Small Intestines Channels

Action Moisturizing the Intestines to relax the bowels, promoting diuresis to relieve edema.

Indications

(1) Dry bowels with constipation. Usually used with Xing Ren (Semen Armeniacae Amarum), Bai Zi Ren (Semen Biotae), etc., as in Wuren Wan (Pill of Five Kinds of Kernels).

(2) Edema, abdominal distension, dysuria, etc. Usually used with Sang Bai Pi (Cortex Mori Radicis), Chi Xiao Dou (Semen Phaseoli) and Bai Mao Gen (Rhizoma Imperatae), as in Yuliren Tang (Semen Pruni Decoction).

Administration 5～12g for making a decoction.

Precautions Contraindicated for insufficiency of the Qi in Middle-jiao, Deficiency of the Spleen-Yang and Kidney-Yang, or Deficiency of the Liver-Yin and Kidney-Yin.

3. Drugs for Purging Heat and Retained Fluid

Drugs of this type are drastic in purgation and can cause serious diarrhea to discharge the retained fluid with defecation, some can also promote diuresis and expel the retained fluid through urination. They are indicated for edema, water retention in the chest and abdomen, accumulation and retention of Phlegm, dyspnea due to retention of Phlegm and fluid and sudden abdominal pain due to obstruction of vital energy.

As these drugs are highly toxic and tend to impair the vital energy, they are suitable only for sthenic syndromes. For prolonged illness when the vital energy is deficient, attention should be paid to protecting the vital energy by applying purgatives first and tonics second or vice versa. For the same reason, attention should also be paid to the processing, dosage, administration and contraindication of those drugs so as to ensure a safe and effective application.

3.1. Gan Sui (Radix Euphorbiae Kansui)

Description The root tuber of Euphorbia kansui T. N. Liou ex T. P. Wang. Family Euphorbiaceae.

Characteristics Bitter and sweet in flavor, cold in nature, toxic, and acting on the Lung, Kidney and Large Intestine Channels.

Action Dispelling fluid by purgation, dispersing mass to relieve edema.

Indications

(1) Systemic edema, fluid retention in the abdomen or in the chest and costal regions. Used alone or with Da Ji (Radix Euphorbiae Pekinensis), Yuan Hua (Flos Genkwa), Hei Chou (Semen Pharbitidis), Mu Xiang (Radix Aucklandiae), etc., as in Zhou Ju Wan

(Bolus for Clearing Away Ascites).

(2) Accumulation and retention of Phlegm, dyspnea due to retention of Phlegm and fluid, chest pain and abdominal pain for the same cause, indigestion and epilepsy due to Phlegm retention. For cough and hypochondriac pain due to Phlegm retention in the chest and costal region, usually used in combination with Da Ji (Radix Euphorbiae), Yuan Hua (Flos Genkwa) and Da Zao (Fructus Ziziphi Jujubae), as in Shi Zao Tang (Ten Jujube Decoction); for fluid retention complicated by Heat in the chest, usually used with Da Huang (Radix et Rhizoma Rhei) and Mang Xiao (Natrii Sulfas), as in Dai Xianxiong Tang (Major Decoction for Removing Phlegm-Heat from Chest); for vomiting, regurgitation and intestine obstruction, usually used with Dai Zhe Shi (Ochra), Mang Xiao (Natrii Sulfas), Gan Jiang (Rhizoma Zingiberis), etc.; for epilepsy due to Phlegm retention in the chest, usually used with Zhu Sha (Cinnabaris) to make Sui Xin Dan (Bolus of Radix Euphorbiae Kansui and Pig's Heart)

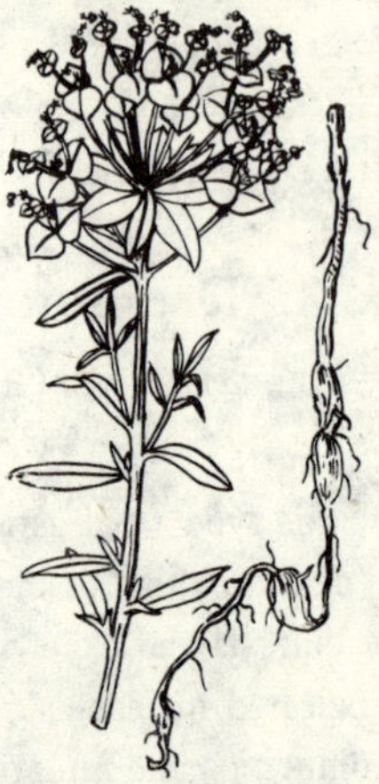

(3) Pyogenic infection. Mix Gan Sui (Radix Euphorbiae Kansui) with water and apply the paste to the affected part.

Administration 0.5～1g for making powder and boluses, not to be decocted; q.s. for external application.

Precautions Not applied to pregnant women or patients of weak constitution. Antagonistic to Gan Cao (Radix Glycyrrhizae).

3.2. Da Ji (Radix Euphorbiae Pekinensis)

Description The root of Euphorbiae pekinensis Rupr. Family Euphorbiaceae; or Knoxia valerianoides Thorel et Pitard. Family Rubiaceae.

Characteristics Bitter and acrid in flavor, cold in nature, toxic, and acting on the Lung, Kidney and Large Intestine Channels.

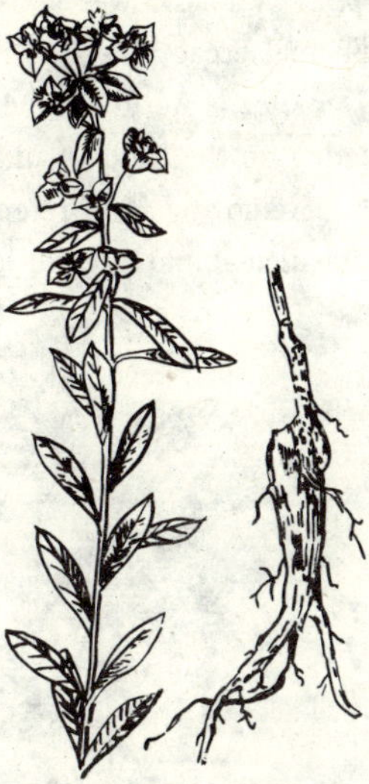

Action Removing water retention, relieving swelling and resolving mass.

Indications

(1) Edema of the face and body, vomiting and regurgitation with dyspnea, retention of water in the chest and abdomen, accumulation of Phlegm and fluid, etc. Used alone or with Gan Sui (Radix Euphorbiae Kansui) and Yuan Hua (Flos Genkwa), as in Shi Zao Tang (Ten Jujube Decoction). In the case of Phlegm accumulation in the chest and costal region resulting in stuffiness sensation in the chest, hypochondriac pain and epilepsy, or pain of the limbs and body due to overflow of Phlegm in the body, Da Ji (Radix Euphorbiae) is dispensed with Gan Sui (Radix Euphorbiae Kansui) and Bai Jie Zi (Semen Sinapis Albae), as in Kong Xian Dan (Pill for Controlling Phlegm).

(2) Pyogenic infection due to Heat pathogen, subcutaneous nodule and scrofula due to accumulation of Phlegm-Fire. Applied externally after being made into a powder and mixed with honey. It can also be applied externally or internally with the mixture of Xiong Huang (Realgar), Shan Ci Gu (Bulbus Cremastrae), etc. as in Zijin Ding (Purplish Gold Lozenge).

Administration 1.5～3g for making a decoction; 0.6～1g for making the powder; q.s. for external application.

Precautions Not applied to patients of weak constitution or during pregnancy. Antagonistic to Gan Cao (Radix Glycyrrhizae).

3.3. Yuan Hua (Flos Genkwa)

Description The flower buds of Daphne genkwa Sieb. et Zucc. Family Thymelaeceae.

Characteristics Acrid and bitter in flavor, warm in nature, toxic, and acting on the Lung, Kidney and Large Intestine Channels.

Action Removing fluid retention, eliminating Phlegm to relieve cough, parasiticidal and effctive for skin diseases.

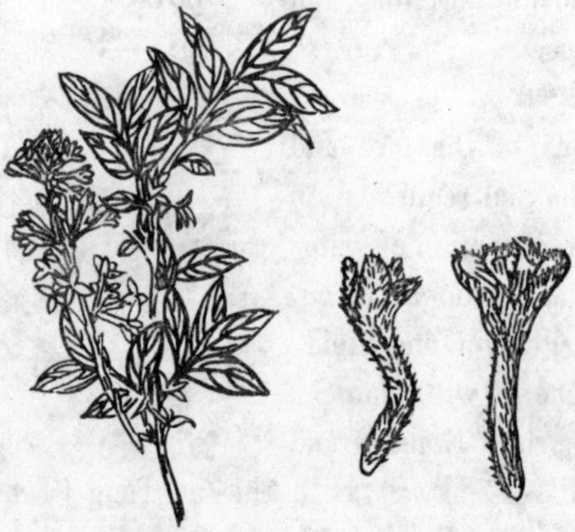

Indications

(1) Edema of the body and face, fluid retention in the abdomen or in the chest and costal region. Used either alone or with Zhi Qiao (Fructus Aurantii), as in Zhiqiao Wan (Bolus of Fructus Aurantii). In the case of Phlegm accumulation and retention in the chest leading to cough, dyspnea and vague pain in the chest and hypochondrium, used together with Gan Sui (Radix Euphorbiae Kansui) and Da Ji (Radix Euphorbiae Pekinensis), as in Shi Zao Tang (Ten Jujube Decoction) ; in the case of constant cough with profuse sputum, boil it with Da Zao (Fructus Ziziphi Jujubae), eat the jujube and the cough will be relieved.

(2) Tinea capitis, scalp infection and neurodermatitis. Powdered and used alone or with powdered Xiong Huang (Realgar) to make an ointment by mixing the powder with lard for external application. In addition, the decoction of Yuan Hua (Flos Genkwa) and Gan Cao (Radix Glycyrrhizae) can be used as a washing lotion for treating chilblain.

Administration 1. 5~3g for making a decoction; 0. 6g for making the powder; q. s. for external application.

Precautions Not applied to patients of weak constitution or during pregnancy. Antagonistic to Gan Cao (Radix Glycyrrhizae).

3. 4. Ba Dou (Fructus Crotonis)

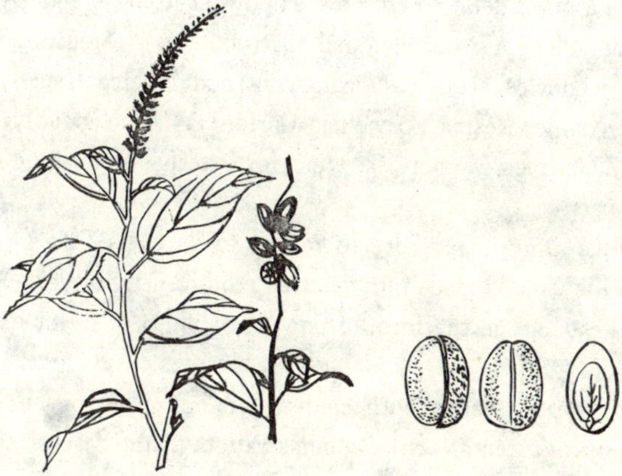

Description The fruit of Croton tiglium L. Family Euphorbiaceae.

Cha acteristics Acrid in flavor,.hot in nature, highly toxic, and acting on the Stomach, Large Intestine and Lung Channels.

Action Relaxing the bowels, dispelling Cold accumulation and fluid retention, eliminating Phlegm and easing throat.

Indications

(1) Food retention due to accumulation of Cold which obstructs the Intestines marked by abdominal distension and pain without bowel movement, and in the severe case, sudden syncope. For treatment, usually used together with Gan Jiang (Rhizoma Zingiberis) and DaiHuang (Radix et Rhizoma Rhei), as in Sanwu Beiji Wan (Bolus of Three Ingredients for Emergency). In the case of accumulation of sthenic Cold in the chest with tenderness and acute pain in the abdomen, usually used with Jie Geng (Radix Platycodi) and Bei Mu (Bulbus Fritillariae Cirrhosae), as in Sanwu Xiaobai San (Minor White Powder of Three Ingredients).

(2) Retention of fluid in the abdomen with abdominal distension. Usually ground with Xing Ren (Semen pruni Armeniacae) into pills for oral administration.

(3) Phlegm retention in the throat which leads to dyspnea, swelling and obstruction of the throat, and suffication. Feed the patient with a bit of defatted croton seed powder to bring about vomiting, so that Phlegm is expelled and obstruction is cleared.

(4) Carbuncles, scofula, subcutaneous nodule, etc. Usually used with Ru Xiang (Resina Boswelliae Carterii), Mo Yao (Myrrha), Mu Bie Zi (Semen Momordicae), etc. for external application of the affected part.

Administration In order to reduce toxicity, Ba Dou (Fructus Crotonis) is usually made into defatted croton seed powder. Oral intake: 0.1～0.3g, in the form of powder or pills; q. s. for external application.

Precautions Taken with cold water; hot gruel or hot water should not be taken after the administration. In the case of nonstop diarrhea after taking the drug, cold decoction of Huang Lian (Rhizoma Coptidis) or cold decoction of mung beans can relieve the symptom. Contraindicated in patients with weak constitution or during pregnancy. Antagonistic to Qian Niu (Semen Pharbitidis).

Wind-Dampness Eliminating Drugs

Drugs capable of eliminating Wind-Dampness from muscles, Meridians, tendons and bones to relieve pain from arthralgia and rheumatism are called Wind-Dampness eliminating drugs.

Drugs of this category are usually acrid and bitter in flavor, warm in nature and are indicated for arthralgia due to Wind-Dampness marked by swelling and pain of the joints with limited movement, spasm of muscles, numbness and hypoesthesia, hemiplegia, flaccidity of the lower limbs and other symptoms.

Clinical application of Wind-Dampness eliminating drugs should be based on actual conditions such as the location and duration of different types of arthralgia-syndrome and appropriate compatible drugs should be selected and used in combination. In the case of invasion of superficies by the pathogenic factors, drugs for relieving superficies-syndromes should be selected; in the case of pathogenic invasion of Meridians, tendons and bones, drugs for activating Blood circulation and regulating Meridians should be selected; while drugs for warming Meridians and dispelling Cold are added to treat Cold Excess syndrome, drugs for eliminating Dampness are added to treat Dampness Excess syndrome, and drugs for strengthening the vital energy are added to treat insufficiency of vital energy.

Since arthralgia-syndromes are mostly chronic, long-time medication is needed and therefore those drugs can be prepared into pills or tincture for convenient administration.

As drugs of this category are usually acrid and dry, they tend to consume Blood and impair Yin and for this reason, they should be applied with caution to Yin Deficiency and Blood insufficiency syndromes.

0. 1. Du Huo (Radix Angelicae Pubescentis)

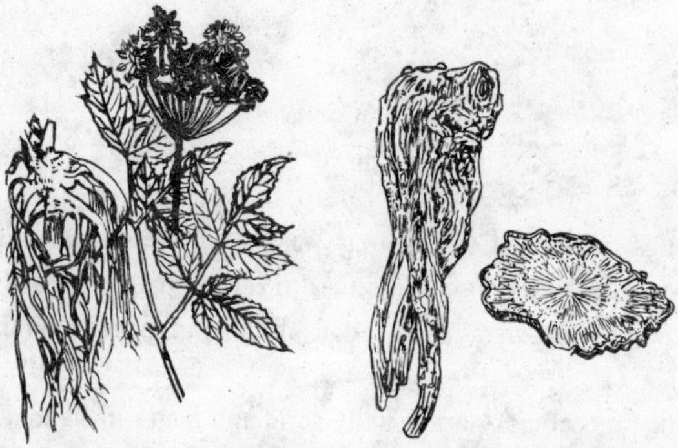

Description The root of Angelicae pubescens Maxim. f. biserrata Shan et Yuan. Family Umbelliferae.

Characteristics Acrid and bitter in flavor, warm in nature, acting on the Kidney and Urinary Bladder Channels.

Action Expelling pathogenic Wind and Dampness, dispersing pathogenic Cold from the superficies and relieving pain.

Indications

(1) Arthralgia due to Wind-Dampness marked by soreness, heaviness and pain of the waist, knees and feet. Usually used with Fang Feng (Radix Ledebouriallae), Xi Xin (Herba Asari), Sang Ji Sheng (Ramulus Loranthi), etc., as in Duhuo Jisheng Tang (Decoction of Radix Angelicae Pubescentis and Ramulus Loranthi).

(2) Fever, chilliness, heaviness and pain of head and body, soreness, heaviness and pain of joints induced by invasion of superficies

by pathogenic Wind-Cold. Usually used with Qiang Huo (Rhizoma seu Radix Noto-pterygii), Chai Hu (Radix Bupleuri), Chuan Xiong (Rhizoma Ligustici Chuanxiong), etc., as in Baidu San (Antitoxic Powder).

(3) Headache, toothache or pruritus of skin with discharge of fluid. For treating headache, usually used with Xi Xin (Herba Asari), Chuan Xiong (Rhizoma Ligustici Chuanxiong), etc., as in Duhuo Xixin Tang (Decoction of Radix Angelicae Pubescentis and Herba Asari); for toothache due to Wind-Fire, used in combination with Shi Gao (Gypsum Fibrosum), Sheng Ma (Rhizoma Cimicifugae), Jiang Can (Bombyx Batryticatus), etc.; for pruritus of Dampness type, used together with Bai Xian Pi (Cortex Dictamni Radicis), Cang Zhu (Rhizoma Atractylodis), Cang Er Zi (Fructus Xanthii), etc.

Administration 3～10g for making a decoction.

Precautions Contraindicated for dryness of the Blood due to Yin Deficiency, asthenic Wind and endogenous Wind.

0.2. Wei Ling Xian (Radix Clematidis)

Description The root and rhizome of Clematis chinensis Osbeck and the other species of the same genus. Family Ranunculaceae.

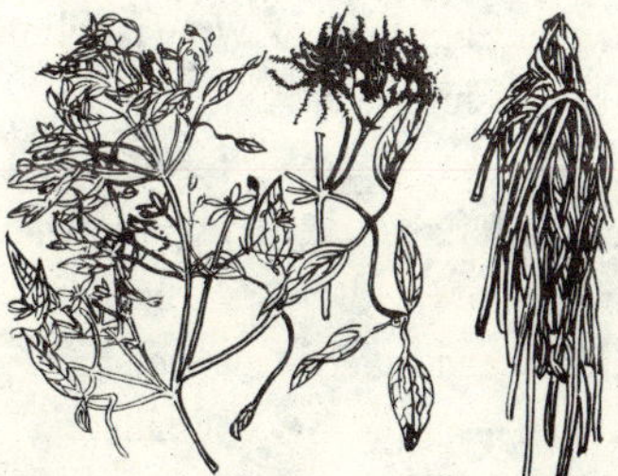

Characteristics Acrid and salty in flavor, warm in nature, acting on the Urinary Bladder Channels.

Action Eliminating pathogenic Wind and Dampness, regulating Collaterals to relieve pain, dispersing Phlegm and stasis, treating fishbone stuck in the throat.

Indications

(1) Pain from arthralgia. Usually used with Chuan Wu (Radix Aconiti), Wu Ling Zhi (Faeces Trogopterorum), Hai Feng Teng (Caulis Piperis Futokadsurae), etc.

(2) Retention of Phlegm in the chest, cough, dyspnea, vomiting, fullness sensation in the abdomen and loss of appetite, etc. Usually used together with Ban Xia (Rhizoma Pinelliae) and Zao Jiao (Spina Gleditsiae), as in Tingtan Suyin Fang (Prescription for Expelling Phelgm and Improving Appetite).

(3) Abdominal pain due to stagnation, mass in the abdomen. Usually used in combination with Dang Gui (Radix Angelicae Sinensis) and Rou Gui (Cortex Cinnamomi).

(4) Fishbone or other bones stuck in the throat. Swallow slowly the decoction of Wei Ling Xian (Radix Clematidis) alone or with vinegar and sugar.

Administration 5～10g for making a decoction; 30g for bone stuck.

Precautions Used with caution for patients of weak constitution.

0. 3. Fang Ji (Radix Stephaniae Tetrandrae)

Description The root of Stephania tetrandra S. Moore (family Menispermaceae), or of Aristolochia fangchi Wu (familv Aristolochiaceae).

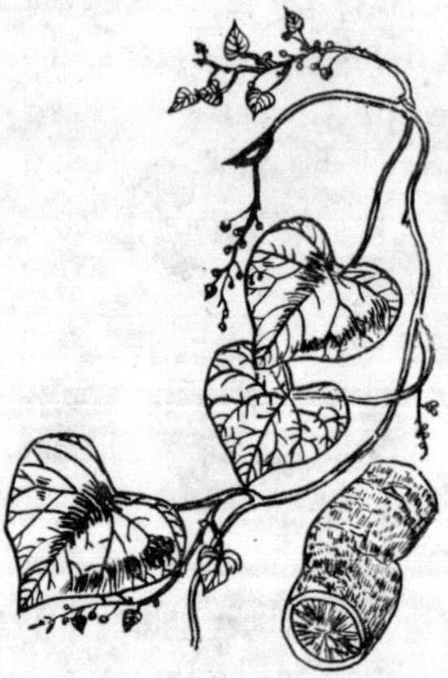

Characteristics Bitter and acrid in flavor, cold in nature, acting on the Urinary Bladder, Kidney and Spleen Channels.

Action Eliminating pathogenic Wind and Dampness, relieving arthralgia pain, promoting diuresis to treat edema.

Indications

(1) Pain from arthralgia. For arthralgia due to Damp-Heat, used with Yi Yi Ren (Semen Coicis), Hua Shi (Talcum), Can Sha (Faeces Bombycis), etc., as in Xuanbi Tang (Decoction for Relieving Arthralgia); for arthralgia due to Damp-Cold, usually used in combi-

nation with Chuan Wu (Radix Aconiti), Gui Xin (tender Ramulus Cinnamomi), Fu Zi (Radix Aconiti Praeparata), etc.; for beriberi with swelling and pain, used with Mu Gua (Fructus Chaenomelis), Niu Xi (Radix Achyranthis Bidentatae), Yi Yi Ren (Semen Coicis), etc.

(2) Dysuria with edema or retention of fluid in the abdomen. In the case of sthenic Heat type, used with Ting Li Zi (Semen Lepidii seu Descurainiae), Jiao Mu (Semen Zanthoxyli), Dai Huang (Radix et Rhizoma Rhei), etc., as in Ji Jiao Li Huang Wan (Pill of Stephania Tetrandrae, Semen Zanthoxyli, Semen Lepidii seu Descurainiae and Radix et Rhizoma Rhei); in the case of asthenic syndrome, usually used with Huang Qi (Radix Astragali seu Hedysari), Bai Zhu (Rhizoma Atractylodis Macrocephalae), Gan Cao (Radix Glycyrrhizae), etc., as in Fangji Huangqi Tang (Decoction of Stephania Tetrandrae and Astragali seu Hedysari).

Administration 5~10g for making a decoction.

Precautions Used with caution for Deficiency of Spleen and Stomach.

0. 4. Qin Jiao (Radix Gentianae Macrophyllae)

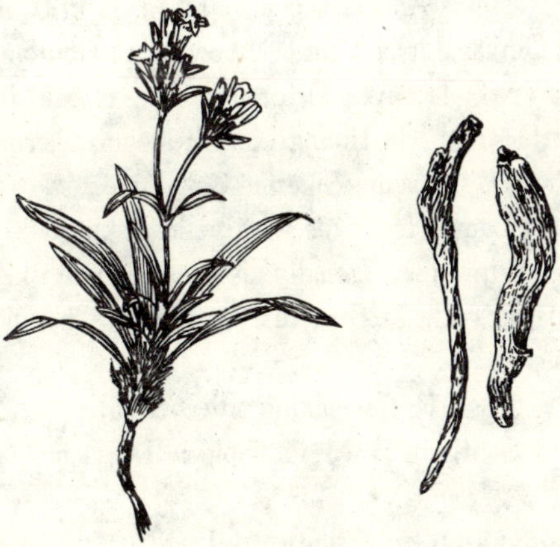

Description Root of Gentiana macrophylla Pall, Gentiana straminea Maxim, Gentiana crassicaulis Duthis et Burk. or Gentiana dahurica Fisch. Family Gentianaceae.

Characteristics Bitter and acrid in flavor, slightly cold in nature, acting on the Stomach, Liver and Gallbladder Channels.

Action Eliminating pathogenic Wind and Dampness, relaxing tendons, regulating Collaterals, clearing away Heat and relieving jaundice.

Indications

(1) Arthralgia pain due to Wind-Dampness, muscular contracture, hemiplagia, etc. For arthralgia of the Cold type, usually used in combination with Du Huo (Radix Angelicae Pubescentis), Sang Ji Sheng (Ramulus Loranthis), etc., as in Duhuo Jisheng Tang (Decoction of Angelicae Pubescentis and Loranthis); for arthralgia of Heat type, used together with Fang Ji (Radix Stephaniae Tetrandrae), Jin Yin Hua (Flos Lonicerae), Zhi Mu (Rhizoma Anemarrhenae), etc.; for apoplexy, used with Qiang Huo (Rhizoma seu Radix Noto-pterygii), Du Huo (Radix Angelicae Pubescentis), Dang Gui (Radix Angelicae Sinensis), etc., as in Da Qinjiao Tang (Major Decoction of Radix Gentiana Macrophyllae).

(2) Hectic fever due to asthnia of viscera. For hectic fever due to Yin Deficiency, usually used with Qing Hao (Herba Artemisiae Annuae), Zhi Mu (Rhizoma Anemarrhenae) and Di Gu Pi (Cortex Lycii Radicis), as in Qinjiao Biejia Tang (Decoction of Gentiana Macrophyllae and Carapax Trionycis); for infantile malnutrition with fever, used together with Hu Huang Lian (Rhizoma Picrorhizae), Ji Nei Jin (Endothelium Corneum Gigeriae Galli), etc.

(3) Jaundice of Damp-Heat type with yellow skin and eyewhite, dysuria with reddish urine. Usually used with Yin Chen (Herba Artemisiae Scopariae), Zhi Zi (Fructus Gardeniae), Che Qian Zi (Semen Plantaginis), etc.

Administration 5～10g for making a decoction.

Precautions Contraindicated for Spleen Deficiency and loose stools.

0.5. Mu Gua (Fructus Chaenomelis)

Description Fruit of Chaenomeles speciosa (Sweet) Nakai or C. sinensis (Thouin) Koehne. Family Rosaceae.

Characteristics Sour in flavor, warm in nature, acting on the Liver and Spleen Channels.

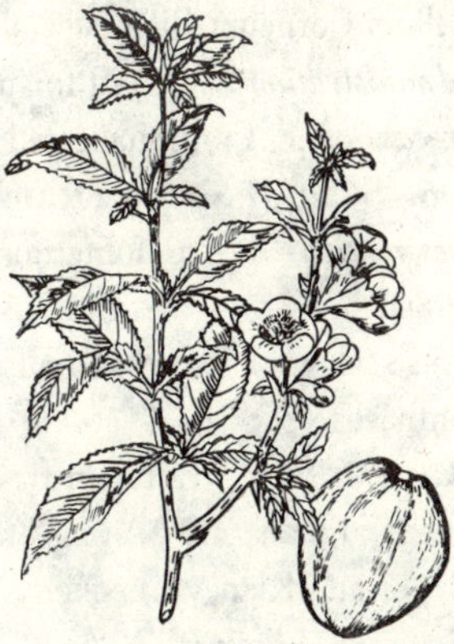

Action Relaxing tendons, regulating Collaterals, eliminating Dampness and improving digestion.

Indications

(1) Arthralgia with pain, contracture of tendons, swelling and pain due to beriberi. In the case of predominance of pathogenic Dampness, usually used with Niu Xi (Radix Achyranthis Bidentatae), Wu Jia Pi (Cortex Acanthopancis Radicis), etc.; in the case of predominance of pathogenic Cold, used with Chuan Wu (Radix Aconiti), Cao Wu (Radix Aconiti Kusnezoffii), etc. For stiff neck, cramp of tendons, inability to move around, used with Ru Xiang (Resina Boswelliae Carterii), Mo Yao (Myrrha), Sheng Di (Radix Rehmanniae), etc., as in Mugua Jian (Fructus Chaenomeles Decoction). For swelling and pain due to beriberi, usually used with Wu Zhu Yu (Fructus Euodiae), Bing Lang (Semen Arecae), etc., as in Jiming San (Cock Crowing Powder).

(2) Vomiting and diarrhea with muscular cramp. In the case of affection of Summer-Dampness marked by vomiting and diarrhea, fullness sensation of the chest, pain and cramp of the abdomen due to predominance of Cold and Dampness complicated by superficies syndromes, used together with Xiang Ru (Herba Elsholtziae seu Moslae), Huo Xiang (Herba Agastachis), etc., as in Xiangru Wan (Bolus of Herba Elsholtziae seu Moslae); in the case of vomiting and diarrhea with severe pain and cramp of the abdomen, used with Can Sha (Faeces Bombycis), Yi Yi Ren (Semen Coicis), Huang Lian (Rhizoma Coptidis), Wu Zhu Yu (Fructus Euodiae), etc., as in Can-Shi Tang (Faeces Bombycis Decoction).

(3) Stagnation of food, indigestion, etc. Usually used with Shan Zha (Fructus Crataegi), Bing Lang (Semen Arecae), Ji Nei Jin (En-

dothelium Corneum Gigeriae Galli),etc.

Administration 6～12g for making a decoction.

Precautions Contraindicated for dysuria and retention of urine.

0. 6. Sang Ji Sheng (Ramulus Loranthi)

Description The foliferous stem and branch of the Taxillus chinensis (D C.) Danser. Family Loranthaceae.

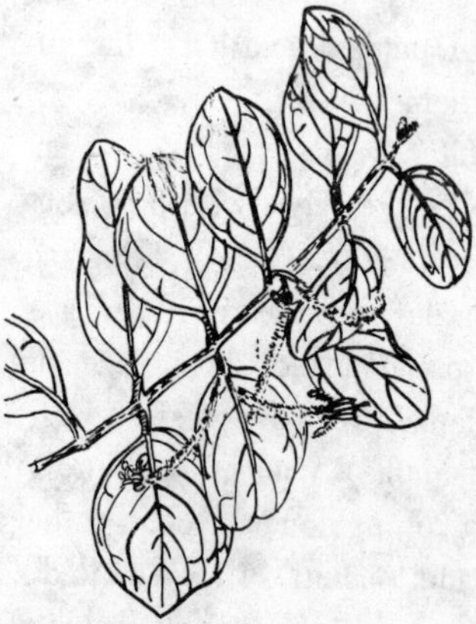

Characteristics Bitter in flavor, neutral in nature, acting on the Liver and Kidney Channels.

Action Eliminating pathogenic Wind and Dampness, tonifying Liver and Kidney, strengthening bones and preventing miscarriage.

Indications

(1) Arthralgia due to pathogenic Wind and Dampness, soreness and pain of waist and knees, weakness of tendons and bones, or hemiplagia, beriberi, etc. For arthralgia, used together with Du Huo (Radix Angelicae Pubescentis), Du Zhong (Cortex Eucommiae), Xi Xin (Herba Asari), etc., as in Duhuo Jisheng Tang (Decoction of Angelicae Pubescentis and Loranthi); for flaccidity of extremities and hemiplegia, usually used with Shu Di (Radix Rehmanniae Praeparata), Gui Ban (Plastrum Testudinis), Niu Xi (Radix Achyranthis Bidentatae), etc.

(2) Threatened abortion, vaginal bleeding during pregnancy or metrorrhagia due to insufficiency of both Liver and Kidney, and unconsolidation of the Chong and Ren Channels. Usually used with Xu Duan (Radix Dipsaci), E Jiao (Colla Corii Asini), Ai Ye (Folium Artemisiae Argyi), etc., as in Sangjisheng San (Ramulus Loranthi Powder).

(3) Dizziness, headache, insomnia and blurred vision. Usually used with Nü Zhen Zi (Fructus Ligustri Lucidi), Du Zhong (Cortex Eu-

commiae), Han Lian Cao(Herba Ecliptae),etc.

Administration 10～20g for making a decoction.

0. 7. Bai Hua She (Bungarus Parvus)

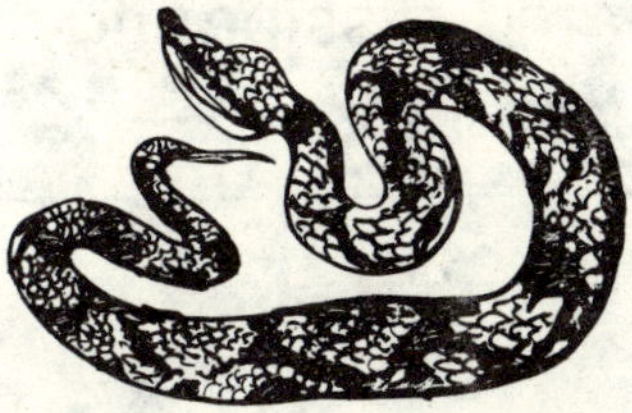

Description The whole body (viscera discarded) of Bungarus multicinctus Blyth. Family Elapidae.

Characteristics Sweet and salty in flavor, warm in nature, toxic,acting on the Liver Meridian.

Action Expelling pathogenic Wind, regulating the Collaterals, relieving convulsion and pain.

Indications

(1) Intractable rheumatism, muscular spasm, deviation of the mouth and eye, numbness of limbs or hemiplegia from apoplexy. Usually used with Qiang Huo (Rhizoma seu Radix Noto-pterygii), Tian Ma (Rhizoma Gastrodiae), Fang Feng (Radix Ledebouriellae),Dang Gui(Radix Angelicae Sinensis),etc. , or used alone by preparing it into cream,medicated wine,pills or powder.

(2) Intractable tinea infection,itching of the skin,scrofula,pyogenic infection,etc. Usually used in combination with Xiong Huang (Realgar),Sheng Dai Huang (Radix et Rhizoma Rhei unprepared), etc. , as in Yanfang Qufeng San (Effective Powder for Eliminating Wind).

(3) Tetanus and infantile convulsion. Used together with Wu Shao She (Zaocys),Wu Gong(Scolopendra),etc. ,as in Ding Ming San (Powder for Life-recovery).

Administration 3～10g for making a decoction; 1～ 1. 5g for taking as a powder.

Precautions Contraindicated for Deficiency of Yin and Blood, or the case of overabundance of Heat bringing about false Wind.

Damp-dissipating Aromatics

Drugs capable of dissipating Dampness and invigorating the function of Spleen and with a aromatic smell are categorized as Damp-dissipating aromatics.

Drugs of this category have a pungent flavor and warm nature, they have the function of regulating the circulation of Qi, eliminating the pathogenic Dampness, invigorating the Spleen and Stomach, and therefore they are indicated for abdominal distension, vomiting, poor appetite, loose stools, lassitude, sweet taste in the mouth, excessive salivation, whitish greasy coat on the tongue due to Dampness invasion of the Spleen and Stomach leading to functional disorder. Some of these drugs can be used to treat Damp-Warm syndromes and syndromes due to Summer-Heat and Dampness.

Compatible drugs should be used in combination according to different types of pathogenic Dampness in clinical application, e. g. for Cold-Dampness, drugs for warming the interior should be used together; for Damp-Heat, drugs for purging Heat and eliminating Dampness should be applied in combination. As Dampness obstructs the normal flow of Qi, and regulating the flow of Qi will help resolve Dampness, drugs of this category are therefore often used together with drugs for promoting the flow of Qi. Besides, they are often dispensed together with drugs for strengthening the Spleen to enhance the Damp-dissipating effect.

As these drugs tend to impair Qi and Ying, care should be taken in applying them to the case of Yin Deficiency and fluid insufficiency or to the case of Deficiency of both Qi and Ying. Also, drugs with a fragrant odour should not be decocted for long lest there should be a loss of efficacy.

0. 1. Cang Zhu (Rhizoma Atractylodis)

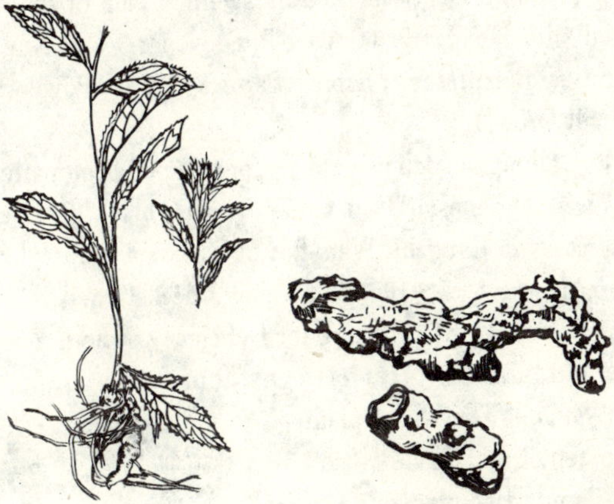

Description The rhizome of Atractylodes lancea (Thunb.) D C., or Atractylodes chinensis (D C.) koidz. Family Compositae.

Characteristics Acrid and bitter in flavor, warm in nature, acting on the Spleen and Stomach Channels.

Action Eliminating Dampness, invigorating the Spleen, dispelling Wind, diminishing cataract to improve eyesight.

Indications

(1) Disturbance of the Middle-jiao due to accumulation of Dampness marked by epigastric distress, abdominal distension, anorexia, nausea and vomiting, lassitude, turbid and greasy tongue coat, etc. Cang Zhu (Rhizoma Atractylodis) is the key drug for eliminating Dampness and invigorating the Spleen, and it is often used together with Hou Po (Cortex Magnoliae Officinalis), Chen Pi (Pericarpium Citri Reticulatae), etc., as in Pingwei San (Powder for Regulating

the Function of Stomach).

(2) Arthralgia-syndrome due to pathogenic Wind-Cold-Dampness, marked by pain of the limbs and joints. Usually used with Qiang Huo (Rhizoma seu Radix Notopterygii), Gui Zhi (Ramulus Cinnamomi), Fang Feng (Radix Ledebouriellae), etc. For affection of pathogenic Wind-Cold-Dampness manifested as headache, anhidrosis and aches in the limbs, used together with Qiang Huo (Rhizoma seu Radix Notopterygii), Fang Feng (Radix Ledebouriellae), etc; for descending of Damp-Heat, marked by swelling pain of the knees, usually used with Huang Bo (Cortex Phellodendri) and Niu Xi (Radix Achyranthis Bidentatae), named Sanmiao San (Powder of Three Wonderful Drugs).

(3) Eye ailments such as external or internal oculopathy, optic atraphy, night blindness. Used alone or with black sesame seed and pork Liver, as in Cangzhu Wan (Pill of Rhizoma Atractylodis).

Administration 5～10g for making a decoction.

Precautions Used with care for Deficiency of both Yin and fluid.

0. 2. Huo Xiang (Herba Agastachis)

Description The whole plant of Pogostemon cablin (Blanco) Benth. Family Labiatae.

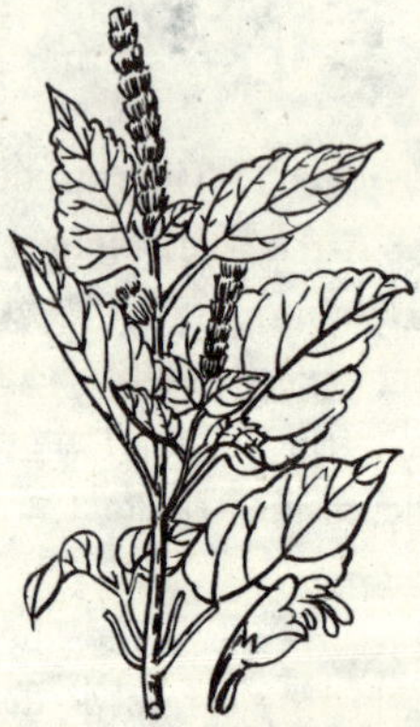

Characteristics Acrid in flavor, slightly warm in nature, acting on the Spleen, Stomach and Lung Channels.

Action Removing Dampness, relieving Summer-Heat and arresting vomiting.

Indications

(1) Disturbance of Middle-jiao due to accumulation of Dampness, marked by epigastric distress, abdominal distension, anorexia, nausea and vomiting. Huo Xiang (Herba Agastachis) is the key drug for removing Dampness and it is often used together with Cang Zhu (Rhizoma Atractylodis), Hou Po

(Cortex Magnoliae Officinalis), Ban Xia (Rhizoma Pinelliae), etc., as in Buhuanjin Zheng Qi San (Priceless Health Restoring Powder).

(2) Affection of exopathogenic Wind-Cold in summer or impairment of the interior by eating uncooked or cold food with manifestations of fever, headache, tight chest, abdominal distension, vomiting and diarrhea. Usually used together with Zi Su (Folium Perillae), Ban Xia (Rhizoma Pinelliae), Hou Po (Cortex Magnoliae Officinalis), etc., as in Huoxiang Zheng Qi San (Powder of Herba Agastachis for Restoring Health). In the case of Summer-Heat with dizziness, tight chest, sticky and greasy sensation in the mouth, used together with Pei Lan (Herba Eupatorii) and Bo He (Herba Menthae) for making a drink by infusing them in the hot boiled water, fresh herb of Huo Xiang (Herba Agastachis) preferable.

(3) Vomiting, especially vomiting induced by pathogenic Dampness in the Spleen and Stomach. Usually used with Ban Xia (Rhizoma Pinelliae). For other kinds of vomiting, compatible drugs should be used in combination, e. g. vomiting due to Damp-Heat should be treated by dispensing it with Huang Lian (Rhizoma Coptidis) and Zhu Ru (Caulis Bambusae in Taeniam); vomiting due to Deficiency of Spleen and Stomach should be treated by dispensing it with Dang Shen (Radix Codonopsis Pilosulae) and Gan Cao (Radix Glycyrrhizae); vomiting due to morning sickness should be treated by dispensing it with Sha Ren (Fructus Amomi), etc.

Administration 5～10g for making a decoction. Double amount for fresh herb. Not decocted for long.

Precautions Used with caution for insufficiency of both Qi and Ying.

0. 3. Hou Po (Cortex Magnoliae Officinalis)

Description The bark of the trunk or root of Magnolia officinalis Rehd. et Wils., or Magnolia officinalis Rehd. et Wils. var. biloba Rehd. et Wils. Family Magnoliaceae.

Characteristics Bitter and acrid in flavor, warm in nature, acting on the Spleen, Stomach, Lung and Large Intestine Channels.

Action Promoting the flow of Qi, eliminating Dampness, removing food stagnation and relieving asthma.

Indications

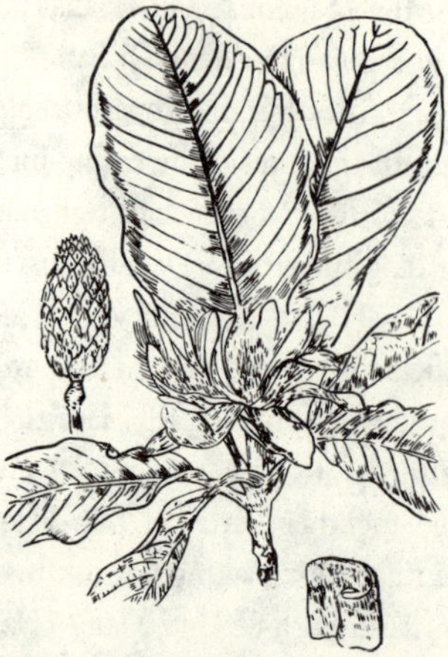

(1) Gastric fullness and abdominal distension due to retention of Dampness, stagnation of indigested food or stagnation of Qi. Hou Po (Cortex Magnoliae Officinalis) is the key drug for dispelling abdominal distension. For stagnation of Dampness in the Middle-jiao marked by abdominal distension, nausea and vomiting, it can be dispensed with Cang Zhu (Rhizoma Atractylodis) and Chen Pi (Pericarpium Citri Reticulatae), as in Pingwei San (Powder for Regulating the Function of Stomach); for accumulation of sthenic Heat leading to constipation, it can be dispensed with Dai Huang (Radix et Rhizoma Rhei), Mang Xiao (Natrii Sulfas) and Zhi Shi (Fructus Aurantii Immaturus), as in Da Cheng Qi Tang (Major Decoction for Purging Down Digestive Qi); for abdominal distension due to Deficiency-Cold, it is used together with Ren Shen (Radix Ginseng), Gan Cao (Radix Glycyrrhizae), Sheng Jiang (Rhizoma Zingiberis Recens), etc.

(2) Cough and asthma with much phlegm due to accumulation of Phlegm-Dampness in the Lung. Usually used together with Ma Huang (Herba Ephedrae), Xing Ren (Semen Armeniacae Amarum), Ban Xia (Rhizoma Pinelliae), etc., as in Houpo Mahuang Tang (Decoction of Cortex Magnoliae Officinalis and Herba Ephedrae).

Administration 3～10g for making a decoction.

Precautions Applied with caution to Qi Deficiency of both Spleen and Stomach.

0.4. Sha Ren (Fructus Amomi)

Description The ripe fruit of Amomum villosum Lour., or Amomum longiligulare Wu. Family Zingiberaceae.

Characteristics Acrid in flavor, warm in nature, acting on the Spleen, Stomach and Kidney Channels.

Action Resolving Dampness to regulate the flow of Qi, warming the Middle-jiao to stop diarrhea, and preventing miscarriage.

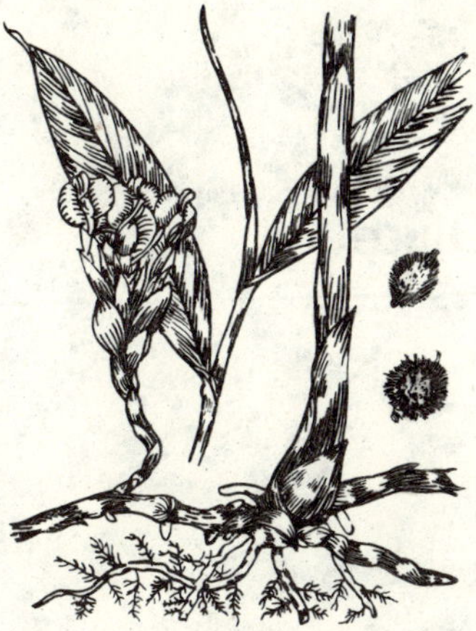

Indications

(1) Epigastric fullness and abdominal distenion, anorexia, nausea, vomiting and diarrhea due to accumulation of Dampness in the Middle-jiao and stagnation of Qi in the Spleen and Stomach. In the case of accumulation of Dampness, usually used with Hou Po (Cortex Magnoliae Officinalis) and Cang Zhu (Rhizoma Atractylodis); in the case of food retention and Qi stagnation, usually used with Mu Xiang (Radix Aucklandiae), Zhi Shi (Fructus Aurantii Immaturus), Bai Zhu (Rhizoma Atractylodis Macrocephalae), etc., as in Xiang Sha Zhi Zhu Wan (Pill of Radix Aucklandiae, Fructus Amomi, Fructus Aurantii Immaturus and Rhizoma Atractylodis Macrocephalae); in the case of Deficiency of Spleen and stagnation of Qi, used together with Dang Shen (Radix Codonopsis Pilosulae), Bai Zhu (Rhizoma Atractylodis), etc., as in Xiang Sha Liujunzi Tang (Decoction of Radix Aucklandiae, Fructus Amomi and Six Noble Ingredients).

(2) Abdominal pain, diarrhea and dysentery due to asthenic Cold of the Spleen and Stomach. Usually used with Gan Jiang (Rhizoma Zingiberis), Fu Zi (Radix Aconiti Praeparata), Rou Dou Kou (Semen Myristicae), etc.

(3) Pernicious vomiting during pregnancy with threatened abortion. Usually used with Bai Zhu (Rhizoma Atractylodis Macrocephalae), Su Geng (Caulis Perillae), Sang Ji Sheng (Ramulus Loranthi), etc.

Administration 3~6g for making a decoction, added late.

Precautions Used with caution for Qi Deficiency and Yin impairment syndromes.

Diuretics

Drugs mainly capable of promoting diuresis and eliminating Dampness are categorized as diuretics.

Drugs of this category can increase the amount of urine and make micturition easy and therefore the pathogenic Dampness in the body can be excreted out through urination. They are mainly indicated for dysuria, edema, water retention in the abdomen, Phlegm retention, diarrhea, stranguria, jaundice, exudative wound, etc.

Most of these drugs are sweet and insipid in flavor, neutral or cold or slightly cold in nature. As "insipid drugs can excrete Dampness", drugs of this type are referred to as insipid drugs for excreting Dampness; while cold drugs can purge Heat and are mostly used for stranguria, these drugs are also known as drugs for inducing diuresis and relieving stranguria.

Drugs of this type should be used in combination with other types of drugs according to different conditions: for edema accompanied with superficies-syndromes, drugs for ventilating the Lung and inducing diaphoresis should be added; for protracted edema with insufficiency of both Spleen-Yang and Kidney-Yang, drugs for warming and tonifying the Spleen and Kidney should be applied together; for excessive Dampness and Heat, drugs for purging Heat and Fire should be dispensed; for impairment of Blood by Heat, drugs for cooling Blood and arresting bleeding should be used in combination.

As application of this type of drugs in large amount for a long time will result in consumption and impairment of Body-Fluid, they should be used with caution for insufficiency of both Yin and Body-Fluid syndromes.

0. 1. Fu Ling (Poria)

Description The sclerotium of the fungus, Poria cocos (Schw.) Wolf. Family Polyporaceae.

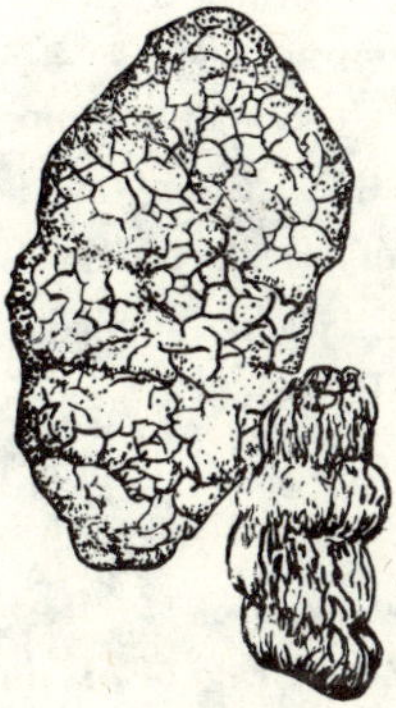

Characteristics Sweet and insipid in flavor, neutral in nature, acting on the Heart, Spleen, Lung and Kidney Channels.

Action Inducing diuresis, excreting Dampness, invigorating the Spleen and tranquilizing the mind.

Indications

(1) Retention of water-Dampness manifested as dysuria, edema, phlegm retention, etc. Usually used together with Zhu Ling (Polyporus Umbellatus), Ze Xie (Rhizoma Alismatis), etc., as in Wuling San (Powder of Five Drugs Including Poria). Since Fu Ling (Poria) is neutral in nature, it can be used for both Damp-Heat and Damp-Cold syndromes when used in combination with relevant drugs. e. g. Damp-Heat syndromes can be treated by applying it with Che Qian Zi (Semen Plantaginis), Mu Tong (Caulis Akebiae), etc.; while Damp-Cold with Fu Zi (Radix Aconiti Praeparata), Gan Jiang (Rhizoma Zingiberis), etc. In the case of vertigo, palpitation, cough and other symptoms induced by Phlegm retention, usually used together with Gui Zhi (Ramulus Cinnamomi), Bai Zhu (Rhizoma Atractylodis Macrocephalae), etc., as in Ling Gui Zhu Gan Tang (Decoction of Poria, Ramulus Cinnamomi, Rhizoma Atractylodis Macrocephalae and Radix Glycyrrhizae).

(2) Lassitude, anorexia and loose stools due to Deficiency of Spleen and weekness of Qi. Usually used with Dang Shen (Radix Codonopsis Pilosulae), Bai Zhu (Rhizoma Atractylodis Macrocephalae) and Gan Cao (Radix Glycyrrhizae), named Sijunzi Tang (Decoction of Four Noble Drugs).

(3) Palpitation and insomnia. In the case of insufficiency of Heart and Spleen, used with Dang Shen (Radix Codonopsis Pilosulae), Long Yan Rou (Arillus Longan), Suan Zao Ren (Semen Ziziphi Spinosae), etc., as in Guipi Tang (Decoction for Invigorating the Spleen and Nourishing the Heart); in the case of Phlegm retention in the interior, used with Shi Chang Pu (Rhizoma Acori Graminei), Yuan Zhi (Radix Polygalae), etc., as in Anshen Dingzhi Wan (Sedative Bolus).

Administration 10~15g for making a decoction.

Precautions Used with caution for Deficiency of both Yin and Body-Fluid.

0. 2. Zhu Ling (Polyporus Umbellatus)

Description The sclerotium of the fungus Polyporus umbellatus (Pers.) Fries. Family Polyporaceae.

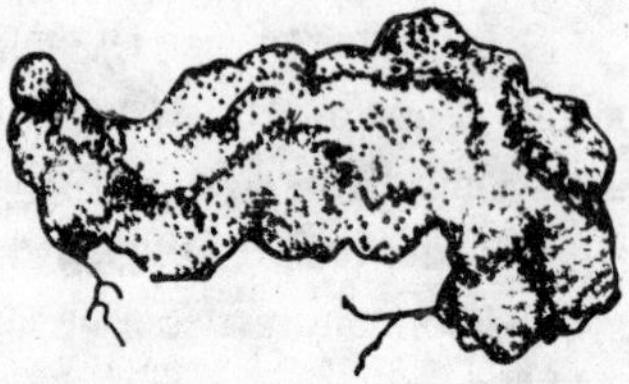

Characteristics Sweet and insipid in flavor, neutral in nature, acting on the Kidney and Urinary Bladder Channels.

Action Inducing diuresis and excreting Dampness.

Indications Dysuria, edema, diarrhea, stranguria with turbid urine, leukorrhagia, etc. Usually used together with Fu Ling (Poria), Ze Xie (Rhizoma Alismatis), etc., as in Siling San (Powder of Four Diuretic Drugs Including Poria). For dysuria due to accumulation of Damp-Heat leading to impairment of Yin, usually used in combination with E Jiao (Colla Corii Asini), Hua Shi (Talcum), etc., as in Zhuling Tang (Decoction of Polyporus Umbellatus).

Administration 5~10g for making a decoction.

Precautions Used with caution for Deficiency of both Yin and Body-Fluid.

0.3. Ze Xie (Rhizoma Alismatis)

Description The tuber of Alisma orientalis (Sam.) Juzep Family Alismataceae.

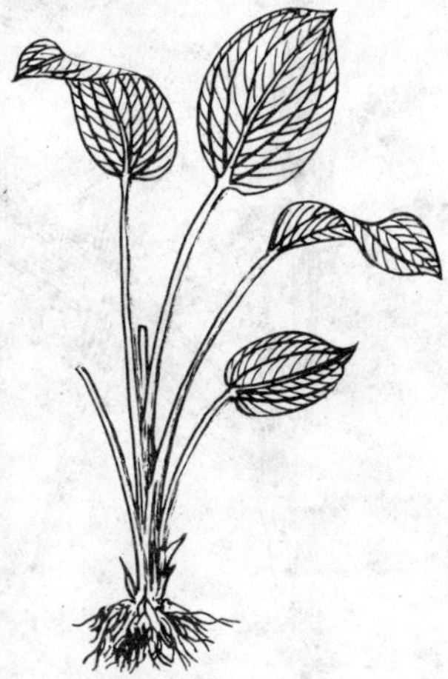

Characteristics Sweet and insipid in flavor, cold in nature, acting on the Kidney and Urinary Bladder Channels.

Action Inducing diuresis, excreting Dampness and removing Heat.

Indications Dysuria, edema, diarrhea, stranguria with turbid urine, leukorrhagia, retention of Phlegm, etc. Being sweet and insipid in flavor, Ze Xie (Rhizoma Alismatis) is capable of excreting Dampness and clearing away Heat, especially Damp-Heat in the Lower-jiao. For edema, dysuria and diarrhea due to excessive Dampness, it is used with Fu Ling (Poria), Zhu Ling (Polyporus Umbellatus), etc., as in Siling San (Powder of Four Diuretic Drugs Including Poria); for Phlegm retention with vertigo, it is used with Bai Zhu (Rhizoma Atractylodis Macrocephalae), named Zexie Tang (Decoction of Rhizoma Alismatis).

Administration 5～10g for making a decoction.

Precautions Application in large dosage will lead to spermatorrhea.

0.4. Yi Yi Ren (Semen Coicis)

Description The ripe seed of Coix lacryma-jobi L. var. ma-yuen (Roman.) Stapf. Family Gramineae.

Characteristics Sweet and insipid in flavor, slightly cold in nature, acting on the Spleen, Stomach and Lung Channels.

Action Inducing diuresis, excreting Dampness, invigorating

Spleen to stop diarrhea, eliminating Dampness to relax muscles, clearing away Heat to drain the pus.

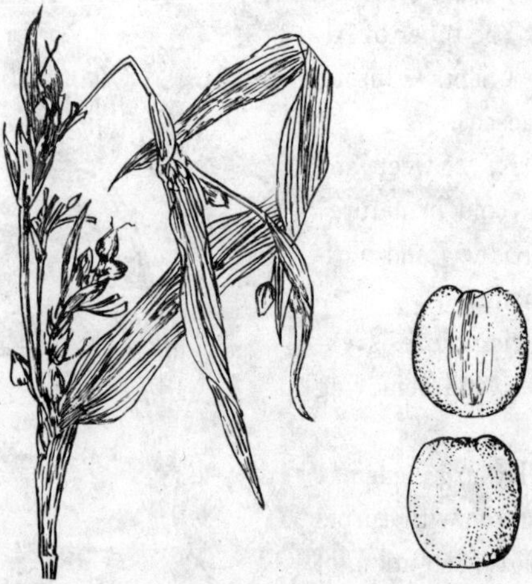

Indications

(1) Dysuria, edema, beriberi with swelling due to Deficiency of Spleen and Excess of Dampness. Usually used with Fu Ling (Poria), Zhu Ling (Polyporus Umbellatus), etc.; or used alone by making a decoction.

(2) Diarrhea, leukorrhagia, etc. due to Spleen Deficiency. Usually used together with Dang Shen (Radix Codonopsis Pilosulae), Bai Zhu (Rhizoma Atractylodis Macrocephalae), Shan Yao (Rhizoma Dioscoreae), etc. For leukorrhagia due to Damp-Heat, used with Huang Bo (Cortex Phellodendri), Che Qian Zi (Semen Plantaginis), Qian Shi (Semen Euryales) etc.

(3) Arthralgia of Wind-Dampness type and muscular rigidity. In the case of cold type, used with Ma Huang (Herba Ephedrae), Xing Ren (Semen Armeniacae Amarum), etc.; in the case of Heat type, used with Fang Ji (Radix Stephaniae Tetrandrae), Sang Zhi (Ramulus Mori), etc. ; in the case of descending of Damp-Heat marked by swelling pain of feet and knees, usually used with Cang Zhu (Rhizoma Atractylodis), Huang Bo (Cortex Phellodendri) and Niu Xi

(Radix Achyranthis Bidentatae), as in Simiao San (Powder of Four Wonderful Drugs).

(4) Dampness febrile diseases. For pathogenic factors invading the Qi system with Dampness heavier than Heat, usually used together with Xing Ren (Semen Armeniacae Amarum), Bai Dou Kou (Fructus Amomi Rotundus), Hua Shi (Talcum), etc., as in Sanren Tang (Decoction of Three Kinds of Seeds).

(5) Pulmonary abscess. Usually used together with Wei Jing (Rhizoma Phragmitis), Tao Ren (Semen Persicae), Dong Gua Ren (Semen Benincasae), etc., as in Weijing Tang (Rhizoma Phragmitis Decoction). For appendicitis, used with Fu Zi (Radix Aconiti Praeparata), Bai Jiang Cao (Herba Patriniae), etc., as in Yiyi Fuzi Baijiang San (Powder of Semen Coicis, Radix Aconiti Praeparata and Herba Patriniae).

Administration 10～30g for making a decoction.

Precautions As the drug is not potent in action, a large dosage of long time application is needed before a satisfactory effect is achieved.

0.5. Che Qian Zi (Semen Plantaginis)

Description The ripe seed of Plantago asiatica L., or Plantago depressa Willd. Family Plantaginaceae.

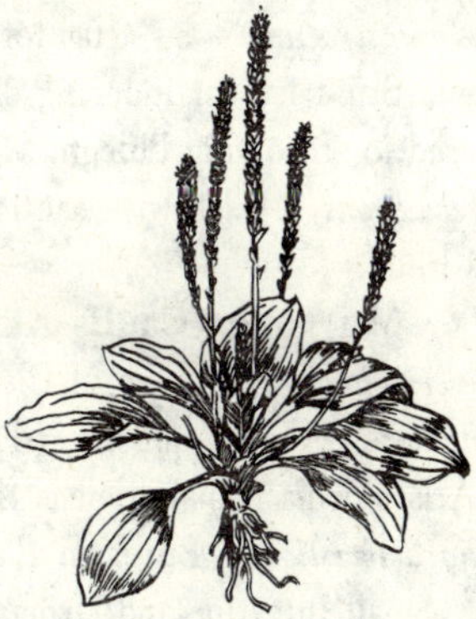

Characteristics Sweet in flavor, cold in nature, acting on the Kidney, Liver and Lung Channels.

Action Inducing diuresis to treat stranguria, excreting Dampness to stop diarrhea, clearing away Heat from the Liver to improve the eyesight, clearing away Heat in the Lung to resolve Phlegm.

Indications

(1) Edema, dysuria or dribbling and painful micturition. Usually used in combination with Mu Tong (Caulis Akebiae), Hua Shi (Talcum), Zhi Zi (Fructus Gardeniae), etc., as in Bazheng San (Powder of Eight Health Restoring Drugs).

(2) Diarrhea due to Summer-Heat and Dampness. Che Qian Zi (Semen Plantaginis) is capable of both inducing diuresis and treating watery diarrhea resulting from excessive Dampness in the body during summer time, and it is usually used with Xiang Ru (Herba Elsholtziae seu Moslae), Fu Ling (Poria), etc., as in Cheqianzi San (Powder of Semen Plantaginis).

(3) Conjunctivitis, cataract, nebula, blurred vision, etc. For conjunctivitis with swelling pain in the eyes due to excessive Heat in the Liver, usually used with Ju Hua (Flos Chrysanthemi), Long Dan Cao (Radix Gentianae), etc.; for chronic cataract with Deficiency of both Liver-Yin and Kidney-Yin, used with Sheng Di (Radix Rehmanniae), Mai Dong (Radix Ophiopogonis) and Gou Qi Zi (Fructus Lycii).

(4) Cough with profuse phlegm due to Heat in the Lung. Usually used with Jie Geng (Radix Platycodi), Xing Ren (Semen Armeniacae Amarum), etc.

Administration 5～10g for making a decoction (wrapped in gauze). Stir-fried for inducing diuresis and arresting diarrhea; unprepared for resolving Phlegm.

Precautions Used with caution for insufficiency of both Yin and Body-Fluid.

0. 6. Mu Tong (Caulis Akebiae)

Description The vine of Clematis armandi Franch. Family Ranunculaceae; Akebia quinata (Thunb.) Decne. (Lardizabalaceae) and Aristolochia manshuriensis Kom. Family Aristolochiaceae.

Characteristics Bitter in flavor, cold in nature, acting on the Heart, Small Intestine and Urinary Bladder Channels.

Action Inducing diuresis to treat stranguria, expelling Heat, promoting lactation and regulating menstruation.

Indications

(1) Damp-Heat in the urinary bladder, scanty and dark urine with

dribbling and painful micturition; or flaming up of Heart-Fire manifested as canker sores, vexation and dark urine, etc. Usually used with Che Qian Zi (Semen Plantaginis), Sheng Di (Radix Rehmanniae), Dan Zhu Ye (Herba Lophatheri), etc., as in Bazheng San (Powder of Eight Health-Restoring Drugs) and Daochi San (Powder for Treating Dark Urine).

(2) Blockage of milk flow after delivery. Used with Wang Bu Liu Xing (Semen Vaccariae), Chuan Shan Jia (Squama Manitis), Tong Cao (Medulla Tetrapanacis), etc. For amenorrhea due to Blood stasis, used with Dan Shen (Radix Salviae Miltiorrhizae) and Niu Xi (Radix Achyranthis Bidentatae).

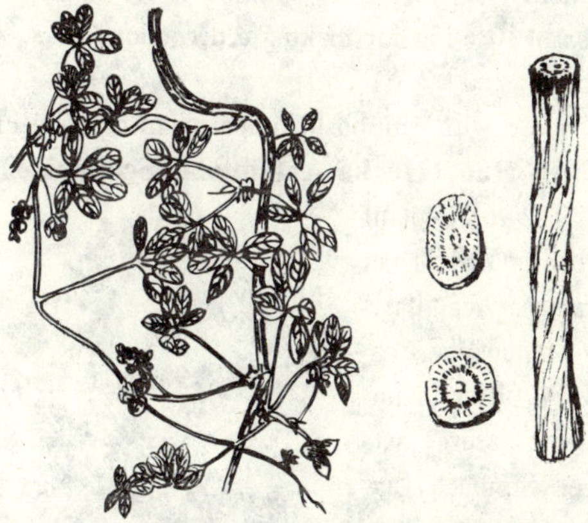

Administration 3~10g for making a decoction.

Precautions Overdosage should be avoided; used with caution during pregnancy.

0.7. Hua Shi (Talcum)

Description The silicate minerals belonging to Talcum group, composed of mainly hydrated magnesium silicate.

Characteristics Sweet and insipid in flavor, cold in nature, acting on the Stomach and Urinary Bladder Channels.

Action Inducing diuresis to treat stranguria, clearing away Summer-Heat, eliminating Dampness to heal skin infection.

Indications

(1) Stranguria of Heat type, dysuria with dribbling and painful urination. Usually used with Mu Tong (Caulis Akebiae) and Che Qian Zi (Semen Plantaginis), as in Bazheng San (Powder of Eight Health-Restoring Drugs). For stranguria caused by urinary stone, used with Jin Qian Cao (Herba Lysimachiae), Hai Jin Sha (Spora Lygodii), etc.

(2) Summer-Heat syndrome with excessive thirst, scanty and dark urine, diarrhea due to Damp-Heat. Used together with Gan Cao (Radix Glycyrrhizae), as in Liuyi San (Six to One Powder).

(3) Exudative skin lesion and eczema. Used alone or together with Huang Bo (Cortex Phellodendri), Ku Fan (Alumen), etc. for external application.

Administration 10～15g for making a decoction; q. s. for external application.

Precautions Used with caution for impairment of Body-Fluid.

0. 8. Yin Chen Hao (Herba Artemisiae Scopariae)

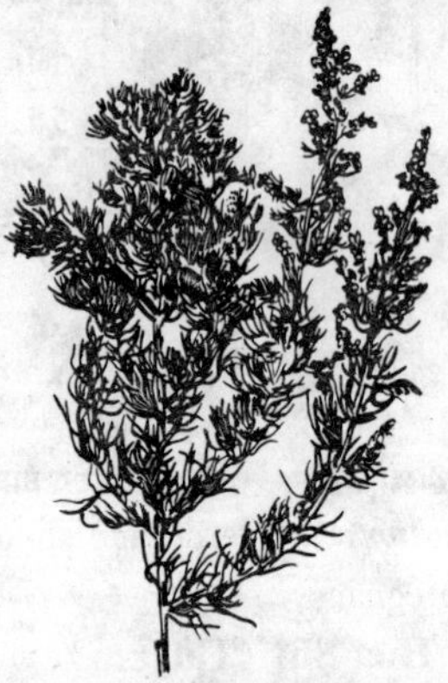

Description The young plant of Artemisia scoparia Waldst. et Kit. or Artemisia capillaris Thunb. Family Compostiae.

Characteristics Bitter in flavor, slightly cold in nature, acting on the Spleen, Stomach, Liver and Gallbladder Channels.

Action Eliminating Damp-Heat, normalizing the function of Gallbladder to treat jaundice.

Indications Jaundice. This drug is exclusively used for treating jaundice. In the case of jaundice induced by Damp-Heat marked by obvious yellow coloration of the skin and eyes, fever and dark urine, used with Zhi Zi (Fructus Gardeniae) and DaiHuang (Radix et Rhizoma Rhei), named Yinchenhao Tang (Decoction of Herba Artemisiae Scopariae); in the case of jaundice induced by Damp-Cold marked by dim yellow coloration of the eyes and skin, poor appetite, epigastric distress, lassitude and chilliness, used with Fu Zi (Radix Aconiti Praeparata), Gan Jiang (Rhizoma Zingiberis), etc., as in Yinchen Sini Tang (Decoction of Herba Artemisiae Scopariae for Restoring Yang).

Administration 10～30g for making a decoction.

Interior-warming Drugs

Drugs capable of warming the interior and dispelling Cold pathogens in the body are referred to as interior-warming drugs.

As drugs of this category are acrid in flavor and hot in nature, they can disperse the Cold pathogens in the interior and restore the Yang-Qi in the body. They are indicated for gastric and abdominal cold pain, vomiting and diarrhea, as well as chilliness, cold limbs, pale complexion, clear and long urination, pale tongue and thready pulse due to weakness of Yang-Qi and excessive Cold in the interior. Some of the drugs in this category have the function of recuperating depleted Yang and rescuing the patient from collapse and therefore they are used for Yang depletion syndromes.

Interior-warming drugs should be used in combination with other types of drugs. e. g. in the case of invasion of exogenous Cold accompanied by superficies-syndrome, diaphoretics should be added; in the case of accumulation of Cold and stagnation of Qi, drugs for regulating the normal flow of Qi should be dispensed; while Cold syndrome induced by Yang Deficiency should be treated by adding warming and tonifying drugs.

As interior-warming drugs are acrid and hot and are liable to induce Fire and cause impairment of Yin, they should be used with caution or avoided for Heat syndromes, Yin Deficiency syndromes or in pregnant women.

0.1. Fu Zi (Radix Aconiti Praeparata)

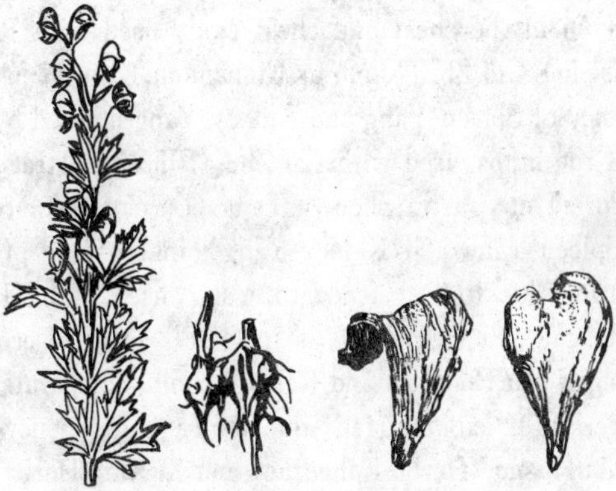

Description The lateral roots of Aconitum carmichaeli Debx. Family Ranunculaceae.

Characteristics Acrid in flavor, hot in nature, poisonous, acting on the Heart, Kidney and Spleen Channels.

Action Recuperating depleted Yang to rescue the patient from collapse, supplementing Fire to strengthen Yang, dispersing Cold to relieve pain.

Indications

(1) Yang depletion syndrome characterized by spontaneous cold sweat, cold limbs with pulse as faint as none. Usually used together with Gan Jiang (Rhizoma Zingiberis), etc., as in Sini Tang (Decoction for Resuscitation).

(2) Yang Deficiency syndromes. In the case of insufficiency of Kidney-Yang marked by chilliness, cold limbs, impotence and frequent urination, used with Rou Gui (Cortex Cinnamomi), Shu Di (Radix Rehmanniae Praeparatae), Shan Zhu Yu (Fructus Corni), etc., as in Shenqi Wan (Bolus for Tonifying the Kidney-Qi); in the case of insufficiency of Spleen-Yang marked by cold pain in the ab-

domen, poor appetite and diarrhea, used with Ren Shen (Radix Ginseng), Bai Zhu (Rhizoma Atractylodis), Gan Jiang (Rhizoma Zingiberis), etc., as in Fuzi Lizhong Wan (Bolus of Radix Aconiti Praeparata for Regulating the Middle-jiao); in the case of insufficiency of Heart-Yang marked by palpitation, shortness of breath, obstruction of Qi in the chest and chest pain, used with Ren Shen (Radix Ginseng), Gui Zhi (Ramulus Cinnamomi), etc.; in the case of insufficiency of Spleen-Yang and Kidney-Yang marked by dysuria, edema of the limbs, used with Bai Zhu (Rhizoma Atractylodis), Fu Ling (Poria), etc., as in Zhenwu Tang (Decoction for Strengthening the Spleen-Yang and Kidney-Yang); in the case of spontaneous sweating due to Deficiency of Yang, used with Huang Qi (Radix Astragali seu Hedysari), as in Qi Fu Tang (Decoction of Radix Astragali seu Hedysari and Radix Aconiti Praeparata); in the case of affection of exopathogens due to Yang Deficiency, usually used with Ma Huang (Herba Ephedrae) and Xi Xin (Herba Asari), as in Mahuang Xixin Fuzi Tang (Decoction of Herba Ephedrae, Radix Aconiti Praeparata and Herba Asari).

(3) Arthralgia caused by Wind-Cold-Dampness marked by joint pains all over the body. Usually used with Gui Zhi (Ramulus Cinnamomi), Bai Zhu (Rhizoma Atractylodis Macrocephalae), Gan Cao (Radix Glycyrrhizae), etc., as in Gancao Fuzi Tang (Decoction of Radix Glycyrrhizae and Radix Aconiti Praeparata).

Administration 3～15g for making a decoction. (It should be decocted 30～60 minutes prior to other drugs.)

Precautions Contraindicated for Heat syndrome, Yin Deficiency syndrome or in pregnant women.

0.2. Gan Jiang (Rhizoma Zingiberis)

Description The rhizome of Zingiber officinale (Willd.) Rosc. Family Zingiberaceae.

Characteristics Acrid in flavor, hot in nature, acting on the Spleen, Stomach, Heart and Lung Channels.

Action Warming the Middle-jiao, recuperating depleted Yang, warming the Lung and resolving Phlegm retention.

Indications

(1) Asthenic Cold of the Spleen and Stomach, marked by cold pain in the abdomen, vomiting, diarrhea, anorexia, etc. Usually used with Ren Shen (Radix Ginseng), Bai Zhu (Rhizoma Atractylodis Macrocephalae), Gan Cao (Radix Glycyrrhizae), etc., as in Lizhong Wan (Pill for Regulating the Function of Middle-jiao). In the case of vomiting and diarrhea due to Stomach-Cold, used with Ban Xia (Rhizoma Pinelliae), as in Banxia Ganjiang San (Powder of Rhizoma Pinelliae and Rhizoma Zingiberis).

(2) Yang depletion syndrome marked by cold limbs and pulse as faint as none. Used with Fu Zi (Radix Aconiti Praeparata) and Zhi Gan Cao (Radix Glycyrrhizae Praeparata), as in Sini Tang (Decoction for Resuscitation).

(3) Retention of Cold Phlegm in the Lung marked by cough, dyspnea, cold appearance, chilly sensation in the back and profuse thin clear sputum. Usually used with Ma Huang (Herba Ephedrae), Xi Xin (Herba Asari), Fu Zi (Radix Aconiti Praeparata), etc., as in Xiao Qinglong Tang (Minor Decoction of Green Dragon).

When dried ginger is stir-fried to slightly black on the surface and brownish yellow inside, it is called Pao Jiang (Rhizoma Zingiberis Praeparata), which is less effective for warming the interior but more effective for warming the Meridians and stopping bleeding than unprepared ginger. It is indicated for bleeding due to asthenic Cold such as hematemesis, hemafecia, metrorrhagia and metrostaxos accompanied by cold hands and feet, pale tongue and thready pulse.

Administration 3~10g for making a decoction.

Precautions Used with caution for Heat syndrome, Yin Deficiency syndrome and in pregnant women.

0.3. Rou Gui (Cortex Cinnamomi)

Description The bark of the trunk and thick branches of Cinnamomum cassia Presl. Family Lauraceae.

Characteristics Acrid and sweet in flavor, hot in nature, acting on the Kidney, Spleen, Heart and Liver Channels.

Action Supplementing Fire to strengthen Yang, dispersing Cold to relieve pain, warming and regulating Meridians.

Indications

(1) Yang-Deficiency syndrome. For insufficiency of Kidney-Yang marked by chilliness, cold limbs, impotence and frequent urination, used with Fu Zi (Radix Aconiti Praeparata), Shu Di (Radix Rehmanniae Praeparata), Shan Zhu Yu (Fructus Corni), etc., as in Shenqi Wan (Bolus for Tonifying the Kidney-Qi); for insufficiency of Spleen-Yang marked by

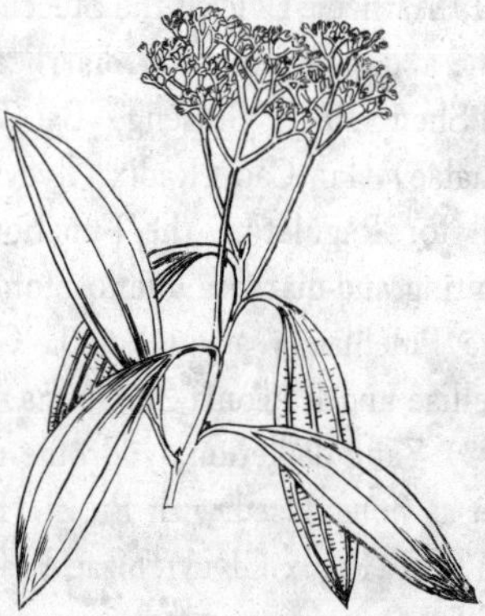

cold pain in the abdomen, poor appetite and diarrhea, usually used with Gan Jiang (Rhizoma Zingiberis), Fu Zi (Radix Aconiti Praeparata), Bai Zhu (Rhizoma Atractylodis Macrocephalae), etc., as in Gui Fu Lizhong Wan (Bolus of Cortex Cinnamomi and Radix Aconiti Praeparata for Regulating the Middle-jiao); for inspiration failure due to Kidney Deficiency marked by dyspnea with inability to lie on the back, cold limbs and sweat on the forehead, usually used with Fu Zi (Radix Aconiti Praeparata), Chen Xiang (Lignum Aquilariae Resinatum) and Wu Wei Zi (Fructus Schisandrae).

(2) All sorts of pain induced by accumulation of Cold and stagnation of Qi. In the case of periumbilical colic and lumbago due to Damp-Cold, used with Du Huo (Radix Angelicae Pubescentis), Sang Ji Sheng (Ramulus Loranthi), Du Zhong (Cortex Eucommiae), etc.; in the case of hernia with pain due to cold, usually used together with Wu Zhu Yu (Fructus Evodiae), Wu Yao (Radix Linderae) and Xiao Hui Xiang (Fructus Foeniculi).

(3) Amenorrhea and menorrhalgia due to pathogenic Cold in the Blood. Used with Gan Jiang (Rhizoma Zingiberis), Dang Gui (Radix Angelicae Sinensis) and Shu Di (Radix Rehmanniae Praeparate), as in Liyin Jian (Decoction for Regulating Yin).

(4) Sores, carbuncles and other external diseases due to pathogenic Cold of Deficiency type in the Qi and Blood systems. For carbuncles of Yin nature manifested as diffused swelling without

sign of rupture and neither red nor hot, it is usually used with Shu Di (Radix Rehmanniae Praeparata), Lu Jiao Jiao (Colla Cornus Cervi), Ma Huang (Herba Ephedrae), etc., as in Yanghe Tang (Yang-activating Decoction); for carbuncles and swellings unhealed long after rupture or unruptured abscesses and swellings, it is used with Huang Qi (Radix Astragali seu Hedysari), Dang Gui (Radix Angelicae Sinensis), etc., as in Tuoli Huangqi Tang (Decoction of Radix Astragali seu Hedysari for Expelling Toxins from Within).

Administration 1～5g for making a decoction, to be added late; 1～2g for making the powder.

Precautions Contraindicated for Yin Deficiency and Fire Excess, or sthenic Heat in the interior, or in women during pregnancy.

0. 4. Wu Zhu Yu (Fructus Evodiae)

Description Nearly matured fruit of Evodia rutaecarpa (Juss.) Benth. Family Rutaceae.

Characteristics Acrid and bitter in flavor, hot in nature, mildly toxic, and acting on the Liver, Spleen and Stomach Channels.

Action Dispelling Cold to relieve pain, soothing the liver to lower the adverse flow of Qi and eliminating Dampness.

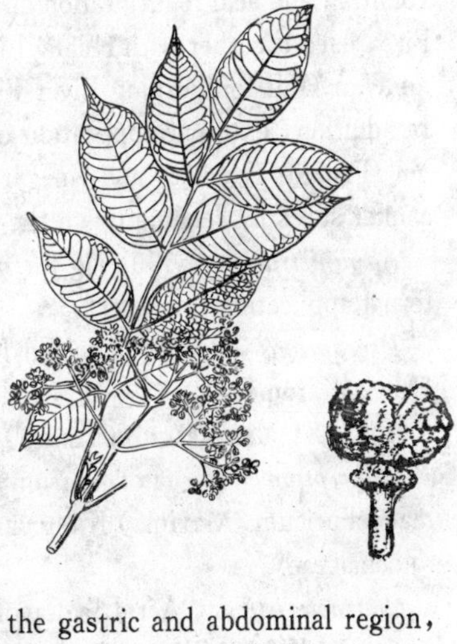

Indications

(1) Pathogenic Cold in the interior. In the case of cold pain in the gastric and abdominal region, used together with Gan Jiang (Rhizoma Zingiberis) and Mu Xiang (Radix Aucklandiae); in the case of chronic diarrhea or diarrhea before dawn due to Deficiency of Spleen-Yang and Kidney-Yang, used with Bu Gu Zhi (Fructus Psoraleae), Rou Dou Kou (Semen Myristieae) and Wu Wei Zi (Fructus Schisandrae), as in Sishen Wan (Pill of Four Miraculous Drugs); in the case of periumbilical colic

due to invasion of Cold, used with Wu Yao (Radix Linderae) and Xiao Hui Xiang (Fructus Foeniculi); for Cold of Deficiency type of Middle-jiao, adverse ascending of Liver-Qi marked by headache and salivation, used with Ren Shen (Radix Ginseng) and Sheng Jiang (Rhizoma Zingiberis Recens), as in Wuzhuyu Tang (Fructus Evodiae Decoction).

(2) Beriberi of Damp-Cold type with pain and swelling. Usually used with Mu Gua (Fructus Chaenomelis), Bing Lang (Semen Arecae), etc., as in Wuzhuyu Mugua Tang (Decoction of Fructus Evodiae and Fructus Chaenomelis).

(3) Vomiting and acid regurgitation. For vomiting and acid regurgitation due to Cold in the Stomach, usually used with Sheng Jiang (Rhizoma Zingiberis Recens) and Ban Xia (Rhizoma Pinelliae); for vomiting and acid regurgitation due to invasion of Stomach by Liver-Fire, used together with Huang Lian (Rhizoma Coptidis), as in Zuojin Wan (Pill for Purging Liver-Fire and Regulating the Stomach). In addition, external application of the paste of powdered Wu Zhu Yu (Fructus Evodiae) and vinegar to the centre of the sole can treat canker sores by sending down the pathogenic Fire.

Administration 1.5～5g for making a decoction; q. s. for external application.

Precautions Contraindicated for Yin Deficiency complicated by Heat syndrome.

0.5. Xi Xin (Herba Asari)

Description Herba of Asarum heterotropoides Fr. Schmidt var. mandshuricum (Maxim.) Kitag. and A. sieboldii Miq. Family Aristolochiaceae.

Characteristics Acrid in flavor, warm in nature, acting on the Lung and Kidney Channels.

Action Dispelling Wind and Cold, relieving pain, warming the Lung to resolve Phlegm retention and waking up the patient from unconsciousness.

Indications

(1) Headache, toothache and arthralgia pain. For treating headache due to Wind-Cold, usually used together with Chuan Xiong

(Rhizoma Ligustici Chuanxiong), Qiang Huo (Rhizoma seu Radix Noto-pterygii), Bai Zhi (Radix Angelicae Dahuricae), etc., as in Chuanxiong Chatiao San (Rhizoma Ligustici Chuanxiong Mixture); for toothache due to Wind-Cold, used either alone or together with Chuan Wu (Radix Aconiti) and Ru Xiang (Resina Boswelliae Carterii) to make a powder and apply it to the af-

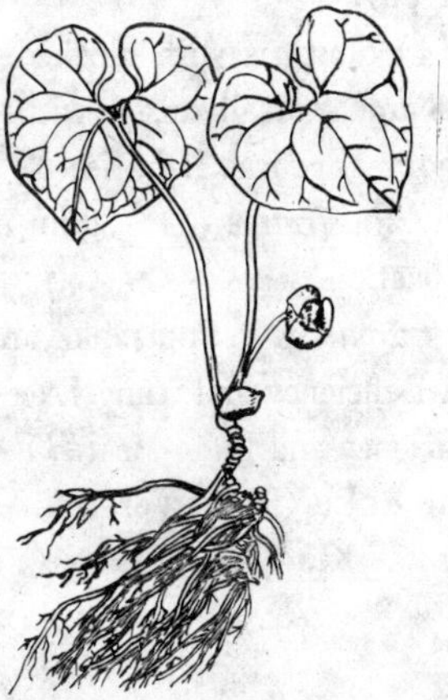

fected place many times a day; for toothache due to Stomach-Fire, usually used with Shi Gao (Gypsum Fibrosum), Huang Qin (Radix Scutellariae), etc; for arthralgia due to Wind-Cold with joint pain, usually used with Qiang Huo (Rhizoma seu Radix Noto-pterygii), Du Huo (Radix Angelicae Pubescentis), Fang Feng (Radix Ledebouriellae), etc.

(2) Affection of exopathogenic Wind-Cold with superficies-syndromes. In the case of severe ache of the body and head, usually used in combination with Qiang Huo (Rhizoma seu Radix Noto-pterygii), Fang Feng (Radix Ledebouriellae), etc., as in Jiuwei Qianghuo Tang (Rhizoma seu Radix Noto-pterygii Decoction of Nine Ingredients); in the case of affection of exopathogens due to Yang Deficiency marked by chilliness, fever, with chilliness severer than fever and deep pulse, usually used with Ma Huang (Herba Ephedrae) and Fu Zi (Radix Aconiti Praeparata), as in Mahuang Fuzi Xixin Tang (Decoction of Herba Ephedrae, Radix Aconiti Praeparata and Herba Asari).

(3) Affection of pathogenic Wind-Cold with Phlegm retention in the Lung manifested by cough and dyspnea with profuse, thin and clear sputum. Usually dispensed with Ma Huang (Herba Ephedrae), Ban Xia (Rhizoma Pinelliae), Gan Jiang (Rhizoma Zingiberis), etc., as in Xiao Qinglong Tang (Minor Decoction of Green

Dragon).

(4) Sinusitis with blocked nose, headache and occasional nasal discharge. Usually used with Xin Yi (Flos Magnoliae), Bai Zhi (Radix Angelicae Dahuricae), Bo He (Herba Menthae), etc.

Administration　1～3g for making a decoction; q. s. for external application.

Precautions　Contraindicated for dizziness and headache due to Yin Deficiency and Yang Excess, or cough and dyspnea due to Yin Deficiency and Lung-Heat. Overdose should be avoided. Antagonistic to Li Lu (Radix Veratri).

0. 6. Xiao Hui Xiang (Fructus Foeniculi)

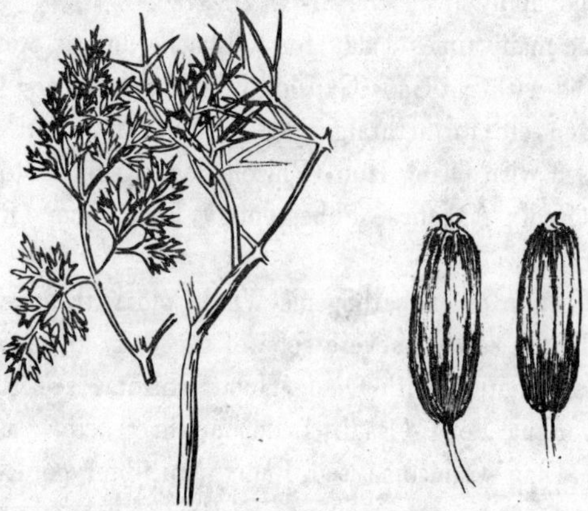

Description　The ripe fruit of Foeniculum vulgare Mill. Family Umbelliferae.

Characteristics　Acrid in flavor, warm in nature, acting on the Liver, Kidney, Spleen and Stomach Channels.

Action　Dispelling Cold to relieve pain and regulating the flow of Qi to normalize the function of Stomach.

Indications

(1) Periumbilical colic of Cold type and orchidoptosis. Usually used with Wu Yao (Radix Linderae), Rou Gui (Cortex Cinnamomi), Chen Xiang (Lignum Aquilariae Resinatum), etc., as

in Nuangan Jian (Decoction for Warming the Liver).

(2) Stomach-Cold with vomiting and poor appetite, distending pain in the gastric and abdominal region. Usually used with Mu Xiang (Radix Aucklandiae), Gan Jiang (Rhizoma Glycyrrhizae), etc.

Administration 3~10g for making a decoction.

Precautions Contraindicated for Yin Deficiency and Heat in the interior.

Qi-regulating Drugs

Drugs whose principal action is regulating the functional activities of Qi and enabling Qi to flow smoothly are referred to as Qi-regulating drugs.

Drugs in this category are mostly fragrant in smell, warm in nature and acrid and bitter in flavor. They are capable of regulating Qi in the Middle-jiao, promoting the flow of Qi to relieve pain, soothing the Liver to resolve stasis and lowering the adverse ascending of Qi to normalize the function of Stomach. These drugs are indicated for Qi stagnation and adverse flow of Qi due to disorder of the functional activities of Qi such as hypochondriac pain, distending pain of the breasts, hernial pain, irregular menstruation and dysmenorrhea induced by stagnation of the Liver-Qi; distending pain of the Stomach and abdomen, belching and acid regurgitation due to stagnation of the Spleen-Qi and Stomach-Qi; stuffiness sensation in the chest and cough due to impairment of the Lung in dispersing and descending Qi; and nausea, vomiting and hiccup due to failure of the Stomach in descending the Stomach-Qi.

Drugs of this category can be selected for use together with other types of drugs in accordance with differences of cases. e. g. in the case of Qi obstruction induced by retention of Phlegm-Dampness in the interior, drugs for removing Dampness and resolving Phlegm should be dispensed; if it is induced by food stagnation, digestive drugs should be used; in the case of accompanying hypofunction of Spleen and Stomach, drugs for invigorating Qi and strengthening Spleen should be used in combination.

Qi-regulating drugs are usually pungent and hot and apt to consume Qi and impair Yin and therefore they should be applied with caution to patients with Yin Deficiency or Qi Deficiency.

0.1. Ju Pi (Pericarpium Citri Reticulatae)

Description The peel of the ripe fruit of Citrus reticulata Blanco and other species of the citrus genus. Family Rutaceae.

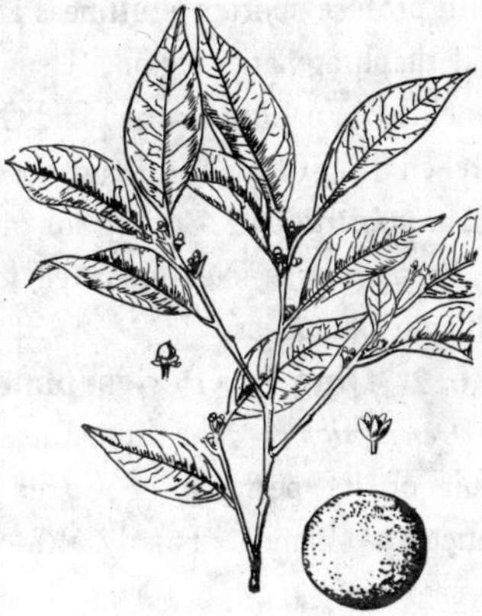

Characteristics Acrid and bitter in flavor, warm in nature, acting on the Spleen and Lung Channels.

Action Regulating Qi, normalizing the function of the Spleen and Stomach, eliminating Dampness and resolving Phlegm.

Indications

(1) Stagnation of Qi in the Spleen and Stomach marked by abdominal distension, belching, vomiting and nausea. Usually used together with Mu Xiang (Radix Aucklandiae), Sha Ren (Fructus Amomi), Zhi Qiao (Fructus Aurantii), etc. In the case of Deficiency of Spleen and Stomach complicated with Qi stagnation, usually used together with Dang Shen (Radix Codonopsis Pilosulae), Bai Zhu (Rhizoma Atractylodis Macrocephalae), Gan Cao (Radix Glycyrrhizae), etc., as in Yigong San (Powder with Wonderful Effect).

(2) Adverse ascending of the Stomach-Qi leading to vomiting and hiccup. Used with Sheng Jiang (Rhizoma Zingiberis Recens), as in Jupi Tang (Decoction of Pericarpium Citri Reticulatae). In the case of Stomach Deficiency with Heat factor, used with Dang Shen (Radix

Codonopsis Pilosulae) and Zhu Ru (Caulis Bambusae in Taeniam), as in Jupi Zhuru Tang (Decoction of Pericarpium Citri Reticulatae and Caulis Bambusae in Taeniam).

(3) Oppressed feeling in the chest, abdominal distension, anorexia, lassitude, diarrhea with thick and greasy tongue coat resulting from retention of Dampness in the Middle-jiao. Usually used with Cang Zhu (Rhizoma Atractylodis), Hou Po (Cortex Magnoliae Officinalis), etc., as in Pingwei San (Peptic Powder).

(4) Retention of Phlegm-Dampness in the Lung marked by cough with profuse sputum, stuffiness and oppressed sensation in the chest and diaphragmatic region. Usually used with Ban Xia (Rhizoma Pinelliae), Fu Ling (Poria) and Gan Cao (Radix Glycyrrhizae), as in Erchen Tang (Two Old Drugs Decoction).

Administration 3~10g for making a decoction.

Precautions Not indicated for cases without Qi stagnation or Phlegm-Dampness.

0. 2. Qing Pi (Pericarpium Citri Reticulatae Viride)

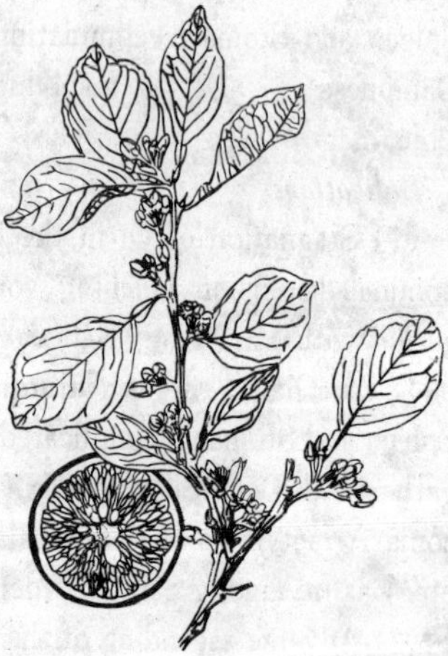

Description The immature fruit or its pericarp of Citrus reticulata Blanco. Family Rutaceae.

Characteristics Bitter and acrid in flavor, warm in nature, acting on the Liver, Gallbladder and Stomach Channels.

Action Soothing the Liver to relieve the stagnation of Qi, dispersing the mass to regulate Qi circulation.

Indications

(1) Stagnation of Liver-Qi marked by costal pain, distending pain of the breasts, swelling pain from hernia and mass in the abdomen. For costal pain, used with Chai Hu (Radix Bupleuri), Xiang Fu (Rhizma Cyperi), Yu Jin (Radix

Currumae),etc.; for distending pain of the breasts with lumps,used together with Xiang Fu (Rhizoma Cyperi), Ju Ye (Folium Citri Reticulatae),etc.;for swelling pain due to mastitis, used with Gua Lou (Fructus Trichosanthis), Jin Yin Hua (Flos Lonicerae), Pu Gong Ying (Herba Taraxaci),etc.; for swelling and pain of hernia, used with Wu Yao (Radix Linderae), Mu Xiang (Radix Aucklandiae), Xiao Hui Xiang (Fructus Foeniculi), etc., as in Tiantai Wuyao San (Powder of Radix Linderae Produced in Tiantai).

(2) Qi stagnation due to indigestion, mass in the abdomen with distending pain. Usually used with Shan Zha (Fructus Crataegi), Mai Ya (Fructus hordei Germinatus), Shen Qu (Massa Fermentata Medicinalis), etc., as in Qingpi Wan (Pill of Per'carpium Citri Reticulatae Viride).

Administration 3~10g for making a decoction.

Precautions Used with caution for Qi Deficiency syndrome.

0.3. Zhi Shi (Fructus Aurantii Immaturus)

Description The immature fruit of Citrus aurantium L., or Citrus sinensis Osbeck. Family Rutaceae.

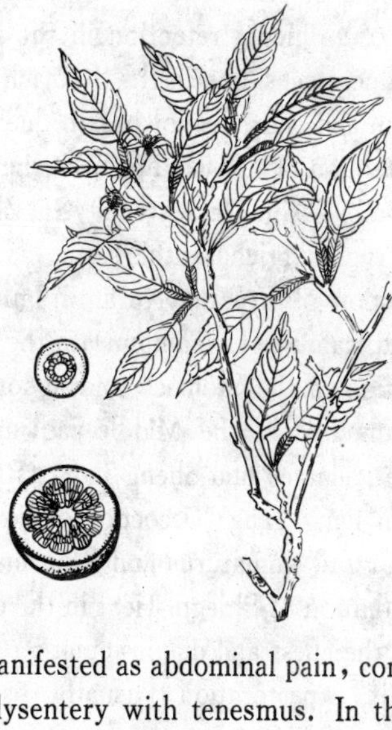

Characteristics Bitter and acrid in flavor, slightly cold in nature, acting on the Spleen, Stomach and Large Intestine Channels.

Action Relieving stagnation of Qi to remove food stagnation and resolving Phlegm to improve digestion.

Indications

(1) Stagnation in the interior and obstruction of the flow of Qi manifested as abdominal pain, constipation as well as diarrhea and dysentery with tenesmus. In the

case of abdominal distension due to food stagnation marked by eructation of fetid odor, used with Shan Zha (Fructus Crataegi), Mai Ya (Fructus Hordei Germinatus), Shen Qu (Massa Fermentata Medicinalis), etc.; in the case of constipation due to accumulation of Heat accompanied with distending pain in the abdomen, usually used with Hou Po (Cortex Magnoliae Officinalis), Dai Huang (Radix et Rhizoma Rhei) and Mang Xiao (Natrii Sulfas), as in Da Chengqi Tang (Major Decoction for Purging Down Digestive Qi); in the case of hypofunction of Spleen and Stomach, indigestion of food and distension of the Stomach and abdomen, used with Bai Zhu (Rhizoma Atractylodis Macrocephalae), as in Zhi Zhu Wan (Pill of Fructus Aurantii Immaturus and Rhizoma Atractylodis Macrocephalae); for accumulation and stagnation of Damp-Heat marked by abdominal pain and constipation, or diarrhea and dysentery with tenesmus, usually used with Dai Huang (Radix et Rhizoma Rhei), Huang Lian (Rhizoma Coptidis), Shen Qu (Massa Fermentata Medicinalis), etc., as in Zhishi Daozhi Wan (Pill of Fructus Aurantii Immaturus for Dispelling Stagnation).

(2) Phlegm retention in the interior marked by distension and fullness sensation in the Stomach and abdomen. In the case of chest pain and shortness of breath due to insufficiency of chest-Yang and retention of turbid Phlegm in the interior, usually used with Xie Bai (Bulbus Allii Macrostemi), Gui Zhi (Ramulus Cinnamomi), Gua Lou (Fructus Trichosanthis), etc., as in Zhishi Xiebai Guizhi Tang (Decoction of Fructus Aurantii Immaturus, Bulbus Allii Macrostemi and Ramulus Cinnamomi); in the case of distension and fullness sensation in the Stomach and abdomen due to stagnation of Phlegm-Dampness in the Middle-jiao, used with Ju Pi (Pericarpium Citri Reticulatae) and Sheng Jiang (Rhizoma Zingiberis Recens), as in Ju Zhi Jiang Tang (Decoction of Pericarpium Citri Reticulatae, Fructus Aurantii Immaturus and Rhizoma Zingiberis Recens); in the case of retention of Phlegm-Heat in the chest marked by stuffiness and pain in the chest and diaphragmatic region with yellow sputum and difficult expectoration, usually used with Huang Lian (Rhizoma Coptidis), Gua Lou (Fructus Trichosanthis) and Ban Xia (Rhizoma

Pinelliae), as in Xiao Xianxiong Tang (Minor Decoction for Relieving Stuffiness in the Chest). In addition, Zhi Shi (Fructus Aurantii Immaturus) can also be used to treat gastroptosis, gastrectasia, prolapse of anus, prolapse of uterus, etc. by dispensing it with Huang Qi (Radix Astragali seu Hedysari), Dang Shen (Radix Codonopsis Pilosulae), Sheng Ma (Rhizoma Cimicifugae), etc.

Administration 3~10g for making a decoction.

Precautions Used with caution for pregnant women.

0. 4. Mu Xiang (Radix Aucklandiae)

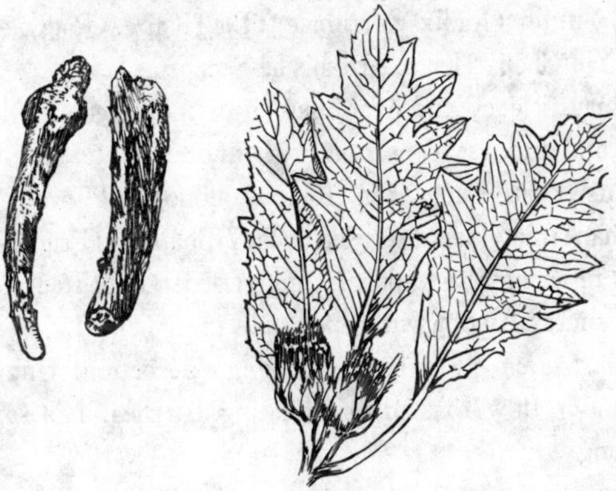

Description The root of Aucklandia lappa Decne. Family Compositae.

Characteristics Acrid and bitter in flavor, warm in nature, acting on the Spleen, Stomach, Large Intestine and Gallbladder Channels.

Action Promoting the flow of Qi, regulating the function of Spleen and Stomach, and relieving pain.

Indications

(1) Qi stagnation in the Stomach and Intestines marked by distending pain in the Stomach and abdomen, indigestion, diarrhea and dysentery with tenesmus, etc. Usually used with Zhi Qiao (Fructus Aurantii), Chuan Lian Zi (Fructus Meliae Toosendan), Yan Hu Suo (Rhizoma Corydalis), etc. In the case of diarrhea and dysentery due to Damp-Heat marked by abdominal pain and tenesmus, used with

Huang Lian (Rhizoma Coptidis), as in Xiang Lian Wan (Pill of Radix Aucklandiae and Rhizoma Coptidis); in the case of diarrhea and dysentery due to retention of indigested food, usually used with Bing Lang (Semen Arecae), Zhi Shi (Fructus Aurantii Immaturus), Dai Huang (Radix et Rhizoma Rhei), etc., as in Muxiang Binglang Wan (Pill of Radix Aucklandiae and Semen Arecae).

(2) Damp-Heat invasion of Liver and Gallbladder, obstruction of Qi circulation marked by distending pain of the chest and hypochondrium, bitter taste in the mouth, yellow coat on the tongue or jaundice, etc. Usually treated by dispensing it with Chai Hu (Radix Bupleuri), Yu Jin (Radix Currumae), Da Huang (Radix et Rhizoma Rhei), Yin Chen (Herba Artemisiae Scopariae).

(3) Insufficiency and hypofunction of the Spleen marked by distension and fullness sensation with anorexia, etc. For treatment, usually used with Dang Shen (Radix Codonopsis Pilosulae), Bai Zhu (Rhizoma Atractylodis Macrocephalae), Sha Ren (Fructus Amomi), etc., as in Xiang Sha Liujunzi Tang (Decoction of Radix Aucklandiae and Fructus Amomi with Six Noble Ingredients).

Administration 3~10g for making a decoction. Unprepared for regulating Qi flow; roasted for arresting diarrhea. Not to be decocted for long.

Precautions Used with caution for Yin Deficiency with excessive Fire.

0.5. Wu Yao (Radix Linderae)

Description The root tuber of Lindera strychnifolia (Sieb. et Zucc.) Vill. Family Lauraceae.

Characteristics Acrid in flavor, warm in nature, acting on the Lung, Spleen, Kidney and Urinary Bladder Channels.

Action Promoting the flow of Qi to relieve pain, warming the Kidney to resolve Cold.

Indications

(1) Accumulation of Cold and stagnation of Qi marked by stuffiness of the chest, distending pain in the chest, costal region and abdomen, periumbilical colic of Cold type and dysmenorrhea. In the case of stuffiness and pain of the chest, used together with Xie Bai

(Bulbua Allii Macrostemi), Yan Hu Suo (Rhizoma Corydalis), Yu Jin (Radix Cirrumae), etc.; in the case of distending pain of the Stomach and abdomen, used with Mu Xiang (Radix Aucklandiae), Zhi Qiao (Fructus Aurantii), Wu Zhų Yu (Fructus Euodiae), etc.; in the case of Cold in the Middle-jiao with Qi stagnation marked by cold pain in the abdomen, usually used together

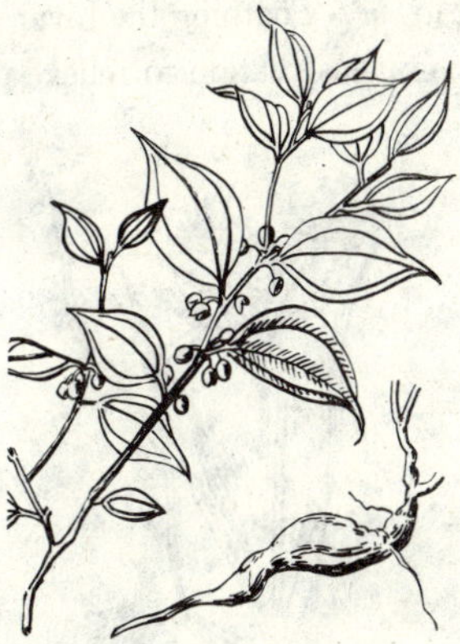

with Chen Xiang (Lignum Aquilariae Resinatum) and Sheng Jiang (Rhizoma Zingiberis Recens), as in Wu Chen Tang (Decoction of Radix Linderae and Lignum Aquilariae Resinatum); in the case of periumbilical colic of Cold type, usually used together with Xiao Hui Xiang (Fructus Foeniculi), Qing Pi (Pericarpium Citri Reticulatae Viride), Mu Xiang (Radix Aucklandiae), etc., as in Tian Tai Wuyao San (Powder of Radix Linderae Produced in Tiantai); in the case of dysmenorrhea, used with Dang Gui (Radix Angelicae Sinensis), Xiang Fu (Rhizoma Cyperi), Mu Xiang (Radix Aucklandiae), etc., as in Wuyao Tang (Decoction of Radix Linderae).

(2) Insufficiency of Kidney-Yang, and Cold of Deficiency type of the urinary bladder which lead to frequent urination, enuresis, etc. For treatment, used together with Yi Zhi Ren (Fructus Alpiniae Oxyphyllae), Shan Yao (Rhizoma Dioscoreae), etc., as in Suoquan Wan (Pill for Decreasing Urination).

Administration 3~10g for making a decoction.

Precautions Contraindicated for Yin Deficiency with excessive Fire.

0. 6. Xiang Fu (Rhizoma Cyperi)

Description The rhizome of Cyperus rotundus L. Family Cyperaceae.

Characteristics Acrid, slightly bitter and sweet in flavor, neutral in nature, acting on the Liver and Triple-jiao Channels.

Action Soothing the Liver to regulate the circulation of Qi, regulating menstruation to relieve pain.

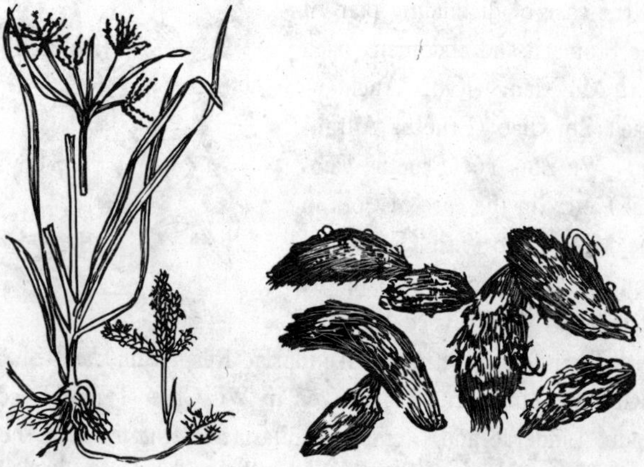

Indications

(1) Distending pain in the chest, costal region and abdomen due to stagnation of the Liver-Qi. For the treatment of distending pain in the hypochondrium and abdomen, used with Chai Hu (Radix Bupleuri), Zhi Qiao (Fructus Aurantii), Chuan Xiong (Rhizoma Ligustici Chuanxiong), etc., as in Chaihu Shugan San (Powder of Radix Bupleuri for Soothing the Liver); in the case of accumulation of Cold and stagnation of Qi manifested as pain in the Stomach and abdomen, usually used with Gao Liang Jiang (Rhizoma Alpiniae Officinari), as in Liang Fu Wan (Pill of Rhizoma Alpiniae Officinari and Rhizoma Cyperi); in the case of periumbilical colic of Cold type, used with Xiao Hui Xiang (Fructus Foeniculi), Wu Yao (Radix Linderae), etc.

(2) Irregular menstruation, dysmenorrhea and distending pain of the breasts. Usually used with Dang Gui (Radix Angelicae Sinensis), Chuan Xiong (Rhizoma Ligustici Chuanxiong), Bai Shao (Radix Paeoniae Alba), etc. In the case of dysmenorrhea accompanied by cold pain in the lower abdomen, usually used with Ai Ye (Folium Artemisiae Argyi), as in Ai Fu Wan (Pill of Folium

Artemisiae Argyi and Rhizoma Cyperi); in the case of lump in the breast and distending pain prior to menstruation, usually used with Chai Hu (Radix Bupleuri), Qing Pi (Pericarpium Citri Reticulatae Viride), Ju Ye (Folium Citri Reticulatae), etc.

Administration 6～12g for making a decoction.

Precautions Used with caution for Qi Deficiency or Heat in the Blood syndromes.

0.7. Xie Bai (Bulbus Allii Macrostemi)

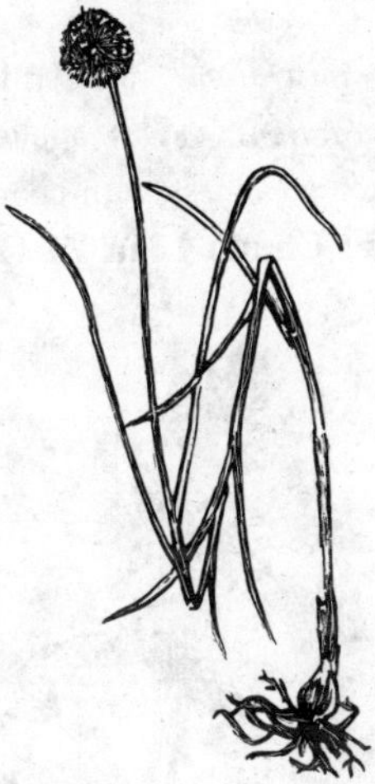

Description The bulb of Allium macrostemon Bge. Family Liliaceae.

Characteristics Acrid and bitter in flavor, warm in nature, acting on the Lung, Stomach and Large Intestine Channels.

Action Relieving the obstruction of Yang-Qi to disperse the accumulated pathogens, and activating the flow of Qi to remove stagnation.

Indications

(1) Obstruction of Qi in the chest with chest pain induced by accumulation of Cold-Phlegm and obstruction of chest-Yang. Xie Bai (Bulbus Allii Macrostemi) is the most important drug for treating obstruction of Qi in the chest, and it is usually used together with Gua Lou (Fructus Trichosanthis), as in Gualou Xiebai Baijiu Tang (Decoction of Fructus Trichosanthis and Bulbus Allii Macrostemi with Wine). In the case of severe stagnation of Qi and obstruction of Phlegm complicated with tight chest and short breath, and cough with profuse sputum, used with Zhi Shi (Fructus Aurantii Immaturus), Hou Po (Cortex Magnoliae Officinalis), etc., as in Zhishi Xiebai Guizhi Tang (Decoction of Fructus Aurantii Immaturus, Bulbus Allii Macrostemi and Ramulus Cinnamomi); in the case of accompanying obstruction by Blood stasis

marked by stabbing pain in the chest and back, used with Dan Shen (Radix Salviae Miltiorrhizae), Hong Hua (Flos Carthami), Chi Shao (Radix Paeoniae Rubra), etc.

(2) Qi stagnation in the Stomach and Intestines marked by diarrhea and dysentery with tenesmus. Usually used with Chai Hu (Radix Bupleuri), Bai Shao (Radix Paeoniae Alba), Zhi Shi (Fructus Aurantii Immaturus), etc.; in the case of accompanying Damp-Heat, used with Huang Lian (Rhizoma Coptidis), Qin Pi (Cortex Fraxini), etc.

Administration 5～10g for making a decoction.

Precautions Not applied to Qi deficency with stagnation or Stomach weakness with poor appetite.

0. 8. Chuan Lian Zi (Fructus Meliae Toosendan)

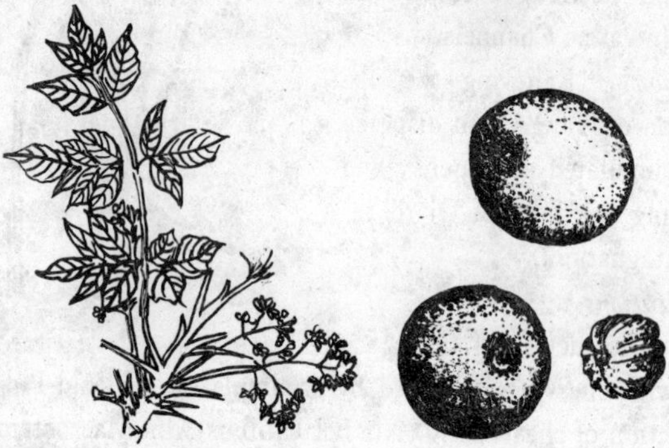

Description Fruit of Melia toosendan Sieb. et Zucc. Family Meliaceae.

Characteristics Bitter in flavor, cold in nature, mildly toxic, and acting on the Liver, Stomach, Small Intestine and Urinary Bladder Channels.

Action Regulating the circulation of Qi to relieve pain, killing parasitis and curing fungus.

Indications

(1) Stagnation of Liver-Qi or discoordination between Liver and Stomach marked by distending pain in the hypochondrium and ab-

domen, hernia with swelling and pain, etc. In the case of stagnation of Liver-Qi with preponderance of Heat, used with Yan Hu Suo (Rhizoma Corydalis), named Jinlingzi San (Powder of Fructus Meliae Toosendan); in the case of periumbilical colic of Cold type, usually used with Xiao Hui Xiang (Fructus Foeniculi), Mu Xiang (Radix Aucklandiae), Wu Zhu Yu (Fructus Euodiae), etc., as in Daoqi Tang (Decoction for Activating the Circulation of Qi).

(2) Abdominal pain due to ascariasis. Usually used together with Shi Jun Zi (Fructus Quisqualis) and Bing Lang (Semen Arecae). In addition, when baked brown and powdered, it can be used to treat tinea capitis by applying the paste made of sesame oil and the powder to the affected place.

Administration 3～10g for making a decoction; q. s. for external application.

Precautions Not applied to asthenic Cold of the Spleen and Stomach.

Digestion-promoting Drugs

Drugs used principally for improving appetite and digestion and removing food stagnation are categorized as digestion-promoting drugs or drugs for improving digestion and removing food stagnation.

Digestion-promoting drugs are mostly sweet in flavor, neutral in nature and are capable of improving digestion, normalizing the function of Stomach, some of them can also invigorate the Spleen. They are mainly indicated for distension, fullness and pain of the Stomach and abdomen, belching, acid regurgitation, nausea, vomiting, irregular bowel movements, etc. due to retention of indigested food. They are also indicated for indigestion due to hypofunction of the Spleen and Stomach.

In clinical application, these drugs should be dispensed with drugs for promoting the circulation of Qi, drugs for resolving Dampness or, drugs for invigorating the function of Spleen, etc. according to the actual condition of the patient, so as to strengthen the effect of improving appetite and digestion and removing food stagnation.

0. 1. Shan Zha (Fructus Crataegi)

Description The ripe fruit of Crataegus cuneata Sieb. et Zucc., or Crataegus pinnatifida Bge. var. major N. E. Br. Family Rosaceae.

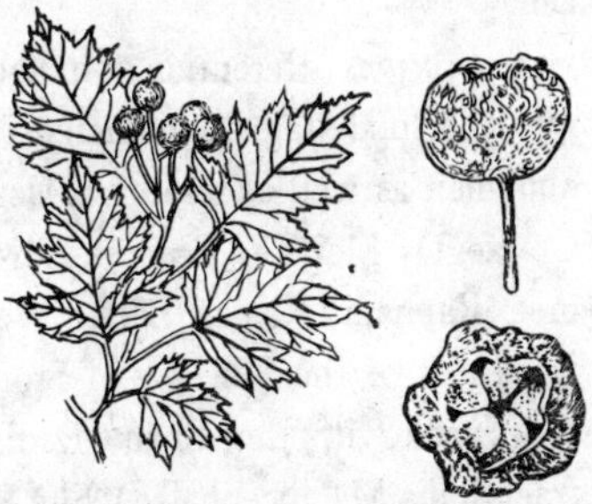

Characteristics Sour and sweet in flavor, slightly warm in nature, acting on the Spleen, Stomach and Liver Channels.

Action Improving digestion, removing food stagnation, activating Blood circulation to disperse Blood stasis.

Indications

(1) Stagnation of indigested meat, abdominal distension and fullness, diarrhea, dysentery or other symptoms induced by food retention. For stagnation of indigested meat, used either alone by making a decoction or together with Qing Pi (Pericarpium Citri Reticulatae Viride) and Mu Xiang (Radix Aucklandiae); for food retention, usually used with Shen Qu (Massa Fermentata Medicinalis), Mai Ya (Fructus Hordei Germinatus) and Lai Fu Zi (Semen Raphani); for diarrhea and dysentery with abdominal pain or pus-and-blood stools, usually stir-fried and used with Huang Lian (Rhizoma Coptidis), Ku Shen (Radix Sophorae Flavescentis), Mu Xiang (Radix Aucklandiae), etc.

(2) Lingering lochia after delivery with Blood retention and abdominal pain, hernia or swelling of testis with bearing-down pain, etc. For Lochiorrhea, used with Yi Mu Cao (Herba Leonuri), Pu Huang (Pollen Typhae), etc., for hernia, used with Ju He (Semen Citri Reticulatae) and Xiao Hui Xiang (Fructus Poeniculi).

Administration 10～15g for making a decoction, large dosage being as much as 30g.

Precautions Over intake of the raw fruit should be avoided.

0.2. Shen Qu (Massa Fermentata Medicinalis)

Description A leavened preparation of the mixture of Semen Armeniacae Amarum, Herba Artemisiae Annuae, Fructus Xanthii, wheat bran and flour.

Characteristics Sweet and acrid in flavor, warm in nature, acting on the Spleen and Stomach Channels.

Action Improving digestion and regulating the function of Stomach.

Indications Retention of indigested food, diarrhea due to impairment by food stagnation, distension and fullness of the Stomach and abdomen as well as anorexia. Usually used with Shan Zha (Fructus Crataegi), Mai Ya (Fructus Hordei Germinatus) and Lai Fu Zi (Semen Raphani), as in Baohe Wan (Lenitive Pill). In the case of weakness of the Spleen and Stomach with poor appetite and lassitude, used with Ren Shen (Radix Ginseng), Bai Zhu (Rhizoma Atractylodis Macrocephalae), Sha Ren (Fructus Amomi), etc. In addition, it can be used as an adjuvant of mineral drugs to help absorption, as in Cizhu Wan (Medicated Leaven Pill).

Administration 6~15g for making a decoction. Stir-fried brown for stopping diarrhea.

Precautions Contraindicated in womem during breast feeding period.

0. 3. Mai Ya (Fructus Hordei Germinatus)

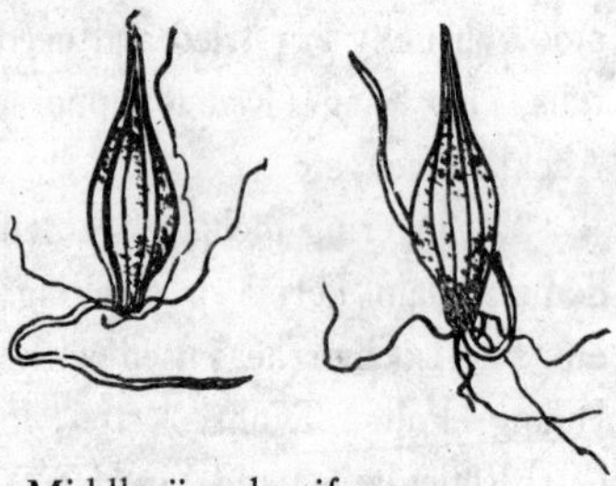

Description The dried germinant fruit of Hordeum vulgare L. Family Gramineae.

Characteristics Sweet in flavor, neutral in nature, acting on the Spleen, Stomach and Liver Channels.

Action Improving appetite and normalizing the function of the Middle-jiao, lactifuge.

Indications

(1) Retention of indigested food, anorexia, distension and fullness of the Stomach and abdomen, or indigestion with poor appetite, etc. This drug is good at removing stagnation of rice, flour and potatoes, and is usually used together with Shan Zha (Fructus Crataegi), Shen Qu (Massa Fermentata Medicinalis), Ji Nei Jin (Endothelium Corneum Gigeriae Galli), etc. In the case of indigestion due to Spleen Deficiency, used with Dang Shen (Radix Codonopsis Pilosulae), Bai Zhu (Rhizoma Atractylodis Macrocephalae), Shan

Yao (Rhizoma Dioscoreae),etc.

(2) Lactifuge for breast feeding women and for galactostasis. Usually made into a decoction for oral intake with half of the unprepared drug and half of the stir-fried one.

Administration 10～15g for making a decoction, a large dosage may be as much as 30～120g.

Precautions Not to be used in breast feeding women.

0. 4. Ji Nei Jin (Endothelium Corneum Gigeriae Galli)

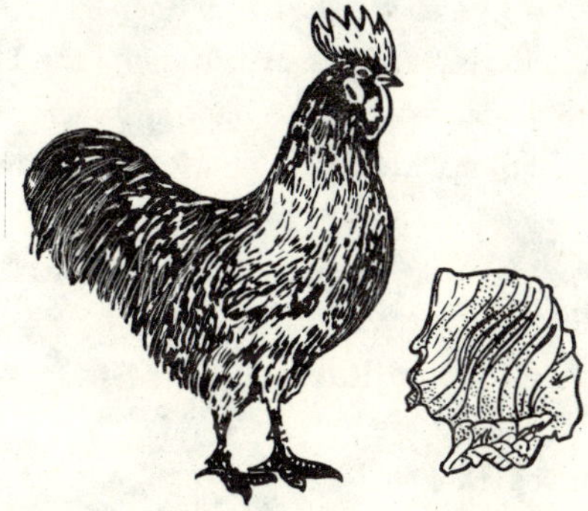

Description The lining membrane of the gizzard of Gallus gallus domesticus Brisson. Family Phasianidae.

Characteristics Sweet in flavor, neutral in nature, acting on the Spleen, Stomach, Small Intestine and Urinary Bladder Channels.

Action Activating the function of the Spleen to improve digestion, treating spontaneous emission and dispelling stone.

Indications

(1) Stagnation of indigested food and infantile dyspepsia and malnutrition. In the mild case of indigestion, used alone in powder form after it is stir-fried to half-burnt; in the case of retention of food with distension and fullness in the Stomach and abdomen, usually used with Shan Zha (Fructus Crataegi), Mai Ya (Fructus Hordei Germinatus), etc.; for infantile dyspepsia and mulnutrition with weakness of the Spleen and Stomach, used with Dang Shen (Radix Codonopsis Pilosulae), Shan Yao (Rhizoma Dioscoreae), Bai Zhu

(Rhizoma Atractylodis Macrocephalae), etc.; for indigestion, poor appetite with abdominal distension and diarrhea, used with Bai Zhu (Rhizoma Atractylodis Macrocephalae) and Gan Jiang (Rhizoma Zingiberis), as in Yipi Bing (Spleen-invigorating Cake).

(2) Enuresis, frequent urination and seminal emission. For enuresis, used with Sang Piao Xiao (Oötheca Mantidis) and Fu Pen Zi (Fructus Rubi); for seminal emission, used with Lian Zi Rou (Semen Nelumbinis), Tu Si Zi (Semen Cuscutae), etc.

(3) Urinary stone and biliary calculus. For the former, used with Jin Qian Cao (Herba Lysimachiae), Hai Jin Sha (Spora Lygodii) and Hu Tao (Juglandis Regiae), as in Sanjin Hutao Tang (Decoction of Three Drugs with Juglandis Regiae); for the latter, used with Dai Huang (Radix et Rhizoma Rhei), Yu Jin (Radix Curcumae), Zhi Zi (Fructus Gardeniae), etc.

Administration 3～10g for making a decoction; 1.5～3g for making the powder.

0.5. Lai Fu Zi (Semen Raphani)

Description The ripe seeds of Raphanus sativus L. Family Cruciferae.

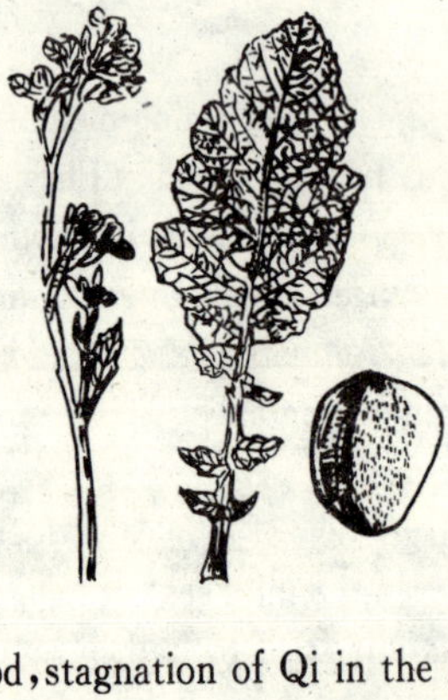

Characteristics Acrid and sweet in flavor, neutral in nature, acting on the Spleen, Stomach and Lung Channels.

Action Improving digestion to remove food stagnation, lowering the adverse flow of Qi to resolve Phlegm.

Indications

(1) Retention of indigested food, stagnation of Qi in the Middle-jiao marked by distension and stuffiness of the Stomach and abdomen, eructation of fetid odor, acid regurgitation or abdominal pain with diarrhea and dysentery, etc. For treatment, usually used in combination with Shan Zha (Fructus Crataegi), Shen Qu (Massa Fer-

mentata Medicinalis), Chen Pi (Pericarpium Citri Reticulatae), etc., as in Baohe Wan (Lenitive Pill). In the case of food stagnation due to Spleen Deficiency, used together with Bai Zhu (Rhizoma Atractylodis Macrocephalae), Shen Qu (Massa Fermentata Medicinalis), Chen Pi (Pericarpium Citri Reticulatae), etc., as in Daan Wan (Pill for Invigorating the Spleen to Improve Digestion).

(2) Retention of excessive Phlegm and saliva manifested as cough, dyspnea with profuse Phlegm of sthenic type. Usually used with Bai Jie Zi (Semen Sinapis Albae) and Su Zi (Fructus Perillae), as in Sanzi Yangqin Tang (Decoction of Three Kinds of Seeds for the Aged). In the case of convulsion and salivation or lockjaw and apoplexy caused by retention of excessive Wind-Phlegm, used with Zao Jiao (Fructus Gleditsiae).

Administration 3～9g for making a decoction.

Precautions Used with caution for Qi Deficiency without food stagnation or Phlegm retention.

Anthelmintics

Drugs with a major effect of expelling or killing parasites are referred to as anthelmintics.

Drugs of this category are indicated for diseases caused by parasites in the intestines, such as ascariasis, enterobiasis, cestodiasis and ancylostomiasis. Through expelling or killing these parasites, it will bring relief to such symptoms as intermittent abdominal pain, anorexia, peculiar food preference, pruritus of the anus as well as emacitation with sallow complexion, large belly without strength, palpitation, edema, etc.

In clinical application of these drugs, such factors as the type of parasites and the constitution of the patient should be taken into consideration, and compatible drugs should be used for improving the appetite, purgation, invigorating the Spleen, etc. In practice, purgation should be applied before or after or simutaneously with tonification in accordance with different cases.

To ensure a good effect, anthelmintics should be taken on an empty stomach. And care should be taken in avoiding overdosage as some of the drugs are toxic. For the weak, the aged and the pregnant women, the drug should be applied with caution.

0. 1. Shi Jun Zi (Fructus Quisqualis)

Description The fruit of Quiqualis indica L. Family Combretaceae.

Characteristics Sweet in flavor, warm in nature, acting on the Spleen and Stomach Channels.

Action Killing and dispelling parasites and removing food stagnation.

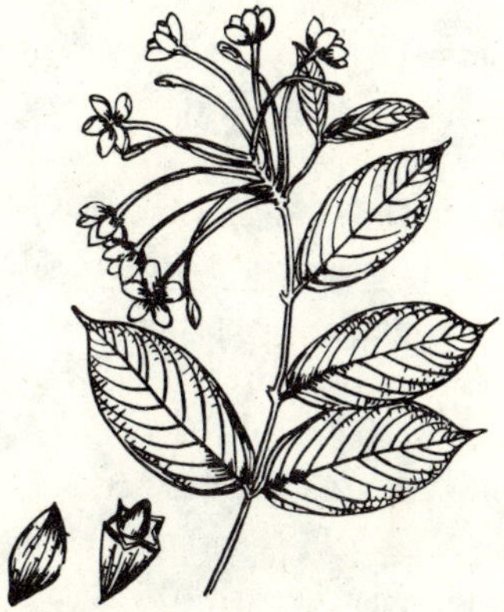

Indications Ascariasis, enterobiasis and infantile mulnutrition. For mild cases, take the stir-fried Shi Jun Zi (Fructus Quisqualis) after chewing it; for the severe cases, dispense it with Bing Lang (Semen Arecae), Ku Lian Pi (Cortex Meliae), etc., as in Shijunzi Wan (Pill of Fructus Quisqualis). In the case of infantile mulnutrition marked by emacitation and indigestion, it is used with Dang Shen (Radix Codonopsis Pilosulae), Bai Zhu (Rhizoma Atractylodis Macrocephalae), Shen Qu (Massa Fermentata Medicinalis), etc.

Administration 6～10g for making a decoction; 1～1.5 grains (stir-fried) per day for each year of age for children to take by chewing, with a total dosage not exceeding 20 grains.

Precautions Tea and overdosage should be avoided during administration.

0.2. Bing Lang (Semen Arecae)

Description The ripe seed of Areca catechu L. Family Palmae.

Characteristics Acrid and bitter in flavor, warm in nature, acting on the Stomach and Large Intestine Channels.

Action Dispelling parasites, removing stagnation, descending the adverse flow of Qi to induce diuresis.

Indications

(1) Many kinds of parasitosis including cestodiasis, fasciolopsiasis, ascariasis, ancylostomiasis and enterobiasis. It is especially effective for dispelling cestodiasis, and it is used with Nan Gua Zi (Semen Cucurbitae) to strengthen the effect. For ascariasis, used with

Qian Niu Zi (Semen Pharbitidis), as in Niu Lang Wan (Pill of Semen Pharbitidis and Semen Arecae).

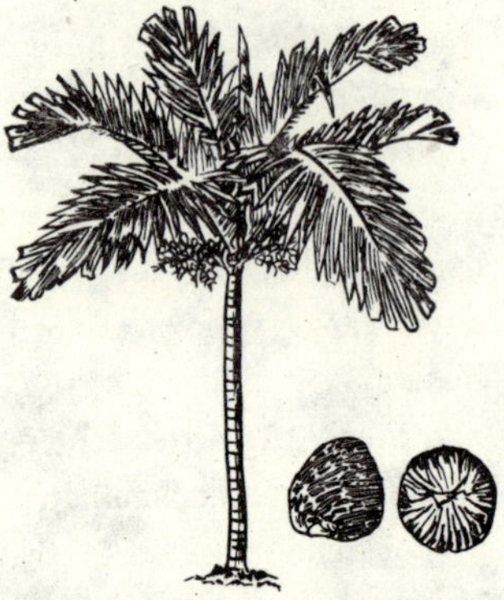

(2) Food retention and Qi stagnation marked by abdominal distension, constipation and dysentery with tenesmus. For food retention, usually used with Mu Xiang (Radix Aucklandiae), Chen Pi (Pericarpium Citri Reticulatae) and Dai Huang (Radix et Rhizoma Rhei), as in Muxiang Binglang Wan (Pill of Radix Aucklandiae and Semen Arecae); for dysentery, used with Huang Lian (Rhizoma Coptidis), etc.

(3) Edema or beriberi. For edema of sthenic type, usually used with Shang Lu (Radix Phytolaccae), Fu Ling Pi (Cortex Poria), Ze Xie (Rhizoma Alismatis), etc., as in Shuzao Yinzi (Decoction for Diuresis); for beriberi with swelling and pain of Damp-Cold type, used with Mu Gua (Fructus Chaenomelis), Wu Zhu Yu (Fructus Euodiae), Chen Pi (Pericarpium Citri Reticulatae), Zi Su (Fructus Perillae), as in Jiming San (Cock Crowing Powder).

Administration 6～15g for making a decoction; when used alone to treat cestodiasis and fasciolopsiasis, the dosage may reach 60～120g.

Precautions Contraindicated for Spleen Deficiency with diarrhea.

0.3. Nan Gua Zi (Semen Cucurbitae)

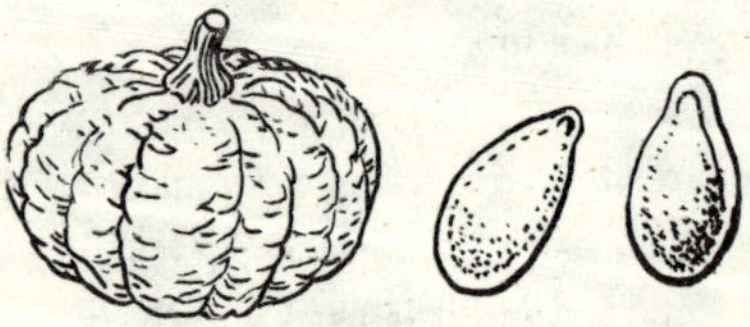

Description The ripe seed of Cucurbita moschata Duch. Family

Cucurbitaceae.

Characteristics Sweet in flavor, neutral in nature, acting on the Stomach and Large Intestine Channels.

Action Killing parasites.

Indications Cestodiasis and ascariasis. For treatment, the patient should first take 60～120g of unprocessed seeds after chewing them, two hours later, take the decoction made of 60～120g of Bing Lang (Semen Arecae), then half an hour after that, take the infusion made of 15g of Mang Xiao (Natrii Sulfas) to help discharge the parasites.

Administration 60～120g for oral intake after chewing.

0.4. Lei Wan (Omphalia)

Description The sclerotium of Omphalia lapidescens Schroet. Family Tricholomataceae.

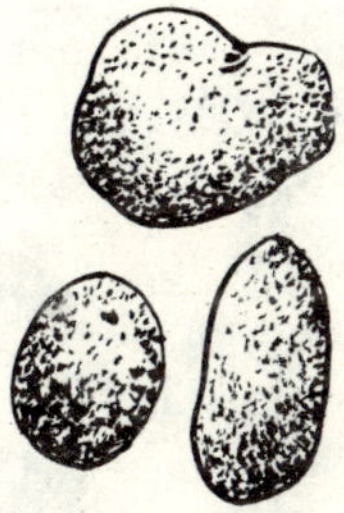

Characteristics Bitter in flavor, cold in nature, mildly toxic, and acting on the Stomach and Large Intestine Channels.

Action Killing parasites and improving digestion.

Indications Mainly indicated for taeniasis, also used for ascariasis and ancylostomiasis. Usually dispensed with Bing Lang (Semen Arecae), Mu Xiang (Radix Aucklandiae), etc. In addition, it can be used for infantile mulnutrition by adding Shi Jun Zi (Fructus Quisqualis), Hu Huang Lian (Rhizoma Picrorhizae), etc., as in Leiwan Dan (Omphalis Pill).

Administration 6～15g made into pills or powder.

Precautions Used with caution for asthenic Cold of the Spleen and Stomach. Avoid exposure to high temperature.

Hemostatics

Drugs with the principal effects for stopping internal and external bleedings of various kinds are referred to as hemostatics

Drugs of this category are capable of stopping bleeding by removing Heat from the Blood, by astringency, by dispersing Blood stasis, or by warming the Meridians respectively. They are indicated for bleedings of various kinds, such as hemoptysis, epistaxis, hematemesis, hematuria, hemafecia, metrorrhagia and metrostaxis, purpura and traumatic bleeding.

Proper hemostatics should be selected according to the different causes of bleeding and actual conditions of the patient. Compatible drugs should be used accordingly. In the case of bleeding due to invasion of Blood by pathogenic Heat, drugs for purging Heat should be dispensed; in the case of bleeding with Blood stasis, drugs for promoting the circulation of Qi and Blood should be added, for bleeding of asthenic Cold nature, drugs for warming Yang and dispelling Cold should be used in combination; for bleeding due to failure of Qi in keeping the Blood within the Blood vessels, drugs for tonifying Qi and Spleen should be used together.

In clinical practice, care should be taken in avoiding side-effect. If there is any sign of Blood stasis, never use drugs for removing Heat from the Blood or astringent hemostatics alone.

0. 1. Xiao Ji (Herba Cephalanoploris)

Description The above ground part of Cephalanoplos segetum (Bge.) Kitam., or Cephalanoplos setosum (Willd.) Kitam. Family Compositae.

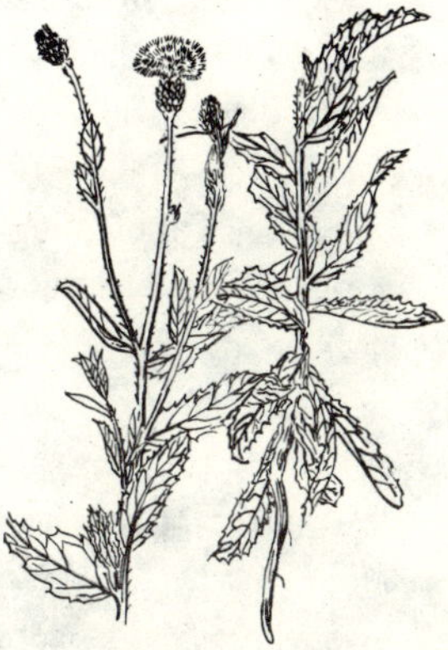

Characteristics Sweet in flavor, cool in nature, acting on the Heart and Liver Channels.

Action Stopping bleeding by dispelling pathogenic Heat from the Blood and curing carbuncles by detoxication.

Indications

(1) Hemoptysis, epistaxis, hematemesis, hematuria, metrorrhagia and metrostaxis due to invasion of Blood by pathogenic Heat. It is especially effective for hematuria. For treatment, usually used together with Pu Huang (Pollen Typhae), Mu Tong (Caulis Akebiae), Hua Shi (Talcum), etc., as in Xiaoji Yinzi (Decoction of Herba Cephalanoploris). In the case of epistaxis due to Blood Heat, the fresh plant can be pounded to paste and made into juice for oral intake.

(2) Pyogenic infection on the body surface induced by Heat-evil. Used alone for internal application or external application by pounding the fresh plant to paste which is then applied to the affected area.

Administration 10～15g of the dried herb or 30～60g of the fresh herb for making a decoction; q. s. for external application.

Precautions Contraindicated for bleeding of asthenic Cold nature.

0. 2. Di Yu (Radix Sanguisorbae)

Description Root of Sanguisorba officinalis L. Family Rosaceae.

Characteristics Bitter and sour in flavor, slightly cold in nature, acting on the Liver, Stomach and Large Intestine Channels.

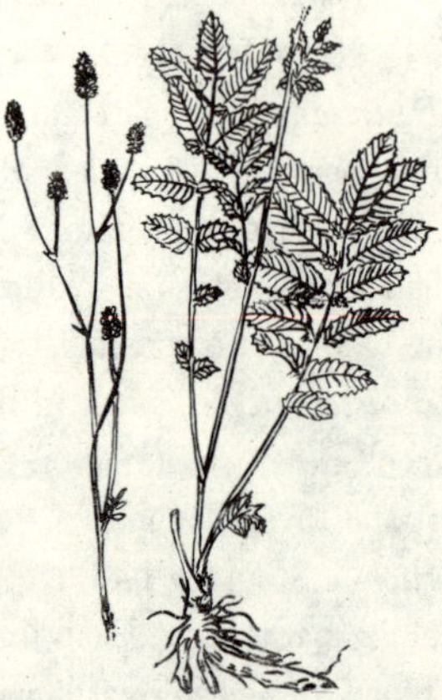

Action Stopping bleeding by clearing away Heat from the Blood and accelerating the healing of sores by detoxication.

Indications

(1) Various kinds of bleeding, especially hemafecia, hemorrhoidal bleeding, dysentery with bloody stool, metrorrhagia and metrostaxis due to Heat invasion of the Blood in the Middle-jiao. For hemafecia and hemorrhoidal bleeding, used together with Huai Hua (Flos Sophorae); for metrorrhagia and metrostaxis, used with Sheng Di (Radix Rehmanniae), Huang Qin (Radix Scutellariae), etc.; for lingering bloody dysentery, usually used with Huang Lian (Rhizoma Coptidis), Mu Xiang (Radix Aucklandiae), Wu Mei (Fructus Mume), etc., as in Diyu Wan (Pill of Radix Sanguisorbae).

(2) Scalds, eczema, etc. It is very effective for treating scalds, usually by applying the mixture of its powder and sesame oil to the affected place; for eczema, gauze soaked in concentrated decoction of Di Yu (Radix Sanguisorbae) is applied to the affected place.

Administration 10～15g for making a decoction; q. s. for external application.

Precautions Not used alone externally for large area of burns.

0.3. Ce Bai Ye (Cacumen Biotae)

Description The tender branch and leaf of Biota orientalis (L.) Endl. Family Cupressaceae.

Characteristics Bitter and astringent in flavor, slightly cold in nature, acting on the Lung, Liver and Large Intestine Channels.

Action Stopping bleeding by clearing away Heat from the Blood, relieving cough by eliminating Phlegm.

Indications

(1) Epistaxis, hematemesis, hemoptysis, hematuria, metrorrhagia and metrostaxis caused by invasion of Heat in the Blood. Usually used with Xiao Ji (Herba Cephalanoploris), Bai Mao Gen (Rhizoma Imperatae), etc. In the case of bleeding of asthenic Cold nature, used with Ai Ye (Folium Artemisiae Argyi), Pao Jiang Tan (carbonized Rhizoma Zingiberis), etc.; in the case of traumatic bleeding, used in powder externally.

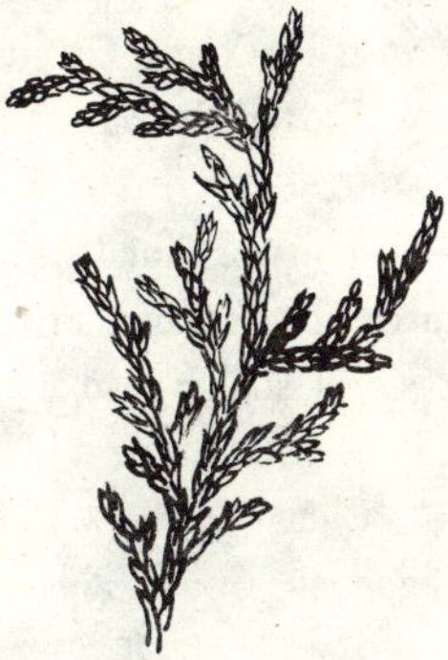

(2) Asthmatic cough with thick sputum due to Lung-Heat. Usually used with Huang Qin (Radix Scutellariae), Jie Geng (Radix Platycodi), etc.

(3) Alopecia or itch of the head. Used externally by soaking it in the wine and applying the wine to the affected area.

Administration 10~15g for making a decoction; q.s. for external use.

Precautions Not used alone for bleeding of asthenic Cold nature.

0. 4. San Qi (Radix Notoginseng)

Description The root of Panax notoginseng (Burk.) Chen. Family Araliaceae.

Characteristics Sweet and slightly bitter in flavor, warm in nature, and acting on the Liver and Stomach Channels.

Action Stopping bleeding by resolving Blood stasis, and relieving pain by activating Blood circulation.

Indications

(1) Various kinds of internal and external bleedings, especially bleeding with Blood stasis. Used alone as a powder for oral intake, or together with Xue Yu Tan (Crini Carbonisatus) and Hua Rui Shi (Ophicalcitum), as in Huaxue Dan (Pill for Resolving Blood Stasis).

(2) Traumatic injury with bruise and pain. Used either internally

or externally, either alone or together with Ru Xiang (Resina Boswelliae Carterii), Mo Yao (Myrrha), etc.

(3) Chest distress and heart pain caused by stagnation of Blood stasis. Usually used with Dan Shen (Radix Salviae Miltiorrhizae), Chuan Xiong (Rhizoma Ligustici Chuanxiong), etc.

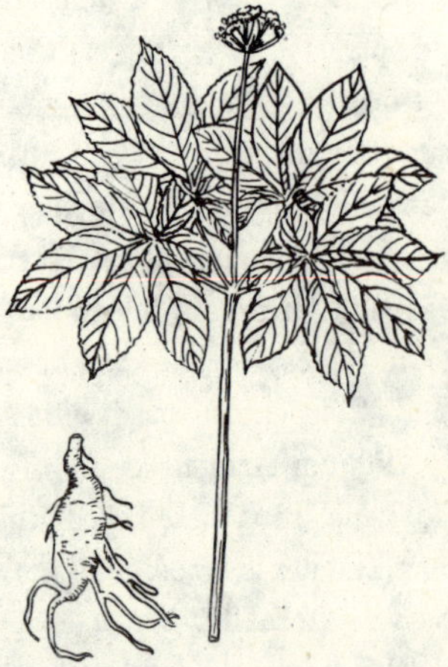

Administration 1～3g for oral intake as a powder; q. s. for external use.

Precautions Used with caution for bleeding due to Yin Deficiency and Fire Excess.

0. 5. Pu Huang (Pollen Typhae)

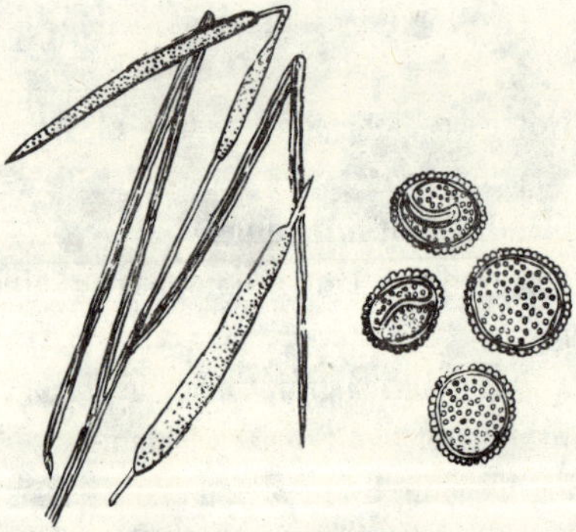

Description The pollen of Typha angustifolia L. Family Typhaceae.

Characteristics Sweet in flavor, neutral in nature, acting on the Liver and Pericardium Channels.

Action Promoting Blood circulation to remove Blood stasis, stopping bleeding by astringency.

Indications

(1) Various bleedings including hemoptysis, epistaxis, hematemesis, hematuria, hemafecia, metrorrhagia, metrostaxis and traumatic bleeding. This drug is characterized by stopping bleeding together with removing Blood stasis and it can be used either alone or together with Xian He Cao (Herba Agrimoniae), Ce Bai Ye (Cacumen Biotae), etc. For traumatic bleeding, used externally by applying its powder to the cut.

(2) Cardiac or abdominal pain, dysmenorrhea and postpartum abdominal pain induced by retention of Blood stasis. Usually used with Wu Ling Zhi (Faeces Trogopterorum), as in Shixiao San (Wonderful Powder for Relieving Blood Stagnation).

(3) Hematuria accompanied by dark urine and painful and difficult urination. Usually used with Sheng Di Huang (Radix Rehmanniae) and Dong Kui Zi (Semen Abutili), as in Puhuang San (Powder of Pollen Typhae).

Administration 3～10g for making a decoction (wrapped in gauze); q. s. for external use.

Precautions Contraindicated in pregnant women.

0. 6. Bai Ji (Rhizoma Bletillae)

Description The rhizome of Bletilla striata (Thunb.) Reichb. f. Family Orchidaceae.

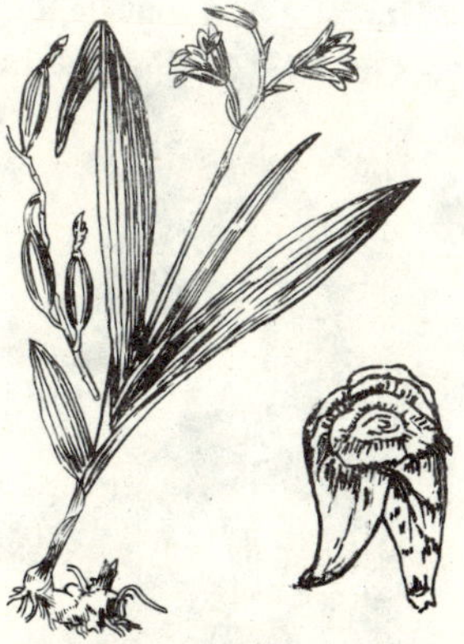

Characteristics Bitter, sweet and astringent in flavor, slightly cold in nature, acting on the Lung, Liver and Stomach Channels.

Action Inducing astringency to stop bleeding, relieving swelling and promoting regeneration of tissue.

Indications

(1) Hemorrhage of the Lung and Stomach as well as traumatic

bleeding. For hemoptysis due to Deficiency of Lung-Yin, usually used with Ou Jie (Nodus Nelumbinis Rhizomatis), E Jiao (Colla Corii Asini) and juice of fresh Sheng Di (Radix Rehmanniae), as in Pipa Wan (Bolus of Folium Eriobotryae); in the case of Stomach hemorrhage, used with Hai Piao Xiao (Os Sepiae), as in Wu Ji San (Powder of Gallus Domesticus); for traumatic bleeding, the powder of Bai Ji (Rhizoma Bletillae) is applied externally.

(2) Sores, carbuncles and other pyogenic infections on the skin, and cracked skin of the hands and feet. The former can be treated by adding Jin Yin Hua (Flos Lonicerae), Chuan Shan Jia (Squama Manitis), Tian Hua Fen (Radix Trichosanthis), etc, as in Neixiao San (Oral Powder for Skin Ailment), in the case of lingering and unhealed ulceration, apply externally with its powder; while the latter can be treated by applying the ointment of its powder and sesame oil to the affected place.

(3) Pulmonary abscess with blood-and-pus mixed sputum, especially at the late stage with decreased sputum. Usually used with Jie Geng (Radix Platycodi), Jin Yin Hua (Flos Lonicerae), Sha Shen (Radix Adenophorae Strictae), etc.

Administration 3～10g for making a decoction; 1. 5～3g of powder for oral use; q. s. for external application.

Precautions Antagonistic to Wu Tou (Radix Aconiti).

0. 7. Ou Jie (Nodus Nelumbinis Rhizomatis)

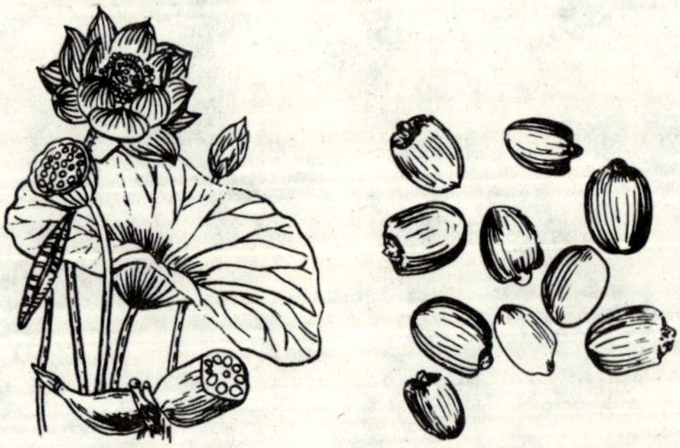

Description The dried node of rhizome of Nelumbo nucefera.

Family Nymphaeaceae.

Characteristics Sweet and astringent in flavor, neutral in nature, acting on the Lung, Liver and Stomach Channels.

Action Inducing astringency to stop bleeding.

Indications Various kinds of bleedings. This drug is good at both inducing astringency to stop bleeding and resolving Blood stasis, and it is especially effective in treating hemoptysis and hematemesis by dispensing with Bai Ji (Rhizoma Bletillae), Ce Bai Ye (Cacumen Biotae), etc.

Administration 10～15g for making a decoction.

Precautions Unprocessed for stopping bleeding by resolving Blood stasis; carbonized for stopping bleeding by inducing astringency.

0.8. Ai Ye (Folium Artemisiae Argyi)

Description The leaf of Artemisia argyi Levl. et Vant. Family Compositae.

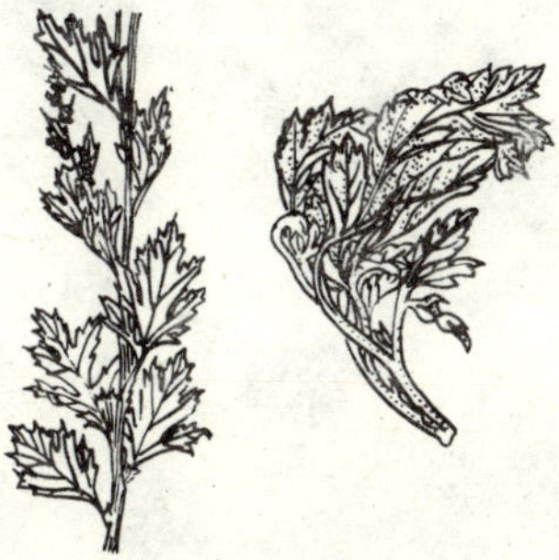

Characteristics Bitter and acrid in flavor, warm in nature, acting on the Liver, Spleen and Kidney Channels.

Action Warming the Channels to stop bleeding, dispelling pathogenic Cold to relieve pain.

Indications

(1) Metrorrhagia, metrostaxis, menorrhagia, etc. due to invasion of asthenic Cold. Usually used together with E Jiao (Colla Corii Asini), Dang Gui (Radix Angelicae Sinensis), etc., as in Jiao Ai Tang (Decoction of Colla Corii Asini and Folium Artemisiae Argyi). In the case of epistaxis and hemoptysis due to invasion of Heat in the Blood, used with fresh Ce Bai Ye (Cacumen Biotae), fresh Sheng Di (Radix Rehmanniae) and fresh lotus leaf, named Sisheng Wan (Bolus of Four Fresh Drugs).

(2) Irregular menstruation, dysmenorrhea, leukorrhagia, cold pain

in the lower abdomen, sterility due to uterine coldness, etc. caused by Deficiency of the Lower-jiao. For treatment, used together with Xiang Fu (Rhizoma Cyperi), Rou Gui (Cortex Cinnamomi) and Wu Zhu Yu (Fructus Euodiae), as in Ai Fu Nuangong Wan (Pill of Folium Artemisiae Argyi and Rhizoma Cyperi for Warming the Uterus).

(3) Eczema and pruritus. Decocted alone for fumigating and washing.

(4) Pain of the limbs and joints due to Cold stagnation. Usually made into moxa stick or cone for acupoint moxibustion.

Administration 3~10g for making a decoction; q. s. for external application.

Precautions Not applied alone for Yin Deficiency with Heat in the Blood.

Drugs for Activating Blood Circulation and Removing Blood Stasis

Drugs with the principal actions of making free passage of Blood in the vessels and promoting the circulation of Blood to resolve Blood stasis are referred to as drugs for activating Blood circulation and removing Blood stasis, among which drugs with strong actions are habitually called potent drugs for removing Blood stasis.

Drugs of this type are mostly acrid in flavor, warm in nature, and capable of promoting Blood circulation to disperse Blood stasis, reducing swelling to relieve pain, regulating menstruation and removing obstruction of Qi and Blood. They are indicated for various syndromes due to obstruction of Blood circulation and retention of Blood stasis in the interior, such as amenorrhea, dysmenorrhea, mass in the abdomen, traumatic injury, suppurative skin infections, arthralgia, etc.

Blood circulates smoothly only when Qi flows normally, and Blood slows down when Qi stagnates, for this reason, drugs for promoting Blood circulation and removing Blood stasis are often used in combination with drugs for promoting the flow of Qi to strengthen their effect. In addition, other compatible drugs should be added in accordance with actual condition of the patient. For example, in the case of Qi stagnation and Blood stasis due to accumulation of pathogenic Cold, drugs for warming the interior should be added; for suppurative skin infections, drugs for purging heat and removing toxins should be added; for mass in the abdomen, drugs for softening and resolving hard masses and Phlegm should be used in combination; for insufficiency of vital Qi, drugs for tonification should be added.

Drugs of this type should not be applied to women with profuse menstruation. For pregnant women, these drugs should be very cautiously given or avoided altogether.

0. 1. Chuan Xiong (Rhizoma Ligustici Chuanxiong)

Description The rhizome of Ligusticum chuanxiong Hort. Family Umbelliferae.

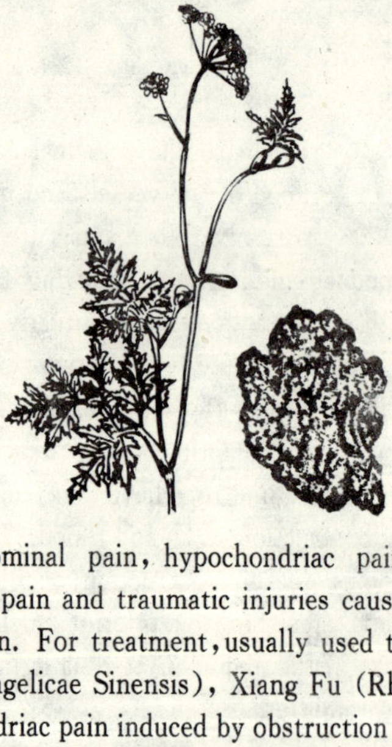

Characteristics Acrid in flavor, warm in nature, acting on the Liver, Gallbladder and Pericardium Channels.

Action Promoting the circulation of both Blood and Qi, and eliminating pathogenic Wind to relieve pain.

Indications

(1) Irregular menstruation, dysmenorrhea, postpartum abdominal pain, hypochondriac pain, suppurative skin infections with pain and traumatic injuries caused by Blood stasis and Qi stagnation. For treatment, usually used together with Dang Gui (Radix Angelicae Sinensis), Xiang Fu (Rhizoma Cyperi), etc. For hypochondriac pain induced by obstruction of Blood circulation due to stagnation of Liver-Qi, used with Chai Hu (Radix Bupleuri), Dang Gui (Radix Angelicae Sinensis), Bai Shao (Radix Paeoniae Alba), etc., as in Chaihu Shugan San (Powder of

Radix Bupleuri for Soothing the Liver);for slow festering skin infections, used with Dang Gui (Radix Angelicae Sinensis),Chuan Shan Jia(Squama Manitis),etc., as in Tounong San (Powder for Promoting Pus Discharge) ; for traumatic injury with Blood stasis, used with Gui Wei (fibrous root of Radix Angelicae Sinensis),Tao Ren (Semen Persicae),etc.

(2) Headache and rheumatic arthralgia. In the case of headache induced by Wind-Cold, used together with Bai Zhi (Radix Angelicae Dahuricae),Xi Xin (Herba Asari),etc., as in Chuanxiong Chatiao San (Chuangxiong Mixture) ; for headache due to Wind-heat, used with Shi Gao (Gypsum Fibrosum), Ju Hua (Flos Chrysanthemi), etc., as in Chuanxiong San (Chuanxiong Powder) ; for headache due to Wind-Dampness, used with Qiang Huo (Rhizoma seu Radix Noto-pterygii), Gao Ben (Rhizoma Ligustici), Fang Feng (Radix Ledebouriellae), etc., as in Qianghuo Shengshi Tang (Dampness Removal Decoction of Rhizoma seu Radix Noto-pterygii);in the case of rheumatic arthralgia and pain of the limbs and joints, used with Xi Xin (Herba Asari), Du Huo (Radix Angelicae Pubescentis), etc.

Administration 3～10g for making a decoction.

Precautions Not used for Yin Deficiency and Fire Excess with red tongue and dry mouth, or profuse menstruation.

0. 2. Dan Shen (Radix Salviae Miltiorrhizae)

Description The root of Salvia miltiorrhiza Bge. Family Labiatae.

Characteristics Bitter in flavor, slightly cold in nature, acting on the Heart, Pericarpium and Liver Channels.

Action Activating Blood circulation to remove Blood stasis, expelling heat from Blood to relieve carbuncles and clearing away vexation to tranquilize the mind.

Indications

(1) Stagnation of Blood marked by amenorrhea, dysmenorrhea, lochiostasis, pain of the Heart and abdomen, and mass in the abdomen. Slightly cold in nature, it is especially effective for Blood stasis complicated by Heat invasion of the Blood. For treating the gynecological diseases mentioned above, it is used with Hong Hua

(Flos Carthami), Tao Ren (Semen Persicae), Yi Mu Cao (Herba Leonuri), etc. ; for pain of the Heart, chest, Stomach and abdomen induced by Blood stasis and Qi stagnation, used with Tan Xiang (Lignum Santali) and Sha Ren (Fructus Amomi), as in Danshen Yin (Decoction of Radix Salvia Miltiorrhizae) ; for mass in the abdomen, used with San Leng (Rhizoma Sparganii), E Zhu (Rhizoma Zedoariae), etc. ; for traumatic injuries with swelling pain, used with Dang Gui (Radix Angelicae Sinensis), Hong Hua (Flos Carthami), Chuanxiong (Rhizoma Ligustici Chuanxiong), etc. ; for arthritis of Heat type, used with Ren Dong Teng (Caulis Lonicerae), Chi Shao (Radix Paeoniae Rubra), Sang Zhi (Ramulus Mori), etc.

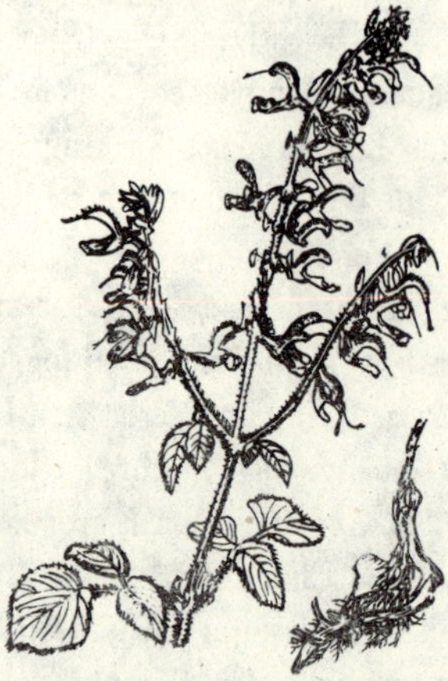

(2) Suppurative skin infections. Usually used with Jin Yin Hua (Flos Lonicerae), Lian Qiao (Fructus Forsythiae), etc.

(3) Vaxation and insomnia. In the case of Heat invasion of the Ying and Blood systems, used with Sheng Di (Radix Rehmanniae), Xuan Shen (Radix Scrophulariae), etc., as in QingYing Tang (Decoction for Clearing Heat in the Ying System); in the case of insufficiency of Blood to nourish the Heart, used with Suan Zao Ren (Semen Ziziphi Spinosae), Bai Zi Ren (Semen Biotae), etc.

Administration 5～15g for making a decoction.

Precautions Antagonistic to Li Lu (Radix Veratri)

0. 3. Tao Ren (Semen Persicae)

Description The kernel of Prunus persica (Linn) Batsch., or Prunus davidiana (Carr.) Franch. Family Rosaceae.

Characteristics Bitter in flavor, neutral in nature, acting on the Heart, Lung and Large Intestine Channels.

Action Activating Blood circulation to resolve Blood stasis, moistening the bowels to relieve constipation.

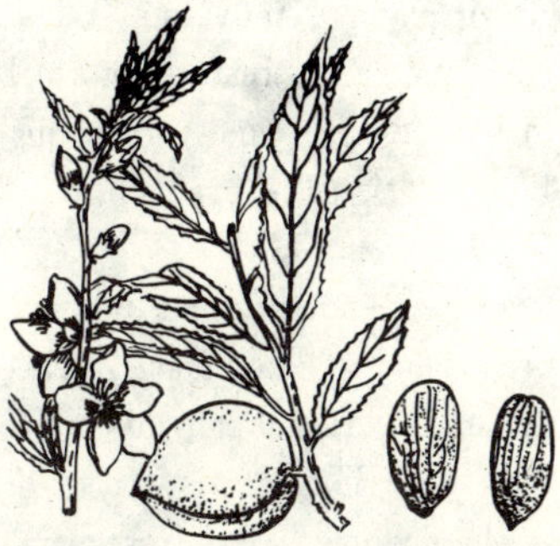

Indications

(1) Amenorrhea and dysmenorrhea due to Blood stasis, postpartum abdominal pain, traumatic injuries and ecchymoma and swelling pain. For treatment, it is usually used with Hong Hua (Flos Carthami), Chuanxiong (Rhizoma Ligustici Chuanxiong), etc., as in Taohong Siwu Tang (Decoction of Four Drugs Including Semen Persicae and Flos Carthami). For traumatic injuries with ecchymoma and swelling pain, used with Hong Hua (Flos Carthami), Dai Huang (Radix et Rhizoma Rhei) prepared with wine, etc., as in Fuyuan Huoxue Tang (Decoction for Recovery and Activating Blood Circulation).

(2) Appendicitis and pulmonary abscess. For the former, used with fresh Lu Gen (Rhizoma Phragmitis), Dong Gua Ren (Semen Benincasae), etc., as in Weijing Tang (Decoction of Rhizoma Phragmitis); for the latter, used with Mu Dan Pi (Cortex Moutan Radicis), Dai Huang (Radix et Rhizoma Rhei), Dong Gua Ren (Semen Benincasae), etc., as in Daihuang Mudanpi Tang (Decoction of Radix et Rhizoma Rhei and Cortex Moutan Radicis).

(3) Constipation due to dryness of the intestines. Usually used with Xing Ren (Semen Armeniacae Amarum), Huo Ma Ren (Fructus Cannabis), etc., as in Runchang Wan (Pill for Moistening the Intestines)

Administration 6～10g (crushed) for making a decoction.

Precautions Contraindicated during pregnancy.

0.4. Hong Hua (Flos Carthami)

Description The tubular corolla of Carthamus tinctorius L. Family Compositae.

Characteristics Acrid in flavor, warm in nature, acting on the Heart and Liver Channels.

Action Activating Blood circulation to restore normal menstruation, and resolving Blood stasis to relieve pain.

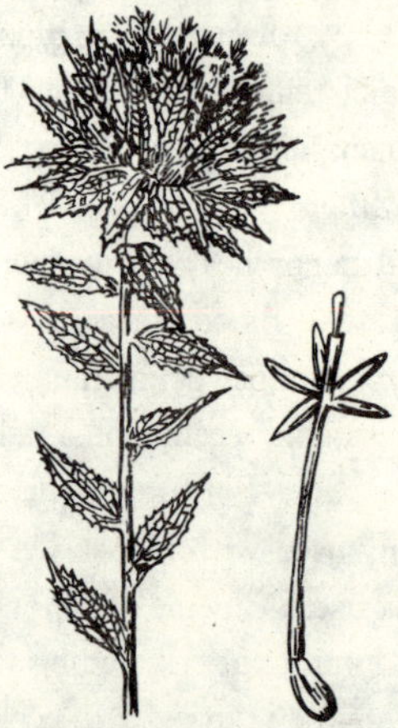

Indications

(1) Amenorrhea and dysmenorrhea due to Blood stasis, postpartum abdominal pain due to retention of Blood stasis, and mass in the abdomen. For treatment, it is used with Tao Ren (Semen Persicae), Dang Gui (Radix Angelicae Sinensis), Chuan Xiong (Rhizoma Ligustici Chuanxiong), etc., as in Taohong Siwu Tang (Decoction of Four Drugs Including Semen Persicae and Flos Carthami).

(2) Traumatic injuries, swelling pain due to Blood stasis and joint pain. Usually used together with Chuan Xiong (Rhizoma Ligustici Chuanxiong), Su Mu (Lignum Sappan), Ru Xiang (Resina Boswelliae Carterii), etc., as in Huoxue Zhitong Tang (Decoction for Activating Blood Circulation and Relieving Pain). It can also be used for suppurative skin infections, usually together with Chi Shao (Radix Paeoniae Rubra), Sheng Di (Radix Rehmanniae), Pu Gong Ying (Herba Taraxaci), etc.

(3) Dark-colored macule induced by stagnation of both Heat and Blood. For treatment, used with Dang Gui (Radix Angelicae Sinensis), Zi Cao (Radix Arnebiae seu Lithospermi), Da Qing Ye (Folium Isatidis), etc., as in Danggui Honghua Yin (Decoction of Radix Angelicae Sinensis and Flos Carthami).

Administration 3～10g for making a decoction.

Precautions Contraindicated for profuse menstruation and during pregnancy.

0.5. Yi Mu Cao (Herba Leonuri)

Description The aerial part of the herb of Leonurus heterophyllus. Family Labiatae.

Characteristics Acrid and bitter in flavor, slightly cold in nature, acting on the Heart, Liver and Urinary Bladder Channels.

Action Activating Blood circulation to remove Blood stasis, and promoting diuresis to relieve edema.

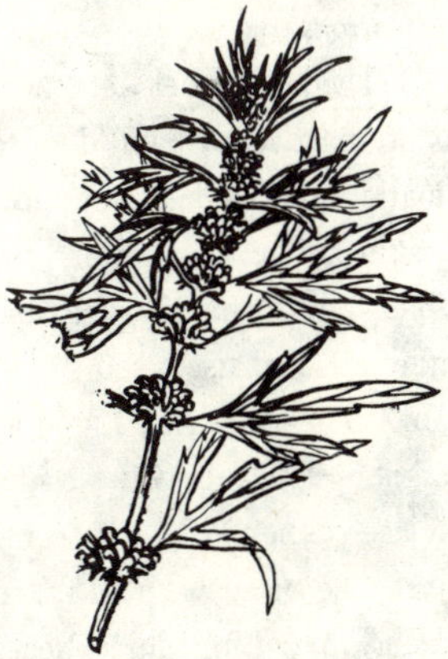

Indications

(1) Irregular menstruation, dysmenorrhea, postpartum abdominal pain, lochiorrhea and uterine bleeding due to retention of Blood stasis, or traumatic injuries, swelling pain, etc. For treatment, it can be decocted with sugar into a soft extract for oral use, i. e. Yimucao Gao (Soft extract of Herba Leonuri); or it can be used with Dang Gui (Radix Angelicae Sinensis), Chi Shao (Radix Paeoniae Rubra), etc., as in Yimu Wan (Pill of Herba Leonuri).

(2) Difficult urination and edema. Used either alone for making a decoction or together with Bai Mao Gen (Rhizoma Imperatae), Fu Ling (Poria), Bai Zhu (Rhizoma Atractylodis Macrocephalae), etc. In addition, this drug is also capable of purging Heat and detoxicating and is used for treating suppurative skin infections and pruritus of urticaria.

Administration 10～30g for making a decoction. When used alone, the dosage may reach 60g. q. s. for external application.

Precautions Not used for Blood Deficiency without Blood stasis.

0. 6. Ru Xiang (Resina Olibani)

Description The resin from the bark of Boswellia carterii Birdw and other species in the same genus. Family Burseraceae.

Characteristics Acrid and bitter in flavor, warm in nature, acting on the Heart, Liver and Spleen Channels.

Action Activating Blood circulation to relieve pain, reducing swelling to promote tissue regeneration.

Indications

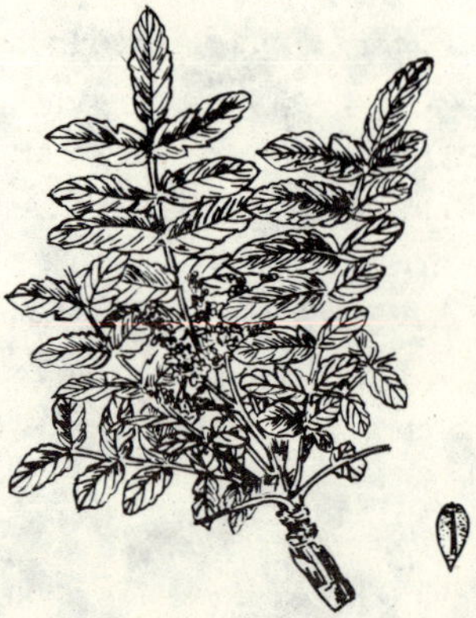

(1) Dysmenorrhea, amenorrhea, stomachache, pain due to traumatic injuries and suppurative skin infections. For the treatment of dysmenorrhea and amenorrhea, it is used with Chuan Xiong (Rhizoma Ligustici Chuanxiong), Dang Gui (Radix Angelicae Sinensis), etc.; for stomachache, used with Mo Yao (Myrrha), Wu Ling Zhi (Faeces Trogopterorum) and Cao Wu (Radix Aconiti Kusnezoffii); for traumatic injuries with swelling and pain, used with Mo Yao (Myrrha), Xue Jie (Resina Draconis), etc., as in Qili San (Anti-bruise Powder); for suppurative skin infections which are hard and painful, used with Mo Yao (Myrrha), Xiong Huang (Realgar), etc.

(2) Rheumatic arthritis with pain and muscular spasm. For treatment, used with Qiang Huo (Rhizoma seu Radix Noto-pterygii), Du Huo (Radix Angelicae Pubescentis), Qin Jiao (Radix Gentianae Macrophyllae), etc.

(3) Slow-healing carbuncles long after the rupture. Usually treated by applying the powder of Mo Yao (Myrrha) and Ru Xiang (Resina Olibani) to the affected place.

Administration 3～10g for making a decoction; q. s. for external use.

Precautions Used with caution for Deficiency and weakness of the Spleen and Stomach. Not applied to pregnant women.

0. 7. Mo Yao (Myrrha)

Description The resin from the bark of Commiphora myrrha Engl. or other species in the same genus. Family Burseraceae.

Characteristics Bitter in flavor, neutral in nature, acting on the Heart, Liver and Spleen Channels.

Action Activating Blood circulation to relieve pain, reducing swelling to promote tissue regeneration.

Indications Traumatic injuries with swelling and pain, stomachache, amenorrhea and dysmenorrhea due to Blood stasis, or suppurative skin infections, slow-healing carbuncles after rupture, etc. It is always used together with Ru Xiang (Resina Olibani) to strengthen the action of activating Blood circulation to relieve pain. Though similar in function to Ru Xiang (Resina Olibani), Mo Yao (Myrrha) is more powerful in removing Blood stasis, while Ru Xiang (Resina Olibani) is good at activating blood circulation to relax the tendons.

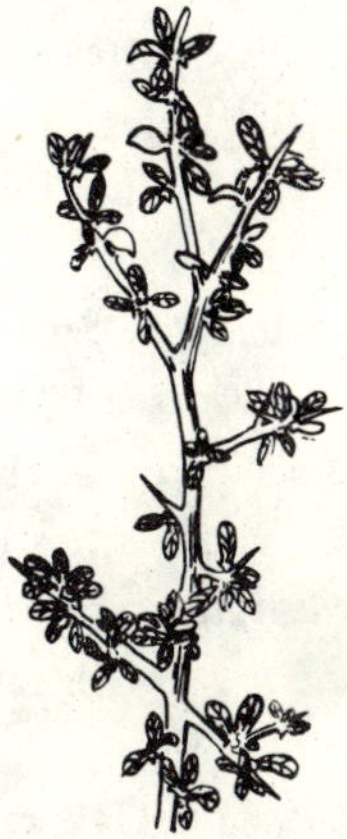

Administration 3～10g for making a decoction; q. s. for external use.

Precautions Used with caution for Deficiency and weakness of the Spleen and Stomach. Not applied to pregnant women. When Ru Xiang (Resina Olibani), and Mo Yao are used together, their dosages should be reduced accordingly.

0. 8. San Leng (Rhizoma Sparganii)

Description The tuber of Sparganium stoloniferum Buch. -Ham. Family Sparganiaceae.

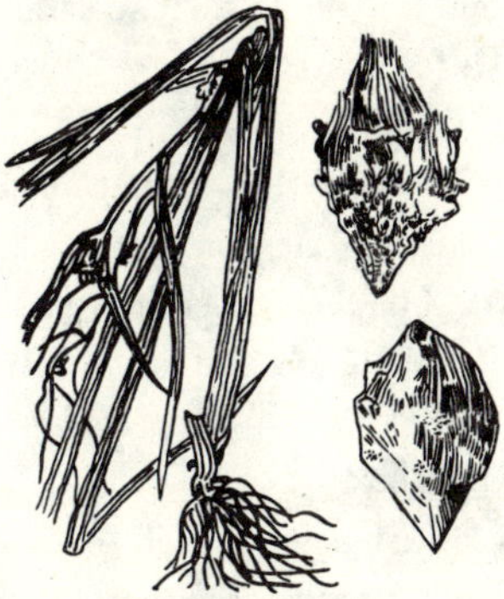

Characteristics Bitter in flavor, neutral in nature, acting on the Liver and Spleen Channels.

Action Removing Blood stasis and activating the circulation of Qi to relieve pain.

Indications

(1) Amenorrhea with abdomi-

nal pain or mass in the abdomen resulting from stagnation of Qi and Blood stasis. For treatment, usually used with E Zhu (Rhizoma Zedoariae) and Chuan Xiong (Rhizoma Ligustici Chuanxiong), as in Sanleng Wan (Pill of Rhizoma Sparganii).

(2) Retention of indigested food due to stagnation of Qi, and distending pain of the Stomach and abdomen. Usually used with E Zhu (Rhizoma Zedoariae), Qing Pi (Pericarpium Citri Reticulatae Viride) and Mai Ya (Fructus Hordei Germinatus), as in Sanleng Jian (Decoction of Rhizoma Sparganii).

Administration 3～10g for making a decoction.

Precautions Contraindicated for menorrhagia and in pregnant women.

0. 9. E Zhu (Rhizoma Zedoariae)

Description The axial rhizome of Curcuma kwangsinensis S. G. Lee et C. F. Liang, C. aromatica Salisb. and C. zedoaria Rosc. Family Zingiberaceae.

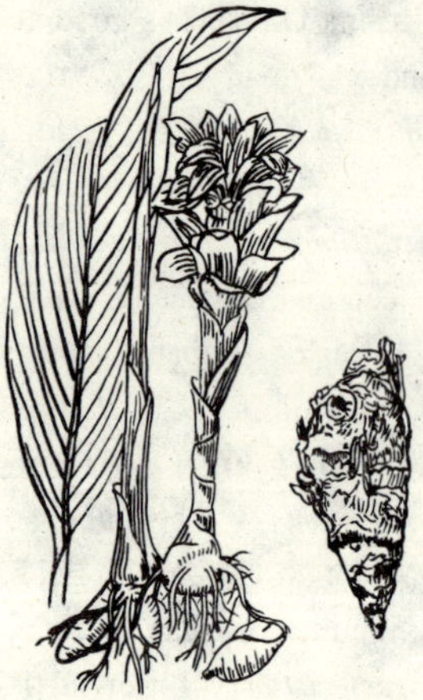

Characteristics Acrid and bitter in flavor, warm in nature, acting on the Liver and Spleen Channels.

Action Removing Blood stasis and activating the circulation of Qi to relieve pain.

Indications

(1) Amenorrhea with abdominal pain and mass in the abdomen due to Qi stagnation and Blood stasis. For the former, it is used together with San Leng (Rhizoma Sparganii), Dang Gui (Radix Angelicae Sinensis), etc.; for the latter, used with San Leng (Rhizoma Sparganii), Bie Jia (Carapax Trionycis), etc.

(2) Distending pain in the Stomach and abdomen due to retention of food. Usually used together with San Leng (Rhizoma Sparganii),

Shan Zha (Fructus Crataegi),etc.

Administration 3～10g for making a decoction.

Precautions Contraindicated for menorrhagia and in pregnant women.

0.10. Yan Hu Suo (Rhizoma Corydalis)

Description The stem tuber of Corydalis turtschaninovii Bess. f. yanhusuo Y.H. Chou et C. C. Hsu. Family Papaveraceae.

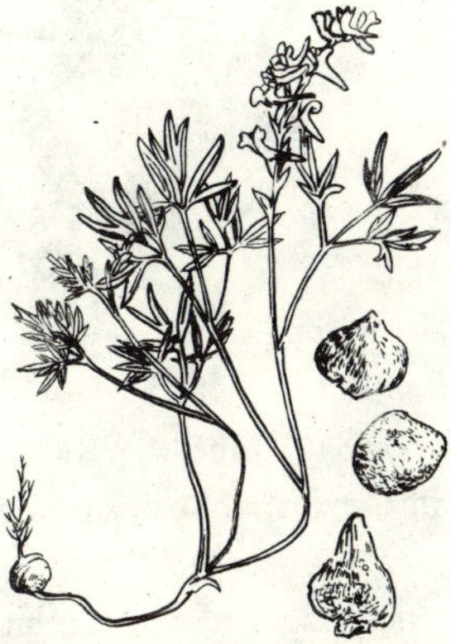

Characteristics Acrid and bitter in flavor, warm in nature, acting on the Heart, Liver and Spleen Channels.

Action Activating the circulation of both Qi and Blood to relieve pain.

Indications Various kinds of pain caused by Qi stagnation and Blood stasis, such as stomachache, abdominal pain, hypochondriac pain, hernial pain, lumbago, joint pain and dysmenorrhea. This drug is effective in treating any kind of pain induced by Qi stagnation and Blood stasis. For treating stomachache and abdominal pain, it is used together with Chuan Lian Zi (Fructus Meliae Toosendan), as in Jinlingzi San (Powder of Fructus Meliae Toosendan); for hernial pain, used with Xiao Hui Xiang (Fructus Foeniculi); for dysmenorrhea, used with Dang Gui (Radix Angelicae Sinensis), Chuan Xiong (Rhizoma Ligustici Chuanxiong), Xiang Fu (Rhizoma Cyperi), etc. for hypochondriac pain, used with Qing Pi (Pericarpium Citri Reticulatae Viride), Xiang Fu (Rhizoma Cyperi), Chuan Xiong (Rhizoma Ligustici Chuanxiong), etc.; while for pain of the joints and limbs, used with Dang Gui (Radix Angelicae Sinensis), Gui Zhi (Ramulus Cinnamomi), Chi Shao (Radix Paeoniae Rubra), etc.

Administration 5～10g for making a decoction; 1.5～3g of powder for oral intake.

Precautions Not applied to Blood Deficiency without Blood stasis.

0. 11. Yu Jin (Radix Curcumae)

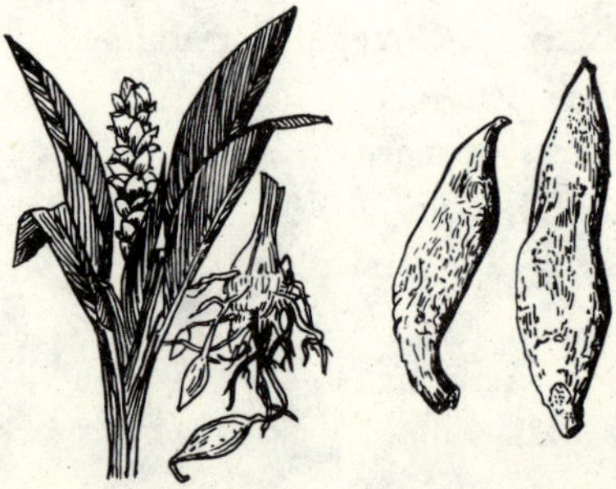

Description The root tuber of Curcuma aromatica Salisb. or Curmuma zedoaria Rosc., or Curcuma longa L. Family Zingiberaceae.

Characteristics Acrid and bitter in flavor, cold in nature, acting on the Heart, Liver and Gallbladder Channels.

Action Activating Blood circulation to relieve pain, promoting the flow of Qi to remove stagnation, clearing away Heat from the Blood, normalizing the Gallbladder to treat jaundice.

Indications

(1) Distending pain of the chest, abdomen and hypochondrium, irregular menstruation, dysmenorrhea and masses in the abdomen resulting from stagnation of Liver-Qi and retention of Blood stasis. For the treatment of distending pain of the chest, abdomen and hypochondrium, it is used together with Chai Hu (Radix Bupleuri), Bai Shao (Radix Paeoniae Alba), Dang Gui (Radix Angelicae Sinensis), etc.; for abdominal pain prior to menstruation due to stagnation of Liver-Qi with Heat invasion, used with Chai Hu (Radix Bupleuri), Dan Pi (Cortex Moutan Radicis), Zhi Zi (Fructus Gardeniae), etc., as in Xuanyu Tongjing Tang (Decoction for Resolving Stagnation to Regulate Menstruation); for masses in the abdomen, used together with Dan Shen (Radix Salviae Miltiorrhizae), Bie Jia (Carapax Trionycis), etc.

(2) Damp-warm syndromes manifested as unconsciousness due to obstruction of the upper orifices by Phlegm-Dampness, or epilepsy and mania due to obstruction of the sense organs in the head by Phlegm-Heat. For the former, used with Shi Chang Pu (Rhizoma Acori Graminei), bamboo juice, etc., as in Changpu Yujin Tang (Decoction of Rhizoma Acori Graminei and Radix Curcumae); for the latter, used with Bai Fan (Alumen), as in Bai Jin Wan (Pill of Alumen and Radix Curcumae).

(3) Hematemesis, epistaxis, hematuria and retrograde menstruation, etc. Usually used with Sheng Di (Radix Rehmanniae), Dan Pi (Cortex Moutan Radicis), Zhi Zi (Fructus Gardeniae), etc.

(4) Jaundice. Used with Jin Qian Cao (Herba Lysimachiae), Yin Chen (Herba Artemisiae Scopariae), etc.

Administration 6～12g for making a decoction.

Precautions Antagonistic to Ding Xiang (Flos Caryophylli).

0.12. Niu Xi (Radix Achyranthis Bidentatae)

Description This drugs includes two kinds of plants: Achyranthes bidentata Blume and Cyathula officinalis Kuan. Family Amaranthaceae.

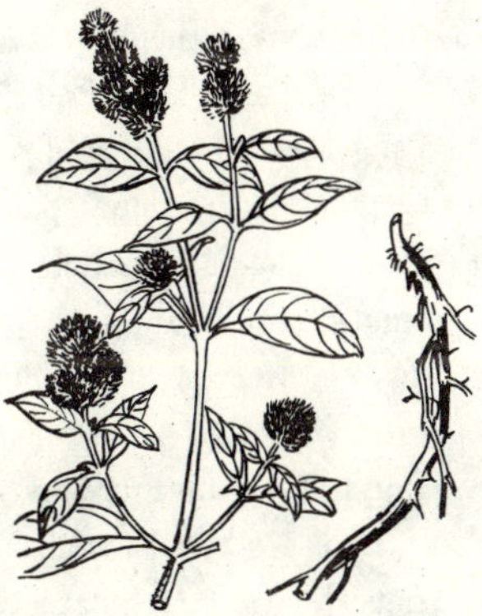

Characteristics Bitter and sour in flavor, neutral in nature, acting on the Liver and Stomach Channels.

Action Activating Blood circulation to remove Blood stasis, reinforcing the Liver and Kidney, strengthening the tendons and bones, and guiding the Blood to flow downwards.

Indications

(1) Dysmenorrhea, amenorrhea, postpartum abdominal pain, irregular menstruation caused by stagnation of Blood stasis, or traumatic injuries. For treatment, it is used with Dang Gui (Radix An-

gelicae Sinensis), Chi Shao (Radix Paeoniae Rubra), Tao Ren (Semen Persicae), etc.

(2) Aching pain of the loins and knees, and weakness of the lower limbs. If the syndromes are caused by descending Damp-Heat, it is used with Cang Zhu (Rhizoma Atractylodis), Huang Bo (Cortex Phellodendri) and Yi Yi Ren (Semen Coicis), as in Simiao San (Powder of Four Wonderful Drugs); if they result from insufficiency of Liver and Kidney, used with Du Zhong (Cortex Eucommiae), Xu Duan (Radix Dipsaci), etc.; if they are due to severe Deficiency with flaccidity of the tendons and bones, usually used with Gui Ban (Plastrum Testudinis), Shu Di (Radix Rehmanniae Praeparata), etc., as in Huqian Wan (Tiger Bone Pill for Checking Exuberance of Yang); if they are induced by pathogenic Wind-Cold-Dampness, used with Du Huo (Radix Angelicae Pubescentis), Sang Ji Sheng (Ramulus Loranthi), Du Zhong (Cortex Eucommiae), etc., as in Duhuo Jisheng Tang (Decoction of Radix Angelicae Pubescentis and Ramulus Loranthi).

(3) Hematuria, difficult and painful urination. Usually used with Hua Shi (Talcum), Tong Cao (Medulla Tetrapanacis), etc., as in Niuxi Tang (Decoction of Radix Achyranthis Bidentatae).

(4) Canker sores, swelling pain of the gums, hematemesis, hematuresis and epistaxis caused by Yin Deficiency and Fire Excess, or vertigo and dizziness due to hyperactivity of Liver-Yang. The former can be treated by adding Shu Di (Radix Rehmanniae Praeparata), Shi Gao (Gypsum Fibrosum), etc., as in Yunü Jian (Decoction of Gypsum Fibrosum); the latter by adding Dai Zhe Shi (Ochra), Long Gu (Os Draconis), Bai Shao (Radix Paeoniae Alba), Xuan Shen (Radix Scrophulariae), etc., as in Zhengan Xifeng Tang (Decoction for Tranquilizing Liver-Wind).

Administration 6～15g for making a decoction.

Precautions Contraindicated in pregnant women and for menorrhagia.

0.13. Chuan Shan Jia (Squama Manitis)

Description The scales of Manis pentadactyla L. Family Mandae.

Characteristics Salty in flavor, slightly cold in nature, acting on the Liver and Stomach Channels.

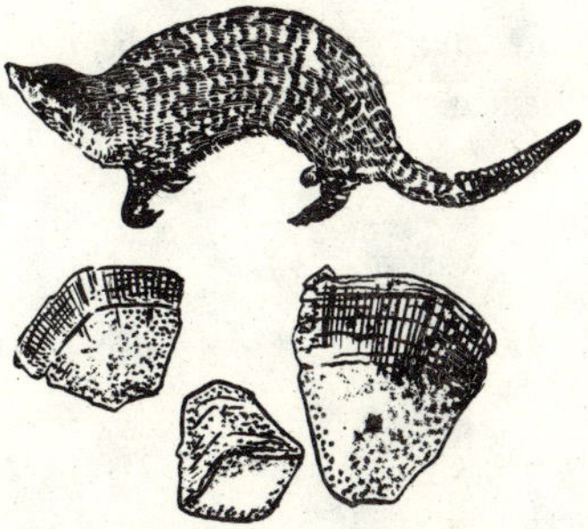

Action Activating Blood circulation to restore normal flow of menstruation, stimulating milk secretion, subduing swelling and promoting the drainage of pus.

Indications

(1) Amenorrhea due to stagnation of Blood, masses in the abdomen and rheumatic arthralgia. For treating amenorrhea due to stagnation of Blood, it is used with Dang Gui (Radix Angelicae Sinensis), Hong Hua (Flos Carthami), etc., as in Chuanshanjia San (Powder of Squama Manitis); for masses in the abdomen, used with San Leng (Rhizoma Sparganii), E Zhu (Rhizoma Zedoariae), etc.; for rheumatic arthralgia, used with Di Long (Lumbricus), Chuan Xiong (Rhizoma Ligustici Chuanxiong), Du Huo (Radix Angelicae Pubescentis), etc.

(2) Galactostasis. Usually used with Wang Bu Liu (Semen Vaccariae). In the case of distension of the breasts due to stagnation of Liver-Qi, used with Chai Hu (Radix Bupleuri) and Qing Pi (Pericarpium Citri Reticulatae Viride); in the case of scanty and thin milk secretion due to insufficiency of Qi and Blood after delivery, used with Huang Qi (Radix Astragali seu Hedysari), Dang Gui (Radix Angelicae Sinensis), etc.

(3) Suppurative skin infections. In the initial stage without pus formation, used with Jin Yin Hua (Flos Lonicerae), Tian Hua Fen (Radix Trichosanthis), etc., as in Xianfang Huoming Yin (Fairy Decoction for Treating Cutaneous Infections); in the case of swelling with pus prior to rupture, used with Zao Ci (Spina Gleditsiae), Dang Gui (Radix Angelicae Sinensis), Huang Qi (Radix Astragali seu Hedysari), etc., as in Tounong San (Powder for Promoting Pus Discharge).

Administration　3～10g for making a decoction; 1～1.5 of powder for oral intake.

Precautions　Contraindicated in pregnant women or for ruptured cutaneous infections.

Expectorants, Antitussives and Antiasthmatics

Drugs whose main action is to remove or resolve Phlegm are referred to as expectorants; while drugs whose main action is to relieve or stop cough and asthma are called antitussives and antiasthmatics respectively. As cough and asthma are usually accompanied with Phlegm, and profuse Phlegm will lead to cough and asthma; on the other hand, as most expectorants have the function of relieving cough and asthma, and most antitussives and antiasthmatics are also capable of resolving Phlegm, and therefore, they are generally referred to as drugs for resolving Phlegm and relieving cough and asthma.

Expectorants are mainly indicated for cough with profuse sputum or dyspnea due to retention of Phlegm, difficulty in expectoration, and diseases induced by Phlegm retention, such as epilepsy, convulsion, goiter, scrofula, deep-rooted carbuncles of Yin nature, etc. Antitussives and anthiasthmatics are chiefly indicated for cough and asthma due to affection of exopathogens or impairment of the functions of internal organs.

In clinical practice, it is important to make a correct choice of the drugs in this category with consideration to the properties of the drugs and the actual condition of the patient, and it is necessary to select other types of drugs to be used in combination so as to enhance the curative effect.

According to their properties, drugs of this category are further divided into three groups: drugs for resolving Cold Phlegm, drugs for resolving Phlegm-Heat, and drugs for relieving cough and asthma.

1. Drugs for Resolving Cold Phlegm

Drugs in this group have the warm and dry properties and are capable of resolving Cold Phlegm and removing Dampness. They are indicated for Cold Phlegm or Damp Phlegm syndromes manifested as cough with whitish, lucid and thin sputum accompanied by stuffiness sensation in the chest and white and smooth tongue coat, etc. In practice, these drugs are usually used in combination with drugs for dispelling Cold and Dampness and invigorating the Spleen. Some of them can also be used to treat ache of the limbs and joints, deep-rooted carbuncles of Yin nature, convulsion, scrofula, etc. induced by obstruction of Meridians by Phelgm.

Characterized by acrid flavor, warm nature and dry and potent properties, these drugs should be applied with caution to patients with dry cough due to Yin Deficiency or those with a history or liability of hemoptysis and hematemesis.

1. 1. Ban Xia (Rhizoma Pinelliae)

Description The stem tuber of Pinellia ternata (Thunb.) Breit. Family Arecae.

Characteristics Acrid in flavor, warm in nature, toxic, and acting on the Spleen, Stomach and Lung Channels.

Action Eliminating Dampness, resolving Phlegm, lowering the adverse ascending of the Qi to stop vomiting, and dispersing masses.

Indications

(1) Cough, profuse sputum, adverse flow of Qi and vertigo due to dysfunction of the Spleen to dispel Dampness and accumulation and retention of Phlegm. For treatment, it is usually used with Chen Pi (Pericarpium Citri Reticulatae), Fu Ling (Poria) and Gan Cao (Radix Glycyrrhizae), as in Erchen Tang (Decoction of Two Old Drugs). For profuse watery sputum of Cold nature, used together with Xi Xin (Herba Asari) and Gan Jiang (Rhizoma Zingiberis), as in Xiao Qinglong Tang (Minor Decoction of Green Dragon); in the case of thick yellowish sputum of Heat nature, used with Gua Lou (Fructus Trichosanthis), Zhi Mu (Rhizoma Anemarrhenae), Huang Qin (Radix Scutellariae), etc.; for vertigo due to adverse ascending of the Phlegm, used with Tian Ma (Rhizoma Gastrodiae), Bai Zhu (Rhizoma Atractylodis Macrocephalae), etc., as in Banxia Baizhu Tianma Tang (Decoction of Rhizoma Pinelliae, Rhizoma Atractylodis Macrocephalae and Rhizoma Gastrodiae).

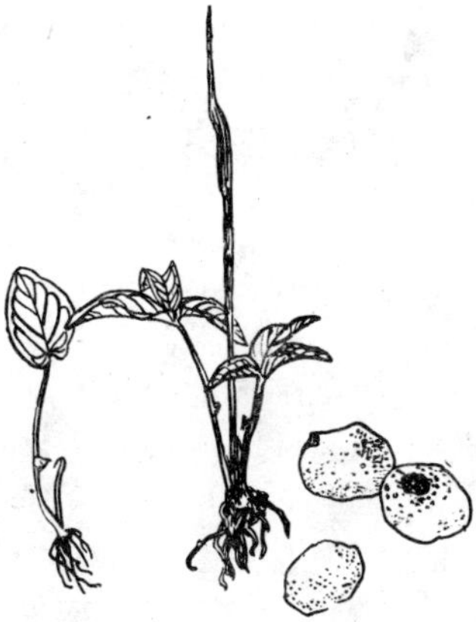

(2) Nausea and vomiting due to adverse ascending of Stomach-Qi. For the treatment of vomiting due to invasion of Stomach by retention of Phlegm-Dampness, it is usually used with Sheng Jiang (Rhizoma Zingiberis Recens), as in Xiao Banxia Tang (Minor Decoction of Rhizoma Pinelliae); for vomiting due to Stomach-Heat, used with Huang Lian (Rhizoma Coptidis), Zhu Ru (Caulis Bambusae in Taeniam) and Ju Pi (Pericarpium Citri Reticulatae), as in Huanglian Jupi Zhuru Banxia Tang (Decoction of Rhizoma Coptidis, Pericarpium Citri Reticulatae, Caulis Bambusae in Taeniam and Rhizoma Pinelliae); for vomiting due to Stomach Deficiency, usually used with Ren Shen (Radix Ginseng) and white honey, named Da Banxia Tang (Major Decoction of Rhizoma Pinelliae); for morning sickness, used

with Su Geng (Caulis Perillae) and Sha Ren (Fructus Amomi).

(3) Stuffiness sensation and distension in the chest, globus hystericus, goiter, subcutaneous nodules, carbuncles and other suppurative skin infections induced by accumulation of Phlegm and Qi. For accumulation of Phlegm and Heat leading to stuffiness sensation and distension of the chest, it is used with Huang Lian (Rhizoma Coptidis) and Gua Lou (Fructus Trichosanthis), as in Xiao Xianxiong Tang (Minor Decoction for Relieving Stuffiness in the Chest); for globus hystericus due to Qi stagnation and Phlegm accumulation, used with Hou Po (Cortex Magnoliae Officinalis) and Su Ye (Folium Perillae), as in Banxia Houpo Tang (Decoction of Rhizoma Pinelliae and Cortex Magnoliae Officinalis); for goiter and subcutaneous nodules, used with Hai Zao (Sargassum), Kun Bu (Thallus Laminariae seu Eckloniae), Zhe Bei Mu (Bulbus Fritillariae Thunbergii), etc.; for suppurative skin infections, made into a paste with its powder and eggwhite for external application to the affected place.

(4) Insomnia due to disorder of the Stomach-Qi. It is used with Chinese sorghum, named Banxia Shumi Tang (Decoction of Rhizoma Pinelliae and Chinese Sorghum).

Administration 5~10g for making a decoction; q. s. for external application.

Precautions Contraindicated for dry cough due to Yin Deficiency, thirst due to impairment of Body-Fluid and bleeding syndromes. Antagonistic to Wu Tou (Radix Aconiti).

1. 2. Tian Nan Xing (Rhizoma Arisaematis)

Description Rhizome of Arisaema erubescens (Wall.) Schott, A. heterophyllum Bl. and Pinellia pedatisecta Schott. Family Areceae.

Characteristics Bitter and acrid in flavor, warm in nature, toxic, and acting on the Lung, Liver and Spleen Channels.

Action Depriving Dampness to resolve Phlegm, eliminating Wind to relieve spasm, dispersing swelling and lumps.

Indications

(1) Cough with profuse sputum and stuffiness sensation and dis-

tension in the chest induced by Damp and pertinacious Phlegm. For treatment, it is used with Ban Xia (Rhizoma Pinelliae), Chen Pi (Pericarpium Citri Reticulatae) and Zhi Shi (Fructus Aurantii Immaturus), as in Daotan Dang (Decoction for Dispelling Phlegm). In the case of cough with thin sputum due to Cold Phlegm, used with Ban Xia (Rhizoma Pinelliae) and Rou Gui (Cortex Cinnamomi), as in Jiang Gui Wan (Pill of Rhizoma Zingiberis and Cortex Cinnamomi); in the case of cough with thick and yellow sputum due to Lung-Heat, used with Huang Qin (Radix Scutellariae), Ban Xia (Rhizoma Pinelliae), etc.

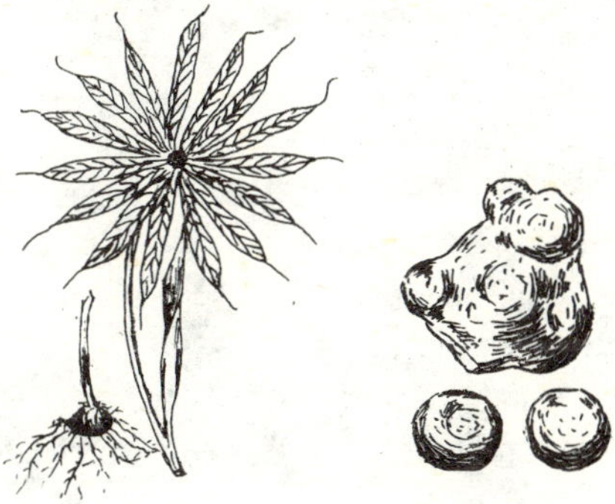

(2) Apoplexy due to accumulation of Phlegm, distortion of the face, epilepsy and tetanus. For apoplexy due to accumulation of Phlegm retention in the Meridians, manifested as dizziness, numbness of the extremities, deviation of the eye and mouth, it is used with Ban Xia (Rhizoma Pinelliae) and Bai Fu Zi (Rhizoma Typphonii); for tetanus with lockjaw and stiff neck and opisthotonos, used with Fang Feng (Radix Ledebouriellae), Bai Fu Zi (Rhizoma Typhonii), Tian Ma (Rhizoma Gastrodiae), etc., as in Yuzhen San (Powder with Marvellous Effect); for epilepsy, used with Quan Xie (Scorpio), Tian Ma (Rhizoma Gastrodiae), etc.

(3) Suppurative skin infections, scrofula, subcutaneous nodules, snake bite, etc. For suppurative skin infections, scrofula and subcutaneous nodules, rubbed with vinegar into a thick paste to be applied

externally; for snake bite, fresh rhizome is crushed into paste for external application, or the powder of Tian Nan Xing (Rhizoma Arisaematis) is mixed with the powder of Xiong Huang (Realgar) and white wine and is applied to the affected area.

Administration 5～10g of prepared drug for making a decoction; 0.3～1g of unprepared drug for making a powder or pills; q.s. for external use.

Precautions Used with caution in pregnant women.

1.3. Bai Jie Zi (Semen Sinapis Albae)

Description The ripe seed of Sinapis alba L., or Brassica juncea (L.) Czern et Coss. Family Cruciferae.

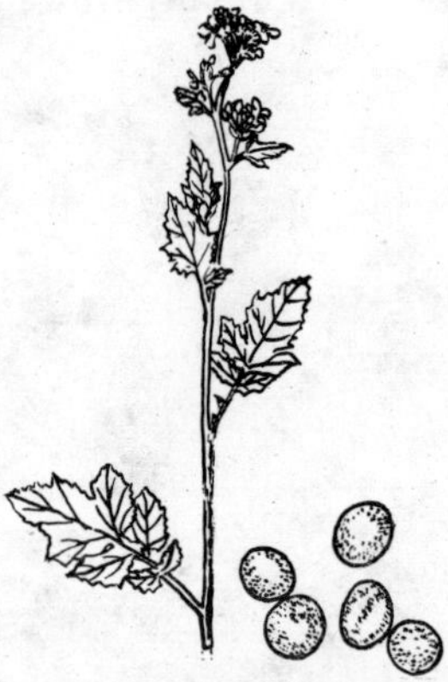

Characteristics Acrid in flavor, warm in nature, acting on the Lung Channel.

Action Resolving Cold Phlegm, dissolving lumps, subduing swelling and regulating Meridians to relieve pain.

Indications

(1) Retention of Cold Phlegm in the Lung marked by cough and asthma with watery sputum, or retention of Phlegm in the chest marked by stuffiness sensation in the chest and pain of the hypochondrium. For the former, it is used with Su Zi (Fructus Perillae) and Lai Fu Zi (Semen Raphani), as in Sanzi Yangqin Tang (Decoction of Three Kinds of Seeds for the Aged); for the latter, used with Gan Sui (Radix Euphorbiae Kansui) and Da Ji (Radix Euphorbiae Pekinensis), as in Kongxian Dan (Pill for Controlling Phlegm-fluid).

(2) Stagnation of Phlegm-Dampness in the Meridians marked by pain and numbness of the joints. Usually used with Mo Yao (Myrrha), Mu Bie Zi (Semen Momordicae), Gui Xin (tender twig of Ramulus Cinnamomi), etc., as in Baijiezi San (Powder of Semen

Sinapis Alba).

(3) Multiple or metastatic abscesses due to Phlegm-Dampness, deep-rooted carbuncles of Yin nature, scrofula and subcutaneous nodules. Usually used with Rou Gui (Cortex Cinnamomi), Lu Jiao Jiao (Colla Cornus Cervi), Shu Di (Radix Rehmanniae Praeparatae), etc., as in Yanghe Tang (Yang-activating Decoction).

Administration 3～10g for making a decoction; q. s. for external application.

Precautions Contraindicated for Yin Deficiency and Fire Excess or Lung Deficiency with chronic cough. Used with caution for allergic skin.

1. 4. Xuan Fu Hua (Flos Inulae)

Description The capitulum of Inula japonica Thunb., or Inula britannica L. Family Compositae.

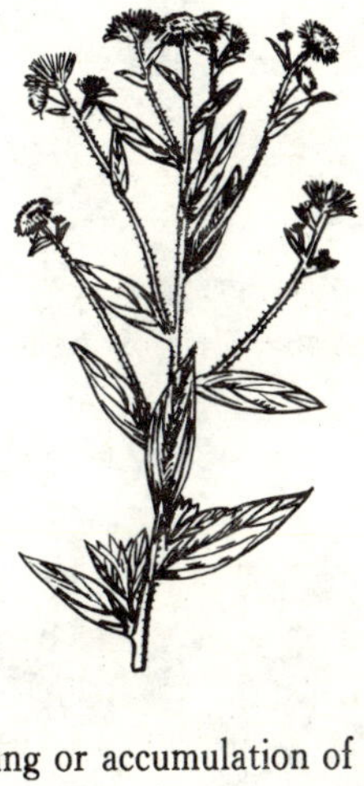

Characteristics Bitter, acrid and salty in flavor, slightly warm in nature, acting on the Lung, Spleen, Stomach and Large Intestine Channels.

Action Eliminating Phlegm, promoting diuresis, and lowering the adverse flow of Qi to stop vomiting.

Indications

(1) Retention of Phlegm in the Lung or accumulation of Phlegm-Dampness in the interior marked by cough and asthma with profuse Phlegm, stuffiness sensation in the chest, etc. For treatment of cough and asthma due to Cold Phlegm complicated by superficies-syndromes, it is used together with Sheng Jiang (Rhizoma Zingiberis), Ban Xia (Rhizoma Pinelliae), Xi Xin (Herba Asari), etc., as in Jinfeicao San (Powder of Flos Inulae); for cough and asthma of sthenic syndrome due to Phlegm-Heat, usually used with Sang Bai Pi

(Cortex Mori Radicis), Jie Geng (Radix Platycodi), Dai Huang (Radix et Rhizoma Rhei),etc. ,as in Xuanfuhua Tang (Decoction of Flos Inulae).

(2) Eructation and vomiting. For eructation and abdominal fullness due to Deficiency of Spleen-Qi and Stomach-Qi and adverse ascending of Phlegm-Dampness, used with Dai Zhe Shi (Ochra), Ban Xia (Rhizoma Pinelliae), Sheng Jiang (Rhizoma Zingiberis Recens) and Ren Shen (Radix Ginseng), as in Xuanfu Daizhe Tang (Decoction of Flos Inulae and Ochra).

Administration 3～10g for making a decoction (wrapped in gauze).

Precautions Contraindicated for Deficiency and descending of Qi or cough due to asthenia of viscera.

2. Drugs for Resolving Heat-Phlegm

Drugs in this group have cold or cool and moisturizing properties, and are capable of resolving Heat-Phlegm or moisturizing the Lung to treat dry cough. They are indicated for cough, thick sputum and difficult expectoration due to Heat-Phlegm or Dry-Phlegm. In application, they are usually used in combination with drugs for clearing away Heat, or drugs for tonifying Yin to moisturize the Lung. Some of them are also used for epilepsy, convulsion, scrofula, multiple or metastatic abscesses, goiter, etc.

These drugs are not to be used for Cold-Phlegm or Deficiency of both Spleen and Stomach.

2. 1. Jie Geng (Radix Platycodi)

Description The root of Platycodon grandiflorum (Jacq.) A. DC. Family Campanulaceae.

Characteristics Bitter and acrid in flavor, neutral in nature, acting on the Lung Channel.

Action Eliminating Phlegm, promoting pus discharge and opening the inhibited Lung energy.

Indications

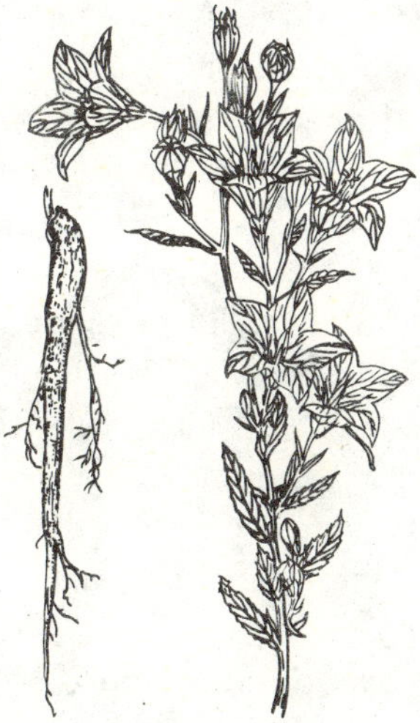

(1) Cough due to affection of exopathogens or Phlegm-Heat. In the treatment of cough due to affection of exopathogens of Wind-Heat type, it is used together with Sang Ye (Folium Mori), Bo He (Herba Menthae), Xing Ren (Semen Armeniacae Amarum), etc., as in Sang Ju Yin (Decoction of Folium Mori and Flos Chrysanthemi); for cough of Wind-Cold type, used with Xing Ren (Semen Armeniacae Amarum), Su Ye (Folium Perillae), Chen Pi (Pericarpium Citri Reticulatae), etc., as in Xing Su San (Powder of Semen Armeniacae Amarum and Folium Perillae); for cough induced by Phlegm-Heat with yellow and thick sputum and difficult expectoration, used together with Gua Lou (Fructus Trichosanthis), Huang Qin (Radix Scutellariae) and Bei Mu (Bulbus Fritillariae Cirrhosae), as in Qingjin Huatan Wan (Bolus for Clearing Away Phlegm from the Lung).

(2) Pulmonary abscess with chest pain, purulent and bloody expectoration and foul, thick yellow sputum. For treatment, it is used together with Gan Cao (Radix Glycyrrhizae), as in Jiegeng Tang (Decoction of Radix Platycodi); it can also be used with Yu Xing Cao (Herba Houttuyniae), Yi Yi Ren (Semen Coicis), Dong Gua Ren (Semen Benincasae), etc.

(3) Sorethroat, aphonia or suppurative infection with no rupture. For the former, used with Gan Cao (Radix Glycyrrhizae), Bo He (Herba Menthae) and Niu Bang Zi (Fructus Arctii), as in Jiawei Gan Jie Tang (Augmented Decoction of Radix Glycyrrhizae and Radix Platycodi), in the case of severe sorethroat due to invasion of Heat, used with Shan Dou Gen (Radix Sophorae Subprostratae), Ban

Lan Gen (Radix Isatidis) and Huang Qin (Radix Scutellariae); for the latter used with Sheng Huang Qi (unprepared Radix Astragali seu Hedysari), Dang Gui (Radix Angelicae Sinensis) and Chuan Shan Jia (Squama Manitis).

Administration 3～10g for making a decoction.

Precautions Used with caution in patients with Yin Deficiency and chronic cough, or with liability of hemoptysis.

2. 2. Chuan Bei Mu (Bulbus Fritillariae Cirrhosae)

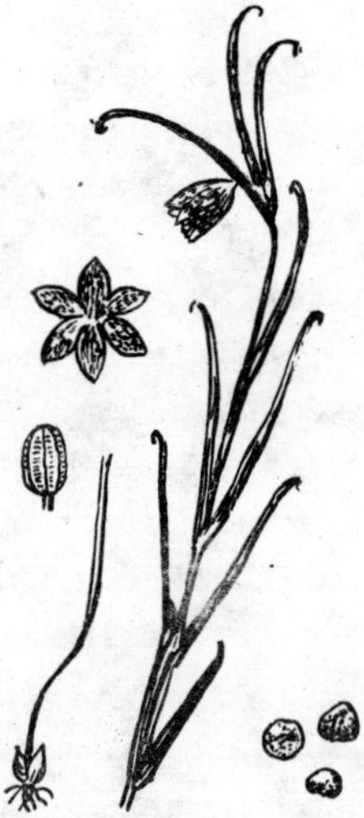

Description The bulb of Fritillaria cirrhosa D. Don, F. unibracteata Hsiao et K. C. Hsia and F. przewalskii Maxim. Family Liliaceae.

Characteristics Bitter and sweet in flavor, slightly cold in nature, acting on the Lung and Heart Channels.

Action Moisturizing the Lung to resolve Phlegm and clearing away Heat to disperse masses.

Indications

(1) Cough with sticky sputum and difficult expectoration caused by Heat-Phlegm and Yin Deficiency with dryness of the Lung. For the treatment of Heat-Phlegm with cough and sticky sputum, it is used with Zhi Mu (Rhizoma Anemarrhenae), named Ermu Wan (Bolus of Bulbus Fritillariae Cirrhosae and Rhizoma Anemarrhenae); for cough with scanty sputum and difficult expectoration due to Yin Deficiency and Dryness of the Lung, used with Mai Men Dong (Radix Ophiopogonis), Sha Shen (Radix Adenophorae Strictae), etc.

(2) Scrofula, subcutaneous nodules, mammary abscess, carbuncles, etc. For scrofula and subcutaneous nodules, it is used together with Xuan Shen (Radix Scrophulariae) and Mu Li (Concha

Ostreae), as in Xiaoluo Wan (Pill for Eliminating Scrofula); for mammary abscess, used with Pu Gong Ying (Herba Taraxaci), Lian Qiao (Fructus Forsythiae) and Tian Hua Fen (Radix Trichosanthis), as in Xiaoyong Sandu Tang (Decoction for Eliminating Abscess and Toxins); for carbuncles, used with Jin Yin Hua (Flos Lonicerae), Ru Xiang (Resina Olibani), Mo Yao (Myrrha), etc., as in Xianfang Huoming Yin (Fairy Decoction for Treating Cutaneous Infection).

Administration 3～10g for making a decoction; 1～1.5g for taking as a powder.

2.3. Gua Lou (Fructus Trichosanthis)

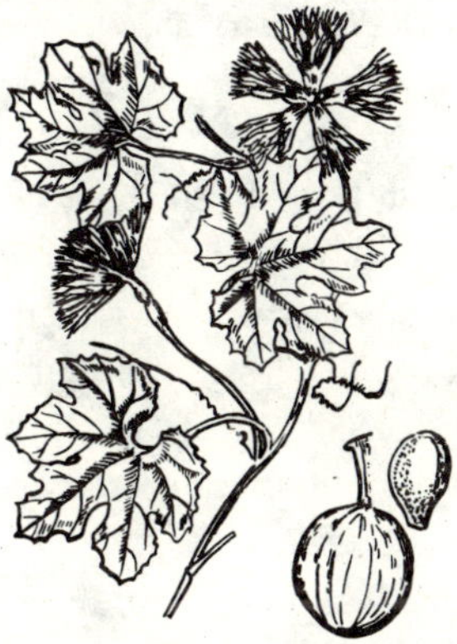

Description The ripe fruit of Trichosanthes Kirilowii Maxim. or Trichosanthes rosthornii Harms. Family Cucurbitaceae.

Characteristics Sweet in flavor, cold in nature, acting on the Lung, Stomach and Large Intestine Channels.

Action Clearing away Heat, resolving Phlegm, promoting the flow of Qi to relieve chest oppression, dispersing lumps and carbuncles, and moistening the intestines to relax the bowels.

Indications

(1) Cough with thick sputum and difficulty in expectoration due to Lung-Heat. For treatment, it is usually used with Zhi Mu (Rhizoma Anemarrhenae) and Zhe Bei Mu (Bulbus Fritillariae Thunbergii). In the case of accumulation of Phlegm-Heat in the interior marked by expectoration of thick, sticky and yellow sputum, oppressed feeling in the chest and constipation, it is treated by using Gua Lou Ren (Semen Trichosanthis) with Huang Qin (Radix Scutellariae), Dan Nan Xing (Arisaema cum Bile), Zhi Shi (Fructus Aurantii Immaturus), etc., as in Qingqi Huatan Wan (Bolus for

Clearing Away Phlegm-Heat).

(2) Chest pain and stuffiness sensation in the chest due to obstruction of Qi or Phlegm-Heat in the chest. For chest pain, used with Xie Bai (Bulbus Allii Macrostemi) and Ban Xia (Rhizoma Pinelliae), as in Gualou Xiebai Banxia Tang (Decoction of Fructus Trichosanthis, Bulbus Allii Macrostemi and Rhizoma Pinelliae); for accumulation of Phlegm-Heat in the chest marked by stuffiness sensation and tenderness in the chest and hypochondrium, usually used with Huang Lian (Rhizoma Coptidis) and Ban Xia (Rhizoma Pinelliae), as in Xiao Xianxiong Tang (Minor Decoction for Relieving Stuffiness in the Chest).

(3) Pulmonary abscess, breast nodules, etc. For pulmonary abscess with purulent and bloody expectoration, used with Jin Yin Hua (Flos Lonicerae), Yu Xing Cao (Herba Houttuyniae), Yi Yi Ren (Semen Coicis), etc.; for breast nodules with swelling and pain, used with Pu Gong Ying (Herba Taraxaci), Ru Xiang (Olibanum) and Qing Pi (Pericarpium Citri Reticularae Viride).

(4) Insufficiency of Body-Fluid in the intestines marked by constipation and dry stools. Usually treated by using Gua Lou Ren (Semen Trichosanthis) with Huo Ma Ren (Fructus Cannabis), Zhi Qiao (Fructus Aurantii), etc.

Administration 10～20g of the whole Gua Lou (Fructus Trichosanthis) or 10～15g of Gua Lou Ren (Semen Trichosanthis) for making a decoction.

Precautions Not applied to Spleen Deficiency with loose stools. Antagonistic to Wu Tou (Radix Aconiti).

2. 4. Zhu Ru (Caulis Bambusae in Taeniam)

Description The mesexine shaved from the stem of Lophatherum gracile Brongn. Family Gramineae.

Characteristics Sweet in flavor, slightly cold in nature, acting on the Lung and Stomach Channels.

Action Clearing away Heat and Phlegm, relieving vexation and vomiting.

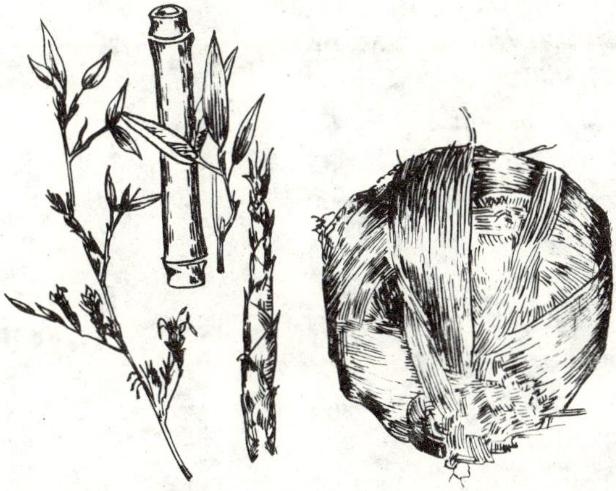

Indications

(1) Cough due to Lung-Heat with yellow and thick sputum or disturbance of the Heart by Phlegm-Fire manifested by vexation. For the treatment of cough due to Phlegm-Heat, it is used with Huang Qin (Radix Scutellariae) and Gua Lou (Fructus Trichosanthis); for accumulation of Phlegm-Heat which transforms into Fire and invades the Heart resulting in vexation, insomnia and palpitation, used with Zhi Shi (Fructus Aurantii Immaturus), Chen Pi (Pericarpium Citri Reticulatae), Ban Xia (Rhizoma Pinelliae), etc. as in Wendan Tang (Decoction for Warming the Gallbladder).

(2) Vomiting due to Stomach-Heat. Usually used with Huang Lian (Rhizoma Coptidis), Chen Pi (Pericarpium Citri Reticulatae) and Ban Xia (Rhizoma Pinelliae), as in Huanglian Jupi Zhuru Banxia Tang (Decoction of Rhizoma Coptidis, Pericarpium Citri Reticulatae, Caulis Bambusae in Taeniam and Rhizoma Pinelliae). In the case of vomiting due to asthenic Heat of the Stomach, used with Ren Shen (Radix Ginseng), Ju Pi (Pericarpium Citri Reticulatae), Sheng Jiang (Rhizoma Zingiberis Recens), etc., as in Jupi Zhuru Tang (Decoction of Pericarpium Citri Reticulatae and Caulis Bambusae in Taeniam).

Administration 6～10g for making a decoction.

Precautions Contraindicated for asthenic Cold of the Spleen and Stomach.

2.5. Hai Zao (Sargassum)

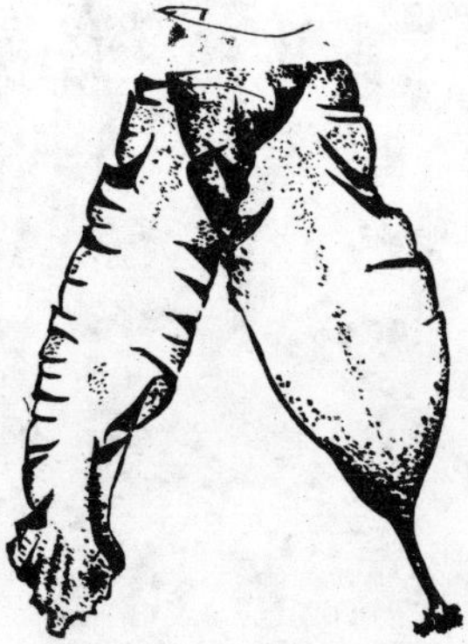

Description The thalline of Sargassum fusiforme (Harv.) Setch. and S. pallidum (Turn.) C. Ag. Family Fueacea.

Characteristics Salty in flavor, cold in nature, acting on the Liver, Stomach and Kidney Channels.

Action Eliminating Phlegm, softening the hard lumps, promoting diuresis and reducing edema.

Indications

(1) Goiter, scrofula and swelling of testis. For treating goiter, it is often used together with Bei Mu (Bulbus Fritillariae Cirrhosae), Kun Bu (Thallus Laminariae seu Eckloniae) and Qing Pi (Pericarpium Citri Reticulatae Viride), as in Haizao Yuhu Tang (Jade-pot Decoction of Sargassum); for scrofula, used with Xia Ku Cao (Spica Prunellae), Xuan Shen (Radix Scrophulariae), Lian Qiao (Fructus Forsythiae), etc., as in Neixiao Luoli Wen (Pill for Oral Administration to Treat Scrofula); for swelling of testis, used either alone or together with Qing Pi (Pericarpium Citri Reticulatae Viride), Ju He (Semen Citri Reticulatae), etc.

(2) Beriberi and edema. Used with Che Qian Zi (Semen Plantaginis), Ze Xie (Rhizoma Alismatis), Zhu Ling (Polyporus Umbellatus), etc.

Administration 10～15g for making a decoction.

Precautions Antagonistic to Gan Cao (Radix Glycyrrhizae)

3. Drugs for Relieving Cough and Asthma

Drugs in this group are mainly capable of nourishing the Lung to relieve cough, lowering the adverse flow of Qi and removing Phlegm to relieve asthma. They are indicated for cough, dyspnea and other symptoms due to disorder of Lung-Qi. Because of the complexity and variation of asthmatic cough syndromes, clinical application of the drugs should be flexible with regard to the actual condition of the patient and they should be used in combination with drugs of other categories.

3. 1. Xing Ren (Semen Armeniacae Amarum)

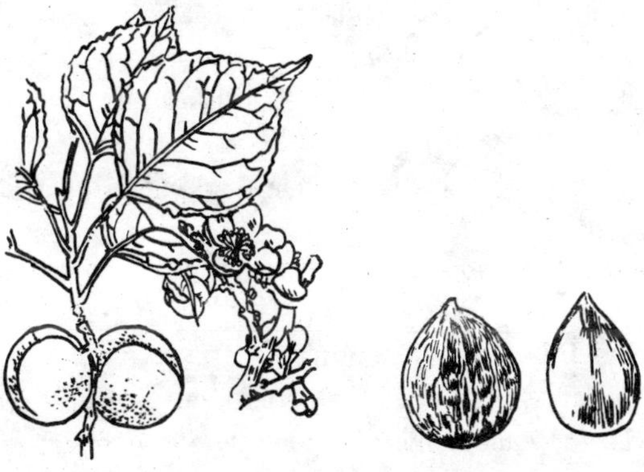

Description The kernel of Prunus armeniaca L. var. ansu Maxim, or Prunus sibirica L., or Prunus mandshurica (Maxim) Koehne., or Prunus armeniaca L. Family Rosaceae.

Characteristics Bitter in flavor, slightly warm in nature, mildly toxic, acting on the Lung and Large Intestine Channels.

Action Stopping cough and asthma, moisturizing the intestines to relax the bowels.

Indications

(1) Cough and asthma. For the treatment of cough due to Wind-Cold invasion, it is used with Su Ye (Folium Perillae), Ban Xia (Rhizoma Pinelliae), Fu Ling (Poria), etc., as in Xing Su San (Powder of Semen Armeniacae Amarum and Folium Perillae); for cough due to Wind-Heat invasion, used with Ju Hua (Flos Chrysanthemi), Sang Ye (Folium Mori), Jie Geng (Radix Platycodi), etc., as in Sang Ju Yin (Decoction of Folium Mori and Flos Chrysanthemi); in the case of cough and dyspnea due to Lung-Heat, used with Shi Gao (Gypsum Fibrosum), Ma Huang (Herba Ephedrae), etc., as in Ma Xing Shi Gan Tang (Decoction of Herba Ephedrae, Semen Armeniacae Amarum, Gypsum Fibrosum and Radix Glycyrrhizae); for cough due to Lung Dryness, used with Sha Shen (Radix Adenophorae Strictae), Chuan Bei Mu (Bulbus Fritillariae Cirrhosae), etc., as in Sang Xing Tang (Decoction of Folium Mori and Semen Armeniacae Amarum).

(2) Dry Intestine with constipation. Usually used with Huo Ma Ren (Fructus Cannabis), Dang Gui (Radix Angelicae Sinensis), Zhi Qiao (Fructus Aurantii), etc., as in Runchang Wan (Pill for Moisturizing the Intestines).

Administration 3~10g for making a decoction (added later than other ingredients in the recipe).

Precautions Overdosage should be avoided. Used with caution for babies.

3. 2. Bai Bu (Radix Stemonae)

Description The dried root tuber of Stemona sessilifolia (Miq.). and S. japonica (Bl.) Miq. Family Stemonaceae.

Characteristics Sweet and bitter in flavor, neutral in nature, acting on the Lung Channel.

Action Moistening the Lung to relieve cough, and killing parasites and lice.

Indications

(1) Short-term or prolonged cough, whooping cough and cough due to pulmonary tuberculosis. For treating severe or prolonged cough, it is used alone or together with other ingredients to make a decoction; for cough due to affection of Cold, used with Jing Jie

(Herba Schizonepetae), Jie Geng (Radix Platycodi), Zi Wan (Radix Asteris), etc., as in Zhisou San (Cough-relieving Powder); for cough due to T. B., used with Mai Men Dong (Radix Ophiopogonis), Sheng Di Huang (Radix Rehmanniae), Shan Yao (Rhizoma Dioscoreae), etc.; for whooping cough, used with Sha Shen (Radix Adenophorae Strictae), Chuan Bei Mu (Bulbus Fritillariae Cirrhosae), Bai Qian (Rhizoma Cynanchi Stauntonii), etc.

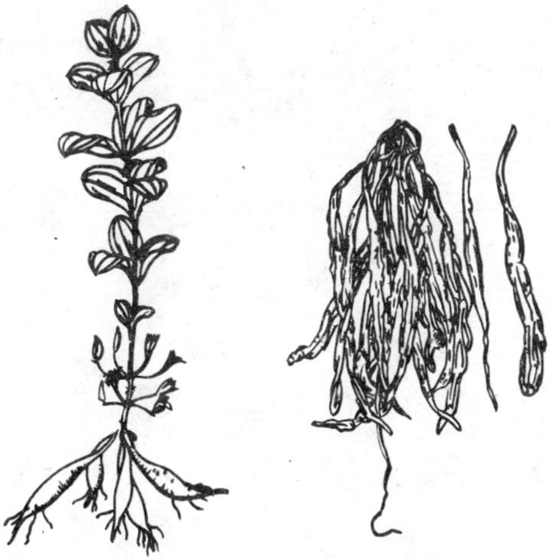

(2) Oxyuriasis, head and body lice. For treating oxyuriasis, the condensed decoction of Bai Bu (Radix Stemonae) is used for enema every evening before sleep, five days as a treatment session; for head and body lice, its decoction is used for external application. In addition, it can be used to treat tinea and vaginal pruritis by fumigating and washing with its hot decoction or the decoction of Huang Bo (Cortex Phellodendri) and Bai Bu (Radix Stemonae).

Administration 5～10g for making a decoction; q. s. for external application.

Precautions Contraindicated for Spleen Deficiency with poor appetite and loose stools.

3. 3. Sang Bai Pi (Cortex Mori Radicis)

Description The root epidermis of Morus alba L. Family

Moraceae.

Characteristics Sweet in flavor, cold in nature, acting on the Lung Channel.

Action Purging Lung-Fire to relieve asthma, promoting diuresis to reduce edema.

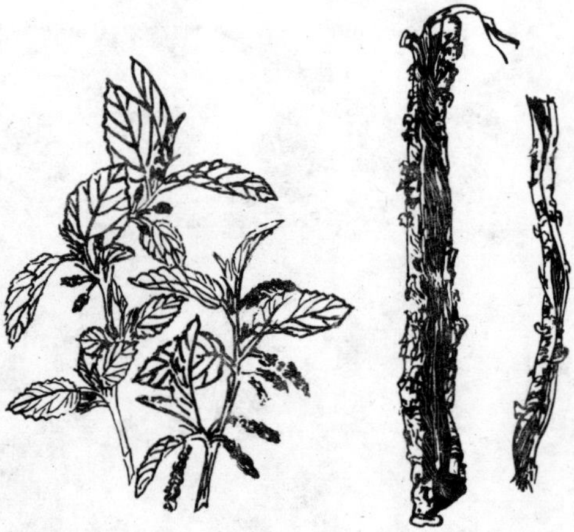

Indications

(1) Cough with profuse sputum due to Lung-Heat and adverse flow of Qi. For treatment, it is used with Di Gu Pi (Cortex Lycii Radicis), Gan Cao (Radix Glycyrrhizae) and Jing Mi (Semen Oryzae), as in Xiebai San (Powder for Expelling Lung-Fire).

(2) Edema and dysuria. Used with Da Fu Pi (Pericarpium Arecae), Fu Ling Pi (Cortex Poria), Sheng Jiang Pi (Cortex Rhizomatis Zingiberis Recens), etc., as in Wupi San (Powder of Five Peels).

Administration 10～15g for making a decoction.

Precautions Contraindicated for Lung-Cold or cough due to affection of exopathogens.

3.4. Su Zi (Fructus Perillae)

Description The ripe fruit of Perilla frutescens (L.) Britt. Family Labiatae.

Characteristics Acrid in flavor, warm in nature, acting on the

Lung and Large Intestine Channels.

Action Relieving cough and asthma, and moisturizing the intestines to relax the bowels.

Indications

(1) Stagnation of Phlegm and adverse flow of Qi manifested as failure to lie flat due to cough and dyspnea, fullness sensation of the chest, abdominal distension, anorexia, constipation, etc. For treatment, it is used together with Bai Jie Zi (Semen Sinapis Albae) and Lai Fu Zi (Semen Raphani), named Sanzi Yangqin Tang (Decoction of Three Kinds of Seeds for the Aged).

(2) Constipation due to Dryness of the Intestines. Used with Huo Ma Ren (Fructus Cannabis), Gua Lou (Fructus Trichosanthis), Xing Ren (Semen Armeniacae Amarum), etc.

Administration 5～10g for making a decoction.

Precautions Contraindicated for chronic cough with Qi Deficiency or loose stools.

3.5. Bai Guo (Semen Ginkgo)

Description The seed of Ginkgo biloba L. Family Ginkgoaceae.

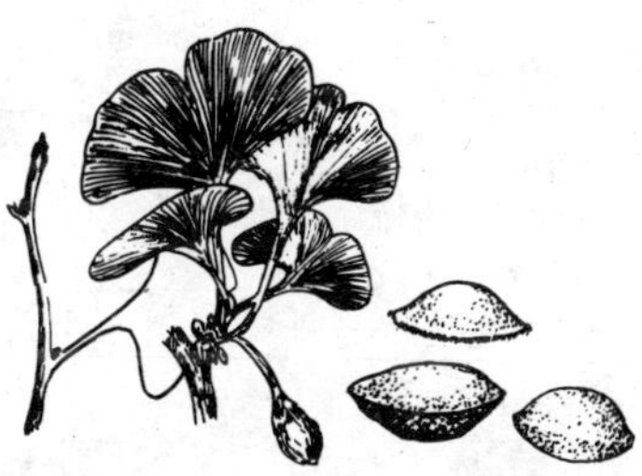

Characteristics Sweet and bitter in flavor, astringent and neutral in nature, mildly toxic, and acting on the Lung Channel.

Indications

(1) Cough, asthma, adverse flow of Qi and profuse Phlegm. For asthma and cough with sputum due to Lung-Cold, it is used with Ma Huang (Herba Ephedrae) and Gan Cao (Radix Glycyrrhizae); for cough and dyspnea with profuse sputum, used with Huang Qin (Radix Scutellariae) and Sang Bai Pi (Cortex Mori Radicis), as in Dingchuan Tang (Decoction for Relieving Asthma).

(2) Whitish and turbid urine and leucorrhagia. For watery leukorrhagia due to Damp-Cold, boiled together with Lian Zi (Semen Nelumbinis), Hu Jiao (Fructus Piperis Nigri) and Wu Gu Ji (Gallus

Domesticus) for eating; as for yellow and thick leukorrhagia due to Damp-Heat, used with Huang Bo (Cortex Phellodendri) and Qian Shi (Semen Euryales), as in Yihuang San (Powder for Eliminating Yellow Leukorrhagia).

Administration 6～10g for making a decoction.

Precautions Overdosage may cause poisoning.

3. 6. Zi Wan (Radix Asteris)

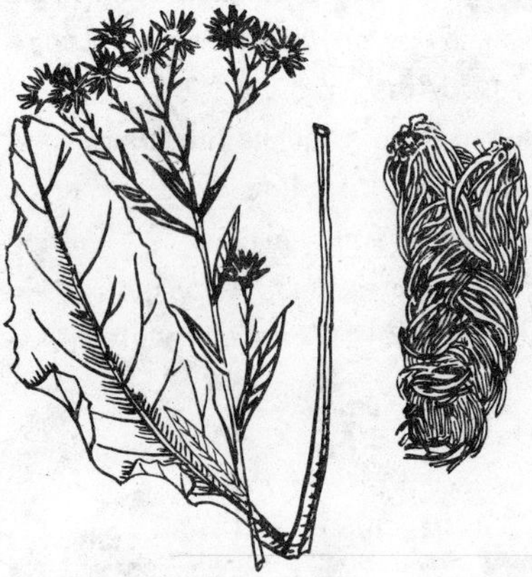

Description The root and rhizome of Aster tataricus L. f. Family Compositae.

Characteristics Acrid and bitter in flavor, warm in nature, acting on the Lung Channel.

Action Relieving cough and resolving Phlegm.

Indications Various types of cough, adverse flow of Qi and difficulty in expectoration. For treating cough due to affection of exopathogens, it is usually used with Jing Jie (Herba Schizonepetae), Bai Qian (Rhizoma Cynanchi Stauntonii), Chen Pi (Pericarpium Citri Reticulatae), etc., as in Zhisou San (Powder for Relieving Cough); for chronic cough, used with Kuan Dong Hua (Flos Farfarae), Bai Bu (Radix Stemonae), etc., as in Ziwan Bai Hua San (Powder of Radix Asteris, Radix Stemonae and Flos Farfarae); for cough with bloody sputum due to insufficiency of Lung-Yin, used with E Jiao (Colla Corii Asini) and Bei Mu (Bulbus Fritillariae Cirrhosae), as in

Ziwan Tang (Decoction of Radix Asteris).

Administration 5~10g for making a decoction.

3. 7. Kuan Dong Hua (Flos Farfarae)

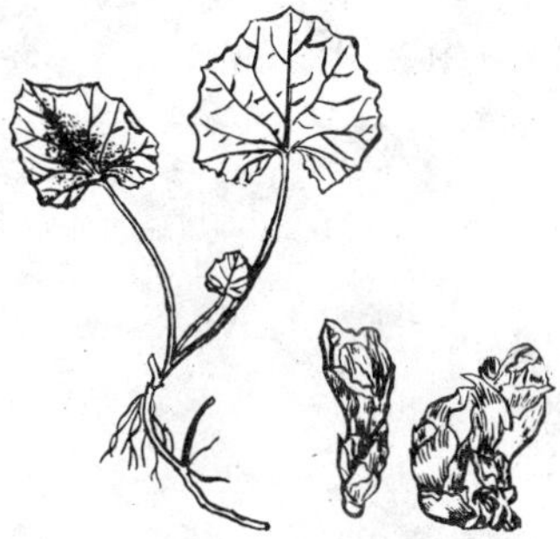

Description The flower bud of Tussilago farfara L. Family Compositae.

Characteristics Acrid in flavor, warm in nature, acting on the Lung Channel.

Action Moiturizing the Lung to relieve cough, lowering the adverse flow of Qi to resolve Phlegm.

Indications Various kinds of cough. For treating cough due to Lung-Cold and adverse flow of Qi, it is used with Zi Wan (Radix Asteris); for cough due to Lung-Heat, used with Zhi Mu (Rhizoma Anemarrhenae), Sang Bai Pi (Cortex Mori Radicis), Xing Ren (Semen Armeniacae Amarum), etc., as in Kuandonghua Tang (Decoction of Flos Farfarae); for cough with bloody sputum due to Lung Deficiency, used with Bai He (Bulbus Lilii), named Bai Hua Wan (Pill of Bulbus Lilii and Flos Farfarae).

Administration 3~10g for making a decoction.

Tranquilizers

Drugs whose principal action is tranquilizing the mind and relieving uneasiness are referred to as tranquilizers.

Tranquilizers exert tranquilizing effects either through sedation or through nourishment of the Heart, and they are indicated mainly for irritability, palpitation, insomnia and forgetfulness due to Excess of Heart-Fire or insufficiency of Heart-Blood, or convulsion, epilepsy and mania due to disturbance of the Heart by Phlegm-Fire.

Drugs of this category can be selected for use according to actual syndromes of the illness and they should be used in combination with appropriate compatible drugs. For instance, Yin Deficiency and Blood insufficiency should be treated by adding drugs for tonifying Blood and strengthening Yin; excessive Heart-Fire should be treated by adding drugs for clearing away Fire from the Heart; as for epilepsy and convulsion, drugs for resolving Phlegm and inducing resuscitation or drugs for eliminating Wind from the Liver should be used as main ingredients with the tranquilizers as the adjuvant.

Heavy tranquilizers of mineral sources should be used together with drugs for tonifying the Stomach and Spleen and they should not be applied for long lest they should cause impairment of Stomach-Qi.

0. 1. Zhu Sha (Cinnabaris)

Description The mineral ore of Cinnabaris (hexagonal system).

Characteristics Sweet in flavor, cold in nature, toxic, and acting on the Heart Channel.

Action Tranquilizing the mind and removing Heat and toxins.

Indications

(1) Irritability, feverish sensation in the chest, palpitation, insomnia, etc. induced by excessive Heart-Fire. For treatment, it is usually used together with Huang Lian (Rhizoma Coptidis), Sheng Di (Radix Rehmanniae), etc., as in Zhusha Anshen Wan (Cinnabaris Sedative Bolus). In the case of palpitation and insomnia due to Blood Deficiency, used with Dang Gui (Radix Angelicae Sinensis), Suan Zao Ren (Semen Ziziphi Spinosae), Bai Zi Ren (Semen Biotae), etc.; for convulsion and epilepsy, used with Hu Po (Succinum), Quan Xie (Scorpio), etc.

(2) Suppurative skin infections, sore throat, etc. For suppurative skin infections, used with Xiong Huang (Realgar) for oral or external administration; for sorethroat and canker sore, used with Bing Pian (Borneolum Syntheticum), Peng Sha (Borax), etc. externally, as in Bing Peng San (Powder of Borneolum Syntheticum and Borax).

Administration 0.3～1g for making a powder or boluses, or ground into powder to be infused for oral use. It can also be mixed with other drugs and then made into decoction. q.s. for external application.

Precautions Overdosage and long-term oral use should be avoided; used with caution for those with abnormal Liver or Kidney functions.

0.2. Long Gu (Os Draconis)

Description The skeleton fossil of prehistoric mammals such as hipparion, elephants, rhinoceros, deer, etc.

Characteristics Sweet and astringent in flavor, neutral and slightly cold in nature, acting on the Heart, Liver and Kidney Channels.

Action Inducing sedation and tranquilization, calming the Liver by suppressing the hyperactivity of Liver-Yang and inducing astringency.

Indications

(1) Restlessness, palpitation, insomnia, dream-disturbed sleep, forgetfulness as well as convulsion, mania, etc. For treatment, it is used with Zhu Sha (Cinnabaris), Mu Li (Concha Ostreae), Suan Zao Ren (Semen Ziziphi Spinosae), etc.

(2) Dizziness, vertigo, irritability, etc. due to Yin Deficiency and Yang excess. Usually used with Mu Li (Concha Ostreae), Bai Shao (Radix Paeoniae Alba), Dai Zhe Shi (Ochra), etc., as in Zhengan Xifeng Tang (Decoction for Tranquilizing Liver-Wind).

(3) Seminal emission, metrorrhagia, metrostaxis, leukorrhagia and sweating of Deficiency type. For treating seminal emission due to Kidney Deficiency, it is used with Sha Yuan Zi (Semen Astragali Complanati), Ji Li (Fructus Tribuli), Jin Ying Zi (Fructus Rosae Laevigatae), Qian Shi (Semen Euryales), etc.; for metrorrhagia and metrostaxis, used with Wu Zei Gu (Os Sepiae), Zong Lü Tan (Trachycarpi Carbonisatus), Huang Qi (Radix Astragali seu Hedysari), etc.; for leukorrhagia, used with Mu Li (Concha Ostreae), Qian Shi (Semen Euryales), Bai Guo (Semen Ginkgo), etc.; for sweating of Deficiency type, used with Huang Qi (Radix Astragali seu Hedysari), Mu Li (Concha Ostreae), etc.

(4) Exudative prurigo and unhealed ulcer. Usually calcined and made into powder for external use.

Administration 15～30g for making a decoction (decocted earlier than other ingredients); q. s. for external application. Unprocessed for calming the Liver; calcined for tranquilization.

Precautions Used with caution for accumulation and stagnation of Damp-Heat.

0. 3. Mu Li (Concha Ostreae)

Description The shell of Ostrea gigas Thunb., or Ostrea talienwhanensis Crosse, or Ostrea rivularis Gould. Family Ostreidae.

Characteristics Salty and astringent in flavor, slightly cold in nature, acting on the Liver, Gallbladder and Kidney Channels.

Action Tranquilizing the mind, calming the Liver by suppressing the hyperactivity of Liver-Yang, softening the hard lump and inducing astringency.

Indications

(1) Palpitation, restlesssnesss, insomnia and forgetfulness. For treatment, it is used with Long Gu (Os Draconis), Gui Zhi (Ramulus Cinnamomi) and Gan Cao (Radix Glycyrrhizae), as in Guizhi Gancao Longgu Muli Tang (Decoction of Ramulus Cinnamomi, Radix Glycyrrhizae, Os Draconis and Concha Ostreae).

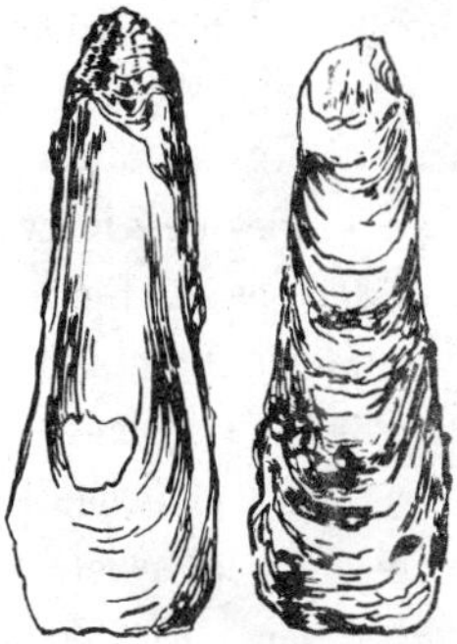

(2) Hyperactivity of Liver-Yang marked by dizziness and vertigo, and stirring of Liver-Wind marked by convulsions of the extremities, etc. For the treatment of Yin Deficiency and Yang Excess with dizziness, vertigo and tinnitus, usually used with Long Gu (Os Draconis), Bai Shao (Radix Paeoniae Rubra), Gui Ban (Plastrum Testudinis), etc., as in Zhengan Xifeng Tang (Decoction for Tranquilizing the Liver-Wind); for late stage febrile diseases with impairment of Yin by Heat and Yin Deficiency and stirring of the Wind, used with Gui Ban (Plastrum Testudinis), Bie Jia (Carapax Trionycis), Di Huang (Radix Rehmanniae), etc., as in Sanjia Fumai Tang (Pulse-Restoring Decoction of Three Shell Drugs).

(3) Goiter, scrofula, masses in the abdomen, etc. Mu Li (Concha Ostreae) is the important drug for those ailments. For the treatment of goiter, it is used with Kun Bu (Thallus Laminariae seu Eckloniae), Hai Zao (Sargassum), Huang Yao Zi (Rhizoma Dioscoreae Bulbiferae), etc., as in Xiaoying Tang (Decoction for Eliminating Goiter); for scrofula, used with Bei Mu (Bulbus Fritillariae Cirrhosae) and Xuan Shen (Radix Scrophulariae), as in Xiaoluo Wan (Bolus for Eliminating Scrofula); for masses in the abdomen due to Blood stasis, used with Dan Shen (Radix Salviae Miltiorrhizae), Bie Jia (Carapax Trionycis), E Zhu (Rhizoma Zedoariae), etc.

(4) Sweating of Deficiency type, seminal emission, leukorrhagia,

metrorrhagia and metrostaxis. For sweating, used with Huang Qi (Radix Astragali seu Hedysari), Ma Huang Gen (Radix Ephedrae), etc., as in Muli San (Powder of Concha Ostreae); for seminal emission due to Kidney Deficiency, used with Lian Xu (Stamen Nelumbinis), Qian Shi (Semen Euryales), Sha Yuan (Semen Astragali Complanati) and Ji Li (Fructus Tribuli), as in Jinsuo Gujing Wan (Golden Lock Pill for Keeping the Kidney Essense); for metrorrhagia, metrostaxis and leukorrhagia, used with Long Gu (Os Draconis), Wu Zei Gu (Os Sepiae), etc.

Administration 15～30g for making a decoction (decocted earlier than other ingredients). Calcined for inducing astringency; unprepared for other uses.

0. 4. Suan Zao Ren (Semen Ziziphi Spinosae)

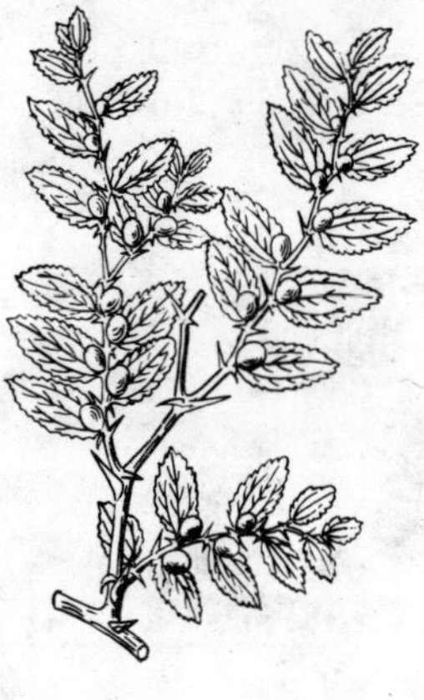

Description The ripe kernel of Ziziphus spinosa Hu. Family Rhamnaceae.

Characteristics Sweet and sour in flavor, neutral in nature, acting on the Heart, Liver, Gallbladder and Spleen Channels.

Action Tonifying the Heart to tranquilize the mind, reinforcing Yin to stop sweating.

Indications

(1) Palpitation, insomnia, dreaminess, forgetfulness, etc. induced by Blood Deficiency in the Heart and Liver. Suan Zao Ren (Semen Ziziphi Spinosae) is the key drug for treating the above syndromes and it is often used together with Bai Zi Ren (Semen Biotae), Dang Gui (Radix Angelicae Sinensis), He Shou Wu (Radix Polygoni Multiflori), etc. For the treatment of Deficiency of Liver accompanied with Heat marked by insomnia and restlessness of Deficiency type, used together with Zhi Mu (Rhizoma Anemarhenae), Fu Ling (Poria), etc., as in Suanzaoren Tang (Decoction of Semen

Ziziphi Spinosae); for insufficiency of Heart and kidney, Yin Deficiency with Heat marked by insomnia and restlessness of Deficiency type, palpitation, forgetfulness, dry mouth, red tongue with scanty coat, used with Bai Zi Ren (Semen Biotae), Sheng Di (Radix Rehmanniae), Xuan Shen (Radix Scropulariae), etc., as in Tianwang Buxin Dan (Cardiotonic Pill).

(2) Spontaneous sweating and night sweating due to weak constitution. Usually used with Mu Li (Concha Ostreae), Shan Zhu Yu (Fructus Corni), Dang Shen (Radix Codonopsis Pilosulae), etc.

Administration 10～15g for making a decoction; 1.5～3g for oral intake of powder before sleep.

Precautions Used with caution for profuse sputum.

0.5. Bai Zi Ren (Semen Biotae)

Description The ripe kernel of Biota orientalis (L.) Endl. Family Cupressaceae.

Characteristics Sweet in flavor, neutral in nature, acting on the Heart, Kidney and Large Intestine Channels.

Action Tonifying the Heart to tranquilize the mind, moisturizing the intestines to relieve constipation.

Indications

(1) Restlessness, insomnia, dreaminess and palpitation induced by failure of Blood in nourishing the Heart. For treatment, it is usually used with Suan Zao Ren (Semen Ziziphi Spinosae), Wu Wei Zi (Fructus Schisandrae), Fu Ling (Poria), etc., as in Yangxin Tang (Decoction for Tonifying the Heart).

(2) Dry intestines with constipation due to Deficiency of Yin and Blood. Usually used with Yu Li Ren (Semen Pruni), Tao Ren (Semen Persicae), etc., as in Wuren Wan (Pill of Kernels of Five Drugs).

Administration 10～15g for making a decoction.

Precautions Used with caution for patients with loose stools or profuse sputum.

0.6. Yuan Zhi (Radix Polygalae)

Description The root of Polygala tenuifolia Willd., or Polygala sibirica L. Family Polygalaceae.

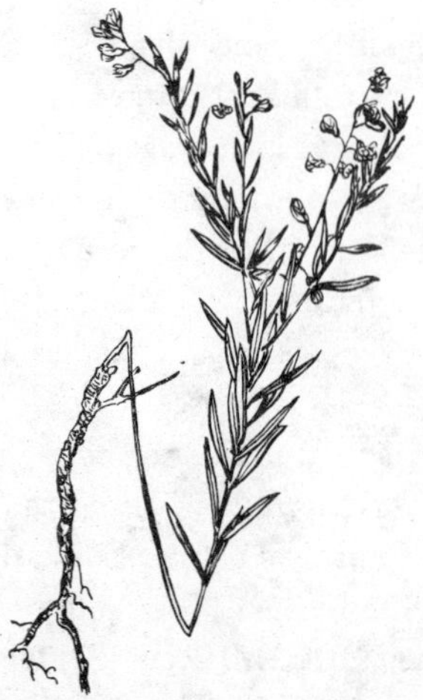

Characteristics Bitter and acrid in flavor, warm in nature, acting on the Heart, Kidney and Lung Channels.

Action Relieving mental distress, tranquilizing the mind, removing Phlegm to induce resuscitation, and reducing swelling of carbuncles.

Indications

(1) Mental distress, palpitation, insomnia and forgetfulness. For treating palpitation and restlessness, used with Zhu Sha (Cinnabaris), Fu Ling (Poria), etc., as in Yuanzhi Wan (Pill of Radix Polygalae); for insomnia and forgetfulness, used with Ren Shen (Radix Ginseng), Shi Chang Pu (Rhizoma Acori Graminei), Fu Ling (Poria), etc., as in Buwang San (Powder for Restoring Memory).

(2) Mental confusion, vague mind or epilepsy, etc. caused by blockage of the Phlegm in the Heart. Used with Shi Chang Pu (Rhizoma Acori Graminei), Yu Jin (Radix Curcumae), etc.

(3) Cough with profuse sputum or thick sputum and difficult expectoration. Used with Jie Geng (Radix Platycodi), Bei Mu (Bulbus Fritillariae Cirrhosae), Gua Lou (Fructus Trichosanthis), etc.

Administration 3～9g for making a decoction.

Precautions Used with caution for gastric ulcer and gastritis.

Drugs for Calming the Liver-Wind

Drugs whose principal action is suppressing the hyperactivity of Liver-Yang and calming the Liver-Wind are included in this category.

Drugs for calming the Liver are chiefly indicated for hyperactivity of Liver-Yang marked by dizziness and vertigo, or stirring up of Liver-Wind marked by epilepsy, convulsion, etc. Some of the drugs can also clear away Heat from the Liver and therefore they are effective for red eyes with swelling and pain, headache, etc.

Drugs in this category should be used in combination with drugs of other categories according to actual condition of the syndrome. For example, Heat Excess leading to up-stirring of Wind should be treated by adding drugs for clearing away Heat in the Blood; Phlegm-Heat with convulsion should be treated by adding drugs for eliminating Heat and Phlegm; Blood Deficiency leading to up-stirring of Wind should be treated by adding drugs for tonifying the Blood; while Yin Deficiency with up-stirring of Wind can be treated by adding drugs for invigorating Yin. Besides, hyperactivity of Liver-Yang or up-stirring of Liver-Wind is usually complicated with mental distress and therefore drugs of this category are often used in combination with tranquilizers.

These drugs are different in property, some are warm in nature and some are cold in nature. Discrimination must be made in the selection of them in order to serve different purposes. Care should be taken in that cold or cool natured drugs should not be used for Spleen Deficiency with chronic convulsion, warm or dry drugs should be applied cautiously for Yin Deficiency and Yang Excess.

0.1. Ling Yang Jiao (Cornu Saigae Tataricae)

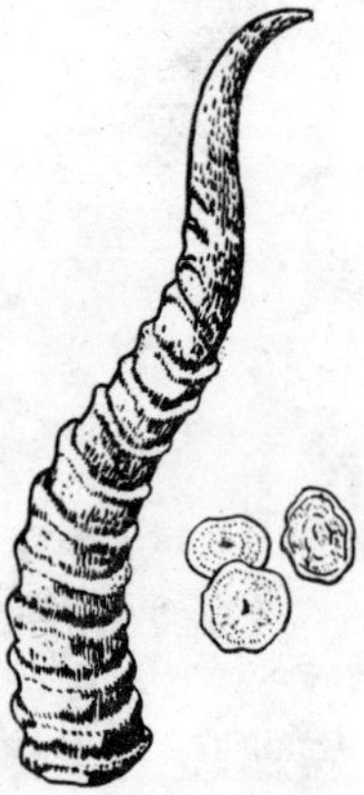

Description The horn of Saiga tatarica L. Family Bovidae.

Characteristics Salty in flavor, cold in nature, acting on the Liver and Heart Channels.

Action Calming the Liver-Wind, clearing away Heat from the Liver to improve eyesight, and removing Heat and toxins.

Indications

(1) Up-stirring of Liver-Wind marked by convulsion and epilepsy. Ling Yang Jiao (Cornu Saigae Tataricae) is the key drug for treating these syndromes, especially when they are induced by intense Heat and it is usually used together with Gou Teng (Ramulus Uncariae cum Uncis), Ju Hua (Flos Chrysanthemi), Sheng Di (Radix Rehmanniae), etc., as in Lingjiao Gouteng Tang (Decoction of Cornu Saigae Tataricae and Ramulus Uncariae cum Uncis).

(2) Hyperactivity of Liver-Yang manifested by dizziness and vertigo. Used with Ju Hua (Flos Chrysanthemi), Shi Jue Ming (Concha Haliotidis), etc.

(3) Epidemic febrile diseases with high fever, unconsciousness, delirium, mania, or skin eruptions with toxic Heat. For treatment, used with Sheng Di (Radix Rehmanniae), Shi Gao (Gypsum Fibrosum), Dan Pi (Cortex Moutan Radicis), etc.

(4) Flaring up of Liver-Fire marked by headache and red eyes.

Usually used with Shi Jue Ming (Concha Haliotidis), Huang Qin (Radix Scutellariae), Long Dan Cao (Radix Gentianae), etc., as in Lingyangjiao San (Powder of Cornu Saigae Tataricae).

Administration 1 ~ 3g for making a decoction (decocted alone and taken after mixing its decoction with the finished decoction of other ingredients); 0.3 ~ 0.5g taken orally of filed powder or ground mixture with water.

Precautions Not used for syndromes without sthenic Fire in the interior.

0.2. Tian Ma (Rhizoma Gastrodiae)

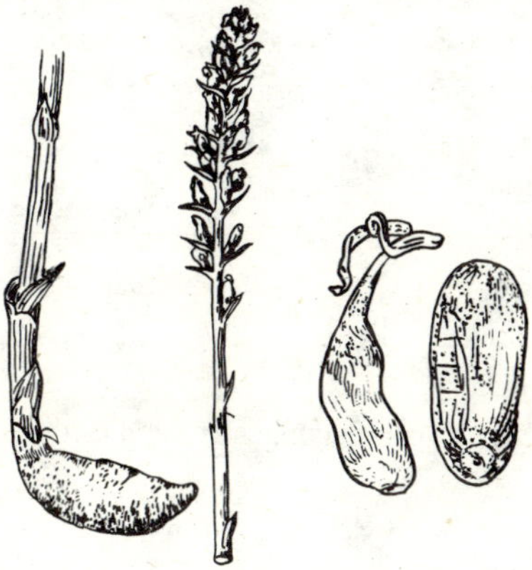

Description The stem tuber of Gastrodia elata Bl. Family Orchidaceae. *Characteristics* Sweet in flavor, neutral in nature, acting on the Liver Channel.

Action Checking the Wind to relieve convulsion, calming the Liver to suppress hyperactivity of Liver-Yang, and removing the obstruction in the Collaterals to relieve pain.

Indications

(1) Up-stirring of Liver-Wind leading to convulsion, fright and epilepsy. For treating infantile convulsion induced by high fever, it is used with Gou Teng (Ramulus Uncariae cum Uncis), Ling Yang Jiao (Cornu Saigae Tataricae), Quan Xie (Scorpio), etc., as in Gouteng Yin (Decoction of Ramulus Uncariae cum Uncis); for chron-

ic infantile convulsion, used with Ren Shen (Radix Ginseng), Bai Zhu (Rhizoma Atractylodis Macrocephalae), Jiang Can (Bombyx Batryticatus), etc., as in Xingpi San (Decoction for Invigorating the Spleen); for tetanus, used with Tian Nan Xing (Rhizoma Arisaematis), Fang Feng (Radix Ledebouriellae), Bai Fu Zi (Rhizoma Typhonii), etc., as in Yuzhen San (Powder with Marvellous Effect).

(2) Vertigo and headache. It is the key drug for treating vertigo and headache and when it is used together with Huang Qin (Radix Scutellariae), Gou Teng (Ramulus Uncariae cum Uncis), Niu Xi (Radix Achyranthis Bidentatae), etc. it can treat vertigo due to hyperactivity of Liver-Yang, as in Tianma Gouteng Yin (Decoction of Rhizoma Gastrodiae and Ramulus Uncariae cum Uncis); when used with Chuan Xiong (Rhizoma Ligustici Chuanxiong), it can treat headache and migraine, as in Tianma Wan (Bolus of Rhizoma Gastrodiae).

(3) Arthralgia of Wind-Dampness type, numbnesss of the limbs, tetraplegia, etc. Used with Qiang Huo (Rhizoma seu Radix Notopterygii), Niu Xi (Radix Achyranthis Bidentatae), Sang Ji Sheng (Ramulus Loranthi), etc.

Administration 3~10g for making a decoction; 1~1.5g for oral use of the powder.

Precautions Contraindicated for headache due to affection of exopathogenic Wind.

0.3. Gou Teng (Ramulus Uncariae cum Uncis)

Description The hooked vine of Uncaria rhynchophylla (Miq.) Jacks., U. macrophylla Wall., and U. hirsuta Havil. Family Rubiaceae.

Characteristics Sweet in flavor, slightly cold in nature, acting on the Liver and Pericardium Channels.

Action Checking the pathogenic Wind to relieve spasm, clearing away Heat to calm the Liver.

Indications

(1) Up-stirring of the Liver-Wind marked by convulsion and epilepsy. For treatment, it is usually used together with Tian Ma (Rhizoma Gastrodiae), Shi Jue Ming (Concha Haliotidis), Quan Xie

(Scorpio),etc. In the case of upstirring of Wind induced by excessive Heat, usually used with Ling Yang Jiao (Cornu Saigae Tataricae), Long Dan Cao (Radix Gentianae), Ju Hua (Flos Chrysanthemi), etc.

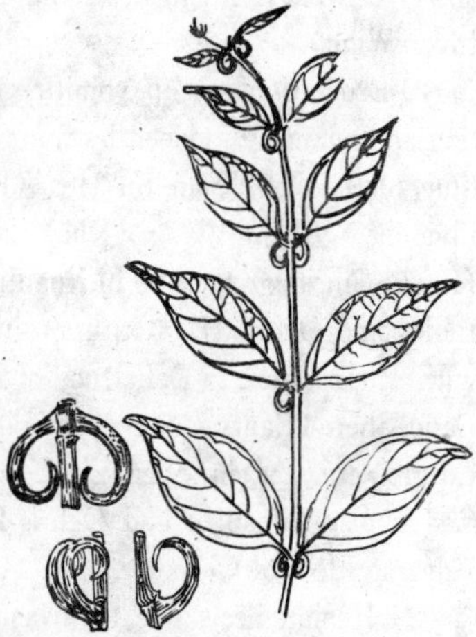

(2) Heat in the Liver Channel with distension and pain in the head, or hyperactivity of Liver-Yang with dizziness and vertigo. For treatment, used with Xia Ku Cao (Spica Prunellae), Huang Qin (Radix Scutellariae), etc. to clear away Liver-Heat; used with Ju Hua (Flos Chrysanthemi), Shi Jue Ming (Concha Haliotidis), etc. to calm the Liver-Yang.

Administration 10～15g for making a decoction. Not to be decocted for too long.

Precautions Contraindicated for headache due to affection of exopathogenic Wind.

0.4. Dai Zhe Shi (Ochra Haematitum)

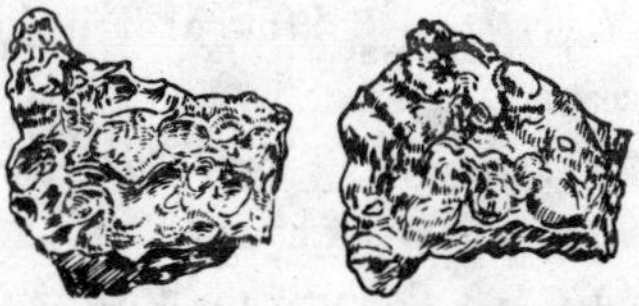

Description The red iron ore of trigonal system ferric trioxide as the chief component.

Characteristics Bitter in flavor, cold in nature, acting on the Liver and Heart Channels.

Action Calming the Liver by suppressing the hyperactivity of Liver-Yang, lowering the adverse flow of Qi, removing Heat from the Blood, and arresting bleeding.

Indications

(1) Dizziness, headache and tinnitus induced by hyperactivity of Liver-Yang. For treatment, it is used together with Long Gu (Os Draconis), Mu Li (Concha Ostreae), Bai Shao (Radix Paeoniae

Alba),etc. ,as in Zhengan Xifeng Tang (Decoction for Tranquilizing Liver-Wind).

(2) Eructation,hiccup,vomiting and asthma. In the case of eructation and vomiting induced by Stomach Deficiency and Phlegm retention, used with Xuan Fu Hua (Flos Inulae), Ban Xia (Rhizoma Pinelliae), Sheng Jiang (Rhizoma Zingiberis Recens), Ren Shen (Radix Ginseng),etc. ,as in Xuanfu Daizhe Tang (Decoction of Flos Inulae and Ochra Haematitum); in the case of adverse flow of Qi with dyspnea due to Deficiency of both Lung and Kidney,used with Dang Shen (Radix Codonopsis Pilosulae), Shan Zhu Yu (Fructus Corni), etc., as in Shen Zhe Zhenqi Tang (Decoction of Radix Codonopsis Pilosulae and Ochra Haematitum for Suppressing the Adverse Flow of Qi).

(3) Hematemesis due to invasion of Heat in the Blood, Usually used with Bai Shao (Radix Paeoniae Alba), Zhu Ru (Caulis Bambusae in Taeniam), Niu Bang Zi (Fructus Arctii), etc. ,as in Hanjiang Tang (Decoction for Stopping Bleeding due to Blood-Heat).

Administration 10～30g for making a decoction (decocted earlier than other ingredients). Unprocessed for checking the adverse flow of Qi and calming the Liver; calcined for stopping bleeding.

Precautions Used with caution in pregnant women.

0. 5. Ci Ji Li (Fructus Tribuli)

Description Fruit of Tribulus terrestris L. Family Zygophyllaceae.

Characteristics Bitter and acrid in flavor, neutral in nature, acting on the Liver Channel.

Action Calming the Liver-Yang, eliminating Wind to treat eye diseases.

Indications

(1) Headache, vertigo, etc. induced by hyperactivity of Liver-Yang. For treatment, it is used together with Zhen Zhu Mu (Concha Margaritifera Usta), Ju Hua (Flos Chrysanthemi), etc.

(2) Chest distress, galactostasis, etc. due to stagnation of Liver-Qi. Usually used with Chai Hu (Radix Bupleuri), Qing Pi (Pericarpium Citri Reticulatae Viride), etc.

(3) Conjunctivitis or cataract, etc. induced by Wind-Heat invasion. Used with Ju Hua (Flos Chrysanthemi), Man Jing Zi (Fructus Viticis), Jue Ming Zi (Semen Cassiae), etc., as in Baijili San (Powder of Fructus Tribuli).

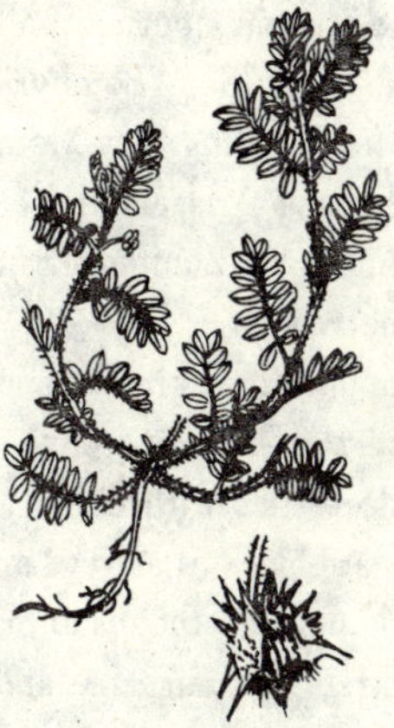

(4) Urticaria with itching. Used with Chan Tui (Periostracum Cicadae), Jing Jie (Herba Schizonepetae), etc.

Administration 6～10g for making a decoction.

Precautions Used with caution for Deficiency of both Qi and Blood or during pregnancy.

0.6. Quan Xie (Scorpio)

Description The dried body of Buthus martensii Karsch. Family Scorpionidae.

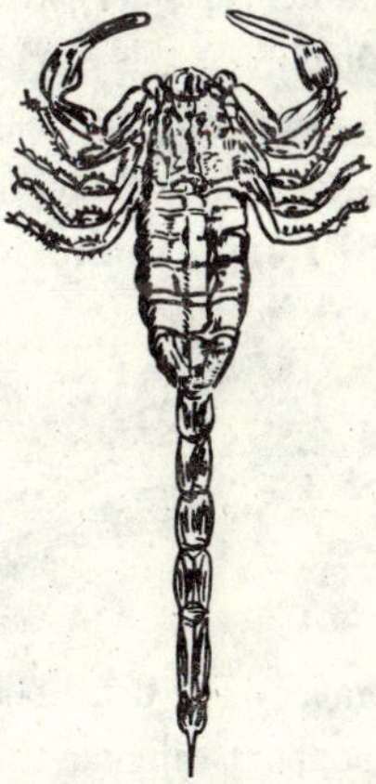

Characteristics Acrid in flavor, neutral in nature, toxic, and acting on the Liver Channel.

Action Calming the Wind to relieve convulsion, detoxicating, resolving lumps, and regulating the collaterals to relieve pain.

Indications

(1) Spasm and convulsion induced by various causes. For treating infantile convulsion, it is used together with Tian Ma (Rhizoma Gastrodiae), Gou Teng (Ramulus Uncariae cum Uncis), Ling Yang Jiao (Cornu Saigae Tataricae), etc.; for chronic infantile convulsion due to Deficiency of the Spleen, used with Dang Shen (Radix

Codonopsis Pilosulae), Bai Zhu (Rhizoma Atractylodis Macrocephalae) and Tian Ma (Rhizoma Gastrodiae); for apoplexy with deviation of the eye and mouth, usually used with Bai Fu Zi (Rhizoma Typhonii) and Jiang Can (Bombyx Batryticatus), named Qianzheng San (Powder for Treating Wry Mouth); for tetanus, used with Tian Nan Xing (Rhizoma Arisaematis), Chan Tui (Periostracum Cicadae), etc., as in Wuhu Zhuifeng San (Five-tiger Powder for Dispelling Pathogenic Wind).

(2) Suppurative skin infections, scrofula, subcutaneous nodules, etc. Roasted crisp and ground to powder to be taken with millet wine, or deep-fried with Zhi Zi (Fructus Gardeniae) in sesame oil till the drugs are black, the dregs are removed from the oil and then yellow wax is put into the oil to make a cream for external application.

(3) Intractable migraine and headache or rheumatic arthralgia. Used either alone by taking its powder orally or together with Wu Gong (Scolopendra), Jiang Can (Bombyx Batryticatus), etc.

Administration 2～5g for making a decoction; 0.5～1g for taking as a powder; q.s. for external application.

Precautions As this drug is toxic, overdosage should be avoided. Used with caution for pregnant women or patients with up-stirring of Wind due to Blood Deficiency.

0.7. Di Long (Lumbricus)

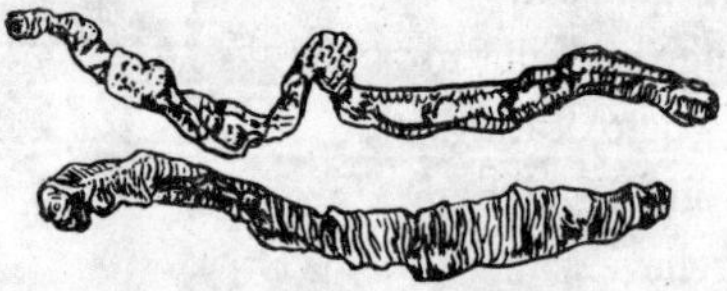

Description The dried body of Pheretima aspergillum (Perrier) or Allolobophora caliginosa (Savigny) trapezoides (Ant. Deges). Family Megascolecidae.

Characteristics Salty in flavor, cold in nature, acting on the Liver, Spleen and Urinary Bladder Channels.

Action Clearing away Heat, calming the Wind, relieving asthma, removing obstruction in the Collaterals and promoting diuresis.

Indications

(1) High fever with fright and convulsion, epilepsy, spasm, etc. For treatment, it is used alone or together with Gou Teng (Ramulus Uncariae cum Uncis), Jiang Can (Bombyx Batryticatus), Ling Yang Jiao (Cornu Saigae Tataricae), etc. In the case of disturbance of the Heart by Phlegm-Fire marked by restlessness and mania, fresh Di Long (Lumbricus) can be dissolved in sugar after being washed for oral use.

(2) Dyspnea with rale in the throat and yellow thick sputum due to excessive Lung-Heat. Usually used with Ma Huang (Herba Ephedrae), Shi Gao (Gypsum Fibrosum), Xing Ren (Semen Armeniacae Amarum), etc.

(3) Arthritis of Heat type marked by red swelling joints with hot pain and limited movement. Usually used with Sang Zhi (Ramulus Mori), Ren Dong Teng (Caulis Lonicerae), Chi Shao (Radix Paeoniae Rubra), etc.; for arthralgia due to Cold-Dampness with limited movement, used with Chuan Wu (Radix Aconiti), Cao Wu (Radix Aconiti Kusnezoffii), etc., as in Xiao Huoluo Dan (Minor Bolus for Activating Energy Flow in the Channels); for Blood stasis due to Qi Deficiency and obstruction in the Meridians manifested by hemiplegia, used with Huang Qi (Radix Astragali seu Hedysari), Dang Gui (Radix Angelicae Sinensis), Hong Hua (Flos Carthami), etc., as in Buyang Huanwu Tang (Decoction for Invigorating Yang and for Recuperation).

(4) Accumulation of Heat marked by anuresis or dribbling and painful micturition. Used either alone or together with Che Qian Zi (Semen Plantaginis), Mu Tong (Caulis Akebiae), etc. In addition, this drug is also effective for detoxication and relieving swellings, it can be used for treating suppurative skin infections by either oral or external application.

Administration 5~15g of dried drug or 10~20g of fresh one for making a decoction; 1~2g of powder for oral use; q. s. for external use.

Drugs for Inducing Resuscitation

Drugs whose principal action is wakening the patient from unconsciousness are referred to as drugs for inducing resuscitation.

Drugs of this category have strong aromatic odor and remarkable action in stimulating the sense organs and restoring consciousness. They are chiefly indicated for unconsciousness, delirium, convulsion, apoplexy, as well as abrupt syncope and loss of consciousness induced by either invasion of Heat in the pericardium or obstruction of the Heart by accumulation of Phlegm and Heat.

Loss of consciousness is observed in two kinds of syndromes: blockage (sthenic) syndrome and prostration (asthenic) syndrome. Drugs of this category can only be used for blockage syndrome, never for prostration syndrome. In addition, blockage syndrome is divided into two types: the Cold type and the Heat type. In clinical practice, compatible drugs should be selected and used in combination, for example, blockage syndrome of Heat type should be treated by adding drugs for clearing away Heat; while that of Cold type by adding drugs for eliminating Cold and activating the flow of Qi.

Drugs for inducing resuscitatiion are only used for emergency and symptomatic relief and therefore they should not be given over a long time. As most drugs are aromatic and their aroma is highly volatile, they are usually used in bolus and powder, only a few can be decocted for a short time.

0. 1. She Xiang (Moschus)

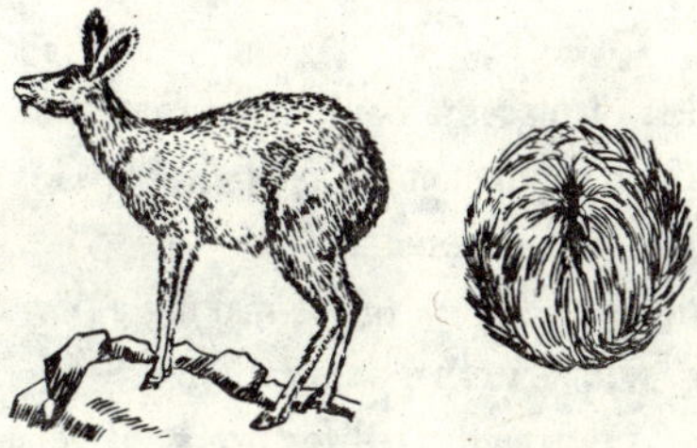

Description The dried secretion in the subumbilical musk cyst of the male musk deer, Moschus berezovskii Flerov, or Moschus sifanicus Przewalski or Moschus moschiferus L. Family Cervidae.

Characteristics Acrid in flavor, warm in nature, acting on the Heart and Spleen Channels.

Action Inducing resuscitation, activating Blood circulation to disperse masses, arresting bleeding and inducing uterine contraction.

Indications

(1) Epidemic febrile diseases with Heat invasion into the pericardium marked by coma, convulsion, syncope induced by Phlegm, apoplexy and epilepsy. For the Heat type, it is used with Niu Huang (Calculus Bovis), Huang Lian (Rhizoma Coptidis), etc., as in Angong Niuhuang Wan (Bolus of Calculus Bovis for Resurrection); for the Cold type, used with Su He Xiang (Storax), Ding Xiang (Flos Syzygii Aromatici), etc., as in Suhexiang Wan (Bolus of Storax).

(2) Suppurative skin infections, mass in the abdomen, amenorrhea, etc. For swelling pain of skin infections, used with Xiong Huang (Realgar), Ru Xiang (Myrrha), etc., as in Xingxiao Wan (Pill for Restoring Consciousness and Subduing Swelling); for mass in the abdomen, and amenorrhea, usually used with San Leng (Rhizoma Sparganii), E Zhu (Rhizoma Zedoariae), Chuan Xiong (Rhizoma Ligustici Chuanxiong), etc.

(3) Sudden gastric or abdominal pain, traumatic injuries, swelling pain due to Blood stasis. For sudden gastric or abdominal pain, used with Mu Xiang (Radix Aucklandiae), Yuan Hu (Rhizoma Corydalis), Chuan Xiong (Rhizoma Ligustici Chuanxiong), etc.; for traumatic injuries, used with Su Mu (Lignum Sappan), Mo Yao (Myrrha), etc.

(4) Retention of placenta or dead fetus in the uterus. Used with Rou Gui (Cortex Cinnamomi), as in Xiang Gui San (Powder of Moschus and Cortex Cinnamomi).

Administration 0.03~0.1g for making a powder or pills; not to be decocted; q.s. for external application.

Precautions Contraindicated for pregnant women.

0.2. Bing Pian (Borneolum Syntheticum)

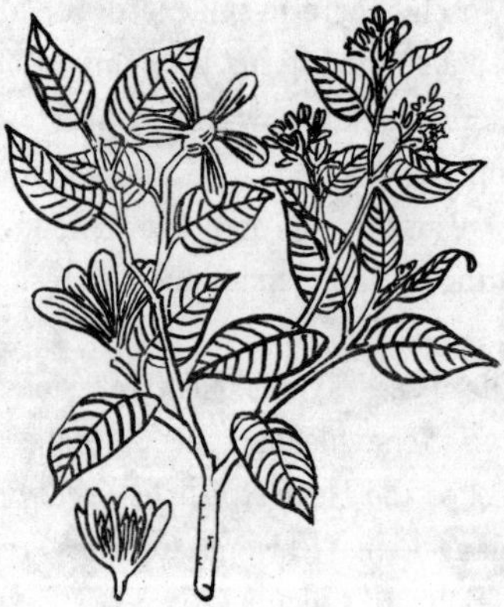

Description The resin of Dryobalanops aromatica Gaertn. f. Family Dipterocarpaceae, or chemically synthesized from camphor and turpentine oil.

Characteristics Acrid and bitter in flavor, slightly cold in nature, acting on the Heart, Spleen and Lung Channels.

Action Inducing resuscitation, clearing Heat and toxins.

Indications

(1) Coma and convulsion of either Heat or Cold type. For treatment, it is used with She Xiang (Moschus), Niu Huang (Calculus

Bovis),etc. ,as in Zhibao Dan (Treasured Bolus).

(2) Various pyogenic infections, eye ailment and sorethroat. For non-healing carbuncles long after the rupture, used with Zhen Zhu (Margarita), Xue Jie (Resina Draconis), etc., as in Shengji San (Powder for Regeneration of Tissue); for canker sores, sorethroat and swelling pain of the eyes, usually used with Peng Sha (Borax) and Zhu Sha (Cinnabaris) for external application after being ground into fine powder, as in Bingpeng San (Powder of Borneolum Syntheticum and Borax).

Administration 0. 03～0. 1g for making a powder or pills; not to be decocted; q. s. for external application.

Precautions Used with caution for pregnant women.

0. 3. Su He Xiang (Storax)

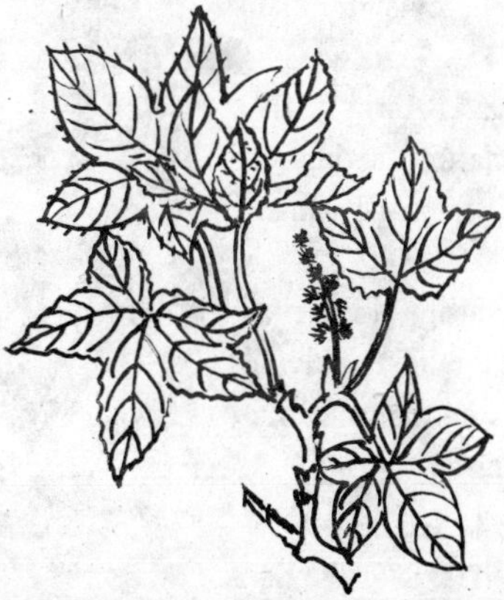

Description The resin obtained from the bark of Liquidambar orientalis Mill. Family Hamamelidaceae.

Characteristics Acrid in flavor, warm in nature, acting on the Heart and Spleen Channels.

Action Inducing resuscitation, eliminating filth and relieving pain.

Indications

(1) Syncope due to Phlegm blockage, coma due to pathogenic Cold blocking the interior. For treatment, it is used with She Xiang

(Moschus), Ding Xiang (Flos Syzygii Aromatici), An Xi Xiang (Benzoinum), etc., as in Suhexiang Wan (Storax Bolus).

(2) Cold pain and stuffiness in the chest and abdomen. Used with Tan Xiang (Lignum Santali), Ru Xiang (Olibanum), etc., as in Guanxin Suhe Wan (Bolus of Storax for Coronary Heart Disease); for precordial pain due to blockage of Phlegm and stagnation of Qi, used with Bing Pian (Borneolum Syntheticum) and the result is satisfactory.

Administration 0.3～1g for making powder or pills, not to be decocted.

Precautions Not used for Heat blockage syndrome

0.4. Shi Chang Pu (Rhizoma Acori Graminei)

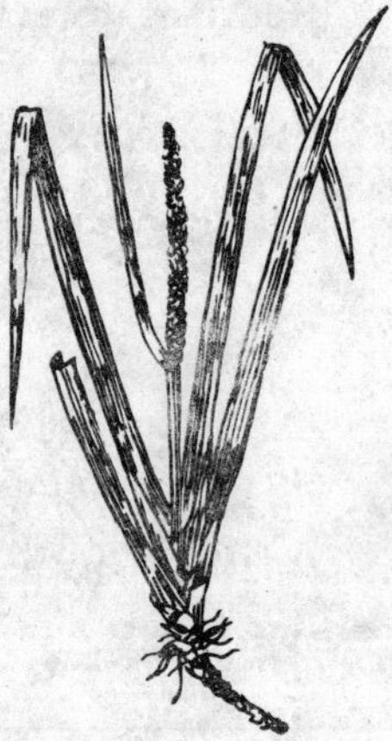

Description The rhizome of Acorus gramineus Soland. Family Areceae.

Characteristics Acrid in flavor, warm in nature, acting on the Heart and Stomach Channels.

Action Inducing resuscitation, calming the mind, resolving Dampness and normalizing the function of Stomach.

Indications

(1) Mental derangement, forgetfulness, tinnitus, etc. induced by retention of Dampness blocking the mind. For treating mental derangement, it is used together with Yu Jin (Radix Curcumae), Ban Xia (Rhizoma Pinelliae), etc.; for forgetfulness, tinnitus and deafness, used with Yuan Zhi (Radix Polygalae), Long Chi (Dens Draconis), etc., as in Anshen Dizhi Wan (Sedative Bolus). It can also be used for treating mania and dementia by adding Zhu Li Zhi (Succus Bambusae), Meng Shi (Lapis Micae Aureus), Zhu Sha (Cinnabaris), etc.

(2) Distension, stuffiness and pain of the chest and abdomen in-

duced by blockage of Dampness and stagnation of Qi. Usually used with Wu Zhu Yu (Fructus Euodiae), Xiang Fu (Rhizoma Cyperi), etc.

(3) Dysentery with inability to take food. Used with Huang Lian (Rhizoma Coptidis), Fu Ling (Poria), etc., as in Kaijin San (Appetizing Powder).

Administration 5～8g for making a decoction.

Precautions Not used for Phlegm-Heat in the interior.

Tonics

Drugs capable of replenishing Qi, Blood, Yin or Yang of the body when they are insufficient, so that to strengthen the body resistance against diseases, and to treat various Deficiency syndromes are referred to as tonics, or drugs for treating Deficiency syndromes.

According to their action and indications, tonics can be divided into four groups: drugs for tonifying Qi, drugs for tonifying Yang, drugs for tonifying Blood and drugs for tonifying Yin, and they are indicated for Qi Deficiency, Yang Deficiency, Blood Deficiency and Yin Deficiency respectively. Because the Qi, Blood, Yin and Yang in the human body are interdependent and interinfluential in pathology, e. g. Deficiency of Qi and Yang denotes insufficiency of the physiological function of the body , Qi Deficiency will lead to Yang Deficiency, similarly, Yang Deficiency is usually accompanied with Qi Deficiency; on the other hand, Blood Deficiency and Yin Deficiency indicate the consumption or impairment of the vital essence—— Blood and Body-Fluid, Blood Deficiency usually lead to Yin Deficiency and Yin Deficiency is always accompanied with Blood Deficiency. For these reasons, drugs for tonifying Qi and Yang, and drugs for tonifying Blood and Yin are often used together for mutual reinforcement. In the case of insufficiency of both Qi and Blood, Deficiency of both Yin and Yang, a therapy of tonifying both Qi and Blood, or both Yin and Yang, should be recommended.

Tonics are used for insufficiency of vital Qi and they should not be applied for sthenic syndromes for fear that an imbalance of Yin and Yang or disorder of Zang-Fu functions may result. However, in cases of coexistence of pathogens and Deficiency of the vital Qi, suitable tonics can be added to drugs for eliminating pathogens in order to enhance the body resistance against diseases.

Generally, tonics should be taken over a long time, so they are usually made into pills or semi-fluid extract for convenient administration. As some tonics may impede digestion, digestion-promo-ting drugs can be used in combination to strengthen the curative effect.

1. Drugs for Reinforcing Qi

Tonics of this group are mostly sweet in flavor, neutral or slightly warm in nature, and they are chiefly indicated for Qi Deficiency syndromes, especially for Deficiency of Spleen-Qi manifested by anorexia, diarrhea, distension and stuffiness in the Stomach and abdomen, listlessness, edema and prolapse of anus, and for Deficiency of Lung-Qi marked by short breath, disinclination to talk, breathlessness after movement, spontaneous sweating, etc. They can also be used for Deficiency of Heart-Qi marked by palpitation, thready and weak pulse, etc.

As Qi can help generate Blood and keep Blood flowing within the vessels, drugs for reinforcing Qi are often used in Blood Deficiency syndromes as well as bleeding due to Qi Deficiency.

Drugs for reinforcing Qi are likely to give rise to accumulation of Qi, and overtake of them may result in distension and fullness in the chest and abdomen and anorexia, to avoid this, they can be used with small amount of drugs for promoting the circulation of Qi and digestion.

1. 1. Ren Shen (Radix Ginseng)

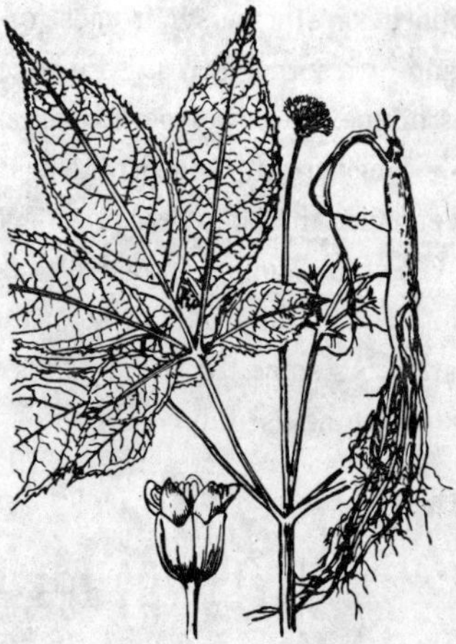

Description The root of Panax ginseng C. A. Mey. Family Araliaceae.

Characteristics Sweet and slightly bitter in flavor, slightly warm in nature, acting on the Spleen and Lung Channels.

Action Replenishing the primordial Qi, restoring pulse, relieving collapse-syndrome, invigorating Spleen and Lung, promoting the production of Body-Fluid to quench thirst, tranquilizing the mind to improve mental power.

Indications

(1) Prostration syndromes due to Qi Deficiency. Ren Shen (Radix Ginseng) is the key drug for treating short breath, listlessness, faint and hardly felt pulse beat, extreme weakness with sign of prostration induced by severe or prolonged illness, massive hemorrhage, hyperemesis or spouting diarrhea. It can be decocted alone, named Dushen Tang (Ginseng Decoction); in the case of prostration with sweat, cold limbs and Yang depletion syndromes, used together with Fu Zi (Radix Aconiti Praeparata), named Shen Fu Tang (Decoction of Radix Ginseng and Radix Aconiti Praeparata); for short breath, thirst with faint and thready pulse due to impairment of Qi and Yin by Heat pathogen, used with Mai Dong (Radix Ophiopogonis) and Wu Wei Zi (Fructus Schisandrae), as in Shengmai San (Powder for Activating Pulse).

(2) Deficiency of Spleen-Qi and Stomach-Qi, lassitude, anorexia, distension and stuffiness in the upper abdomen, vomiting, diarrhea, etc. For treatment, it is used with Bai Zhu (Rhizoma Atractylodis Macrocephalae), Fu Ling (Poria) and Zhi Gan Cao (Radix Gly-

cyrrhizae Praeparata), named Si Junzi Tang (Decoction of Four Noble Drugs); in the case of Spleen Deficiency with Heat invasion characterized by loose stools or diarrhea, used with Bai Zhu (Rhizoma Atractylodis Macrocephalae), Bian Dou (Semen Dolichoris Album), Fu Ling (Poria), etc., as in Shen Ling Baizhu San (Powder of Radix Ginseng, Poria and Rhizoma Atractylodis Macrocephalae).

(3) Deficiency of Lung-Qi marked by short breath, spontaneous sweating, listlessness, weak and faint pulse, etc. For treatment, usually used with Hu Tao (Juglandis Regiae), Ge Jie (Gecko), etc., as in Renshen Hutao Tang (Decoction of Radix Ginseng and Juglandis Regiae), or Renshen Gejie San (Powder of Radix Ginseng and Gecko).

(4) Thirst due to impairment of Body-Fluid, or diabetes. For treating febrile disease with impairment of both Qi and Body-Fluid, fever, thirst, profuse sweating and big and weak pulse, used with Shi Gao (Gypsum Fibrosum), Zhi Mu (Rhizoma Anemarrhenae), etc., as in Baihu Jia Renshen Tang (White Tiger Decoction with Radix Ginseng); for diabetes, used with Sheng Di (Radix Rehmanniae), Tian Hua Fen (Radix Trichosanthis), etc.

(5) Deficiency of both Qi and Blood marked by palpitation, insomnia, forgetfulness, listlessness, etc. Usually used with Dang Gui (Radix Angelicae Sinensis), Suan Zao Ren (Semen Ziziphi Spinosae), Long Yan Rou (Arillus Longan), etc., as in Guipi Tang (Decoction for Invigorating the Spleen and Tonifying the Heart).

(6) Syndromes induced by Deficiency of both Qi and Blood, or Blood Deficiency syndromes. For the former, used with Shu Di (Radix Rehmanniae Praeparata), as in Liangyi Gao (Extract for Treating Both Qi and Blood); for the latter, used with Dang Gui (Radix Angelicae Sinensis), Long Yan Rou (Arillus Longan), etc. In addition, when used with Yang tonics like Lu Rong (Cornu Cerri Pantotrichum), it can treat impotence; when used for weak constitution with affection of exopathogens or with purgation, the drug can help resist diseases to eliminate pathogens.

Administration 5～10g for making a decoction (decocted alone with small fire and its decoction is mixed with that of other ingredients for oral use); 1～2g, 2～3 times a day for oral intake of its powder; for rescuing patients with prostration syndromes, a large dose of 15～30g can be decocted and taken in separate doses.

Precautions Contraindicated for sthenic syndromes and Heat syndromes without Deficiency of the vital Qi. Antagonistic to Li Lu (Radix Veratri), Wu Ling Zhi (Faeces Trogopterorum) and Zao Jia (Fructus Gleditsiae). Tea and turnips should be avoided during medication.

1. 2. Dang Shen (Radix Codonopsis Pilosulae)

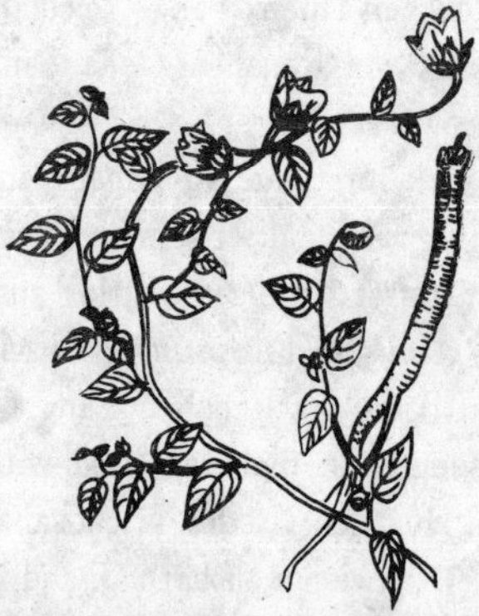

Description The root of Codonopsis pilosula (Franch.) Nannf. Family Campanulaceae.

Characteristics Sweet in flavor, neutral in nature, acting on the Spleen and Lung Channels.

Action Invigorating the Spleen, replenishing Qi, tonifying Blood and promoting the production of Body-Fluid.

Indications

(1) Poor appetite, diarrhea, lassitude and weakness induced by insufficiency of Spleen-Qi. For treatment, it is usually used with Bai Zhu (Rhizoma Atractylodis Macrocephalae), Fu Ling (Poria) and Gan Cao (Radix Glycyrrhizae).

(2) Deficiency of Lung-Qi marked by cough, dyspnea, short breath, weak and low voice, etc. aggravated with movement. Usually used with Huang Qi (Radix Astragali seu Hedysari), Wu Wei Zi (Fructus Schisandrae), etc.

(3) Impairment of Qi and Body-Fluid marked by short breath and thirst. Used with Mai Dong (Radix Ophiopogonis), Wu Wei Zi (Fructus Schisandrae), etc.

(4) Deficiency of Blood marked by sallow complexion, dizziness and palpitation. Usually used with Dang Gui (Radix Angelicae Sinensis), Shu Di (Radix Rehmanniae Praeparata), Bai Shao (Radix

Paeoniae Alba), Ji Xue Teng (Caulis Spatholobi), etc. In addition, it can be used together with drugs for superficies-syndromes and purgatives for treating affection of exopathogens with weak constitution and constipation with Deficiency of vital Qi.

This drug is similar to Ren Shen (Radix Ginseng) and it may replace Ren Shen (Radix Ginseng) in most cases. Yet Dang Shen (Radix Codonopsis Pilosulae) is not as powerful as Ren Shen (Radix Ginseng) in replenishing Qi and therefore, it should not be used for Qi Deficiency with sign of prostration.

Administration 10～30g for making a decoction. It can also be made into powder and boluses.

Precautions Not applied to Heat syndromes or Yin Deficiency and Yang Excess. Antagonistic to Li Lu (Radix Veratri).

1. 3. Xi Yang Shen (Radix Panacis Quinquefolii)

Description The dried root of Panax quinquefolium. Family Araliaceae.

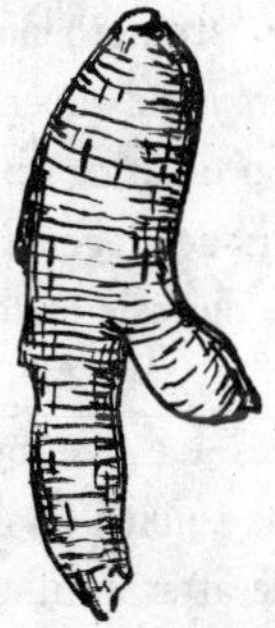

Characteristics Bitter and slightly sweet in flavor, cold in nature, acting on the Heart, Lung and Kidney Channels.

Action Replenishing Qi, tonifying Yin, clearing away Fire and promoting the production of Body-Fluid.

Indications

(1) Yin Deficiency with Fire Excess marked by asthmatic cough with bloody sputum. For treatment, it is used with Mai Dong (Radix Ophiopogonis), E Jiao (Colla Corii Asini), etc.

(2) Febrile diseases with impairment of both Qi and Yin marked by vexation, lassitude and thirst. Usually used with fresh Sheng Di (Radix Rehmanniae), fresh Shi Hu (Herba Dendrobii), etc.

(3) Insufficiency of Body-Fluid marked by dry mouth and thirst. Used alone for making a decoction.

Administration 3～6g for making a separate decoction to be taken after mixing it with that of other ingredients.

Precautions Contraindicated for Cold and Dampness invasion of the Stomach. Antagonistic to Li Lu (Radix Veratri).

1. 4. Huang Qi (Radix Astragali seu Hedysari)

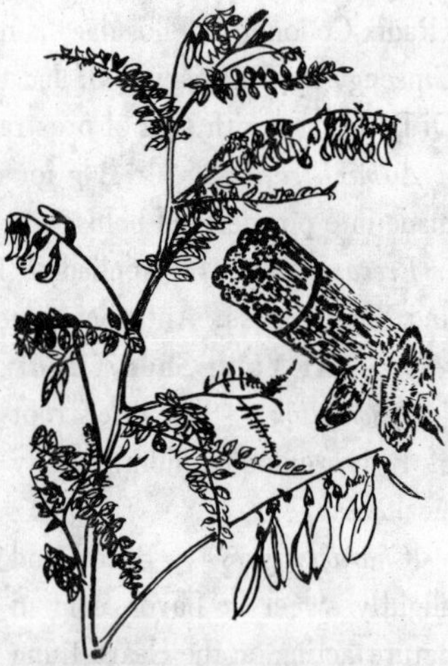

Description The dried root of Astragalus membranaceus Bge. var. mongholicus (Bge.) Hsiao or Astragalus membranaceus (Fisch.) Bge. Family Leguminosae.

Characteristcs Sweet in flavor, slightly warm in nature, acting on the Spleen and Lung Channels.

Action Tonifying Qi, lifting the sunken Yang, strengthening the defensive energy and superficial resistance, promoting pus discharge and tissue regeneration, and inducing diuresis to relieve edema.

Indications

(1) Syndromes induced by Deficiency of both Spleen-Qi and Lung-Qi or by the sunken Qi of the Middle-jiao. For general weakness and lassitude after an illness, it is used with Ren Shen (Radix Ginseng), as in Shen Qi Gao (Extract of Radix Ginseng and Radix Astragali seu Hedysari); for Deficiency of Spleen-Qi with poor appetite and diarrhea, used together with Bai Zhu (Rhizoma Atractylodis Macrocephalae); for Deficiency of both Qi and Yang marked by chilliness and profuse sweating, used with Fu Zi (Radix Aconiti Praeparata), as in Qi Fu Gao (Extract of Radix Astragali seu Hedysari and Radix Aconiti Praeparata); for sinking of Qi of Middle-jiao with prolonged diarrhea and prolapse of anus, of uterus or of viscera, used with Ren Shen (Radix Ginseng), Bai Zhu (Rhizoma A-

tractylodis Macrocephalae), Sheng Ma (Rhizoma Cimicifugae), etc., as in Buzhong Yiqi Tang (Decoction for Reinforcing Middle-jiao and Replenishing Qi).

(2) Qi Deficiency with Blood insufficiency, bleeding due to Qi Deficiency or Qi Deficiency with Blood stasis. For treating impairment of the interior due to overstrain, fever, spontaneous sweating and weak pulse induced by Deficiency of both Qi and Blood, it is used with Dang Gui (Radix Angelicae Sinensis) to tonify Qi and Blood, as in Danggui Buxue Tang (Decoction of Radix Angelicae Sinensis to Tonify Blood); for hemafecia, metrorrhagia or metrostaxis caused by Deficiency and failure of Qi in keeping the Blood flowing within the vessels, usually used with Ren Shen (Radix Ginseng), Bai Zhu (Rhizoma Atractylodis Macrocephalae) and Long Yan Rou (Arillus Longan); for numbness of the limbs due to Qi Deficiency and Blood stasis, used with Gui Zhi (Ramulus Cinnamomi), Bai Shao (Radix Paeoniae Alba), etc., as in Huangqi Guizhi Wuwu Tang (Decoction of Five Drugs Including Radix Astragali seu Hedysari and Ramulus Cinnamomi); for hemiplegia after apoplexy with full consciousness and feeble pulse, used with Dang Gui (Radix Angelicae Sinensis), Hong Hua (Flos Carthami), Tao Ren (Semen Persicae), etc., as in Buyang Huanwu Tang (Decoction for Invigorating Yang and for Recuperation).

(3) Spontaneous sweating or night sweat due to general weakness. Usually used with Mu Li (Concha Ostreae), Ma Huang Gen (Radix Ephedrae), etc., as in Muli San (Powder of Concha Ostreae); for Deficiency of the superficies with spontaneous sweating, chilliness, feeble pulse and susceptibility to common cold, used with Bai Zhu (Rhizoma Atractylodis Macrocephalae) and Fang Feng (Radix Ledebouriellae), as in Yupingfeng San (Jade Screen Powder); for night sweat due to Yin Deficiency with Heat invasion, used with Sheng Di (Radix Rehmanniae), Huang Bo (Cortex Phellodendri), etc., as in Danggui Liuhuang Tang (Decoction of Radix Rehmanniae with Six Yellow Ingredients).

(4) Non-rupture carbuncles or slow-healing carbuncles long after the rupture. For the former, used with Dang Gui (Radix Angelicae

Sinensis), Chuan Shan Jia (Squama Manitis), etc., as in Tounong San (Powder for Promoting Pus Discharge); for the latter, used with Ren Shen (Radix Ginseng), Dang Gui (Radix Angelicae Sinensis), etc., as in Shiquan Dabu Tang (Decoction of Ten Powerful Tonics).

(5) Edema of the limbs and face, dysuria, etc. induced by dysfunction of the Spleen in transport due to Qi Deficiency. Usually used with Fang Ji (Radix Stephaniae Tetrandrae), Bai Zhu (Rhizoma Atractylodis Macrocephalae), etc., as in Fangji Huangqi Tang (Decoction of Radix Stephaniae Tetrandrae and Radix Astragali seu Hedysari). In addition, it can be used for treating diabetes due to Deficiency of Qi and Body-Fluid by adding Sheng Di (Radix Rehmanniae), Mai Dong (Radix Ophiopogonis), Tian Hua Fen (Radix Trichosanthis), etc.

Administration 10～15g or 30～60g in the large dosage for making a decoction. Processed for replenishing Qi and lifting Yang; and unprocessed for other uses.

Precautions It should not be used in the following circumstances: sthenic superficies-syndromes with excessive pathogenic factors, Qi stagnation with blockage of Dampness, retention of indigested food, Yin Deficiency with Yang Excess, onset of carbuncles or Excess of Heat pathogen long after the rupture of carbuncles.

1.5. Bai Zhu (Rhizoma Atractylodis Macrocephalae)

Description The rhizome of Atractylodes macrocephala Koidz. Family Compositae.

Characteristics Bitter and sweet in flavor, warm in nature, acting on the Spleen and Stomach Channels.

Action Replenishing Qi and Spleen, eliminating Dampness by promoting diuresis, stopping sweating and preventing miscarriage.

Indications

(1) Poor appetite, loose stools, distension and fullness of the Stomach and abdomen, lassitude, etc. induced by Deficiency of Spleen-Qi and Stomach-Qi and failure of the Spleen to transport and transform nutrients. For treatment, it is used together with Ren Shen (Radix Ginseng), Fu Ling (Poria) and Gan Cao (Radix Glycyrrhizae), as in Sijunzi Tang (Decoction of Four Noble Drugs); in

the case of Deficiency-Cold of Spleen and Stomach marked by Cold pain in the Stomach and abdomen and diarrhea, usually used with Ren Shen (Radix Ginseng), Gan Jiang (Rhizoma Zingiberis) and Zhi Gan Cao (Radix Glycyrrhizae Praeparata), as in Lizhong Tang (Decoction for Regulating the Function of Middle-jiao); in the case of retention of food, anorexia, distension and stuffiness in the Stomach and abdomen due to Spleen Deficiency, used together with Zhi Shi (Fructus Aurantii Immaturus), as in Zhi Zhu Wan (Pill of Fructus Aurantii Immaturus and Rhizoma Atractylodis Macrocephalae).

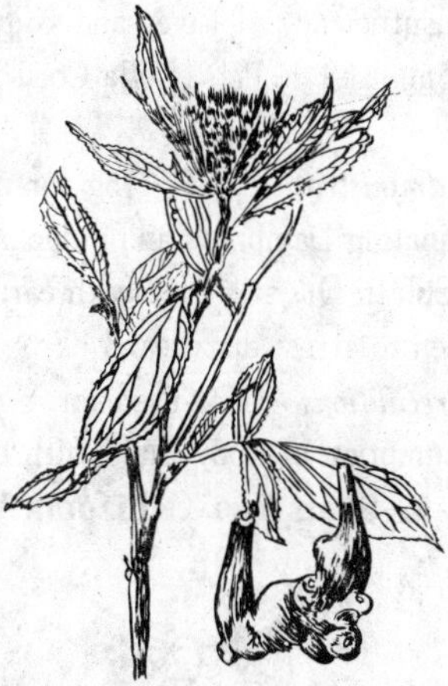

(2) Phlegm retention and edema due to Spleen Deficiency and retention of Water-Dampness. For Phlegm retention with fullness and stuffiness of the chest and hypochondrium, and vertigo, usually used with Gui Zhi (Ramulus Cinnamomi), Fu Ling (Poria) and Gan Cao (Radix Glycyrrhizae), named Ling Gui Zhu Gan Tang (Decoction of Poria, Ramulus Cinnamomi, Rhizoma Atractylodis Macrocephalae and Radix Glycyrrhizae); for retention of Water-Dampness marked by edema of the body and limbs and dysuria, used with Fu Ling (Poria) and Ze Xie (Rhizoma Alismatis), as in Siling San (Powder of Four Drugs Including Poria).

(3) Spontaneous sweating due to Deficiency of the superficies. Usually used with Huang Qi (Radix Astragali seu Hedysari), Fu Xiao Mai (Fructus Tritici Levis), etc.

(4) Threatened abortion due to Deficiency of the Spleen-Qi. In the case of accompanying internal Heat, used with Huang Qin (Radix Scutellariae); in the case of accompanying Qi stagnation with abdominal distension, used with Su Geng (Caulis Perillae), Sha Ren (Fructus Amomi), etc.; in the case of excessive fetus movement due

to insufficiency of Liver and Kidney, used with Du Zhong (Cortex Eucommiae), E Jiao (Colla Corii Asini), Xu Duan (Radix Dipsaci), etc.

Administration 5～15g for making a decoction. Processed for eliminating Dampness and inducing diuresis; stir-fried for replenishing Spleen-Qi; stir-fried with earth or baked brown for replenishing Spleen to arrest diarrhea.

Precautions Not used for Yin Deficiency with internal Heat or consumption of Body-Fluid with thirst.

1. 6. Shan Yao (Rhizoma Dioscoreae)

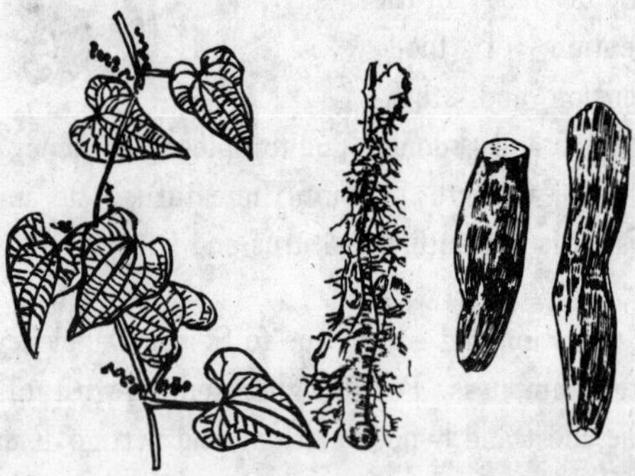

Description The rhizome of Dioscorea opposita Thunb. Family Dioscoreaceae.

Characteristics Sweet in flavor, neutral in nature, acting on the Spleen, Lung and Kidney Channels.

Action Replenishing Spleen and Stomach, promoting the production of Body-Fluid to nourish Lung, strengthening Kidney to arrest spermatorrhea.

Indications

(1) Deficiency of the Spleen and Stomach, poor appetite, loose stools or diarrhea. For treatment, it is used with Ren Shen (Radix Ginseng), Bai Zhu (Rhizoma Atractylodis Macrocephalae), Fu Ling (Poria), etc., as in Shen Ling Baizhu San (Powder of Radix Ginseng, Poria and Rhizoma Atractylodis Macrocephalae).

(2) Cough and dyspnea due to Lung Deficiency. Usually used with Dang Shen (Radix Codonopsis Pilosulae), Mai Dong (Radix Ophiopogonis), Wu Wei Zi (Fructus Schisandrae), etc.; in the case of cough and dyspnea induced by Deficiency of both Lung and Kidney, used together with Shu Di (Radix Rehmanniae Praeparata), Wu Wei Zi (Fructus Schisandrae), etc., as in DuQi Wan (Qi-converging Pill).

(3) Seminal emission, leukorrhagia, frequent urination, etc. due to Kidney Deficiency. For seminal emission due to Kidney Deficiency, used with Shu Di (Radix Rehmanniae Praeparata), Shan Zhu Yu (Fructus Corni), etc., as in Liuwei Dihuang Wan (Bolus of Six Drugs Including Radix Rehmanniae Praeparata); for frequent urination due to Kidney Deficiency, used with Yi Zhi Ren (Fructus Alpiniae Oxyphyllae) and Wu Yao (Radix Linderae), as in Suoquan Wan (Pill for Decreasing Urination); for profuse leucorrhea complicated by Spleen Deficiency and excessive Dampness, used with Bai Zhu (Rhizoma Atractylodis Macrocephalae) and Che Qian Zi (Semen Plantaginis), as in Wandai Tang (Decoction for Treating Leukorrhagia); for leukorrhagia complicated by Damp-Heat, used with Huang Bo (Cortex Phellodendri), etc., as in Yihuang Tang (Decoction for Treating Yellow Leucorrhea); for leukorrhagia due to inconsodidation of the Kidney-Qi, used with Shu Di (Radix Rehmanniae Praeparata), Shan Zhu Yu (Fructus Corni), Tu Si Zi (Semen Cuscutae), etc.

(4) Diabetes or consumption of Body-Fluid and Yin manifested as dysphoria with smothery sensation and thirst. For diabetes, used together with Huang Qi (Radix Astragali seu Hedysari), Ge Gen (Radix Puerariae), Tian Hua Fen (Radix Trichosanthis), Zhi Mu (Rhizoma Anemarrhenae), etc., as in Yuye Tang (Decoction for Diabetes); for thirst due to consumption of Body-Fluid, used with Mai Dong (Radix Ophiopogonis), Yu Zhu (Rhizoma Polygonati Odorati), etc.

Administration 10～30g or 60～250g in a large dosage for making a decoction; 6～10g for oral use of the powder. Processed for replenishing Yin and promoting the production of Body-Fluid; stir-fried for invigorating the Spleen to stop diarrhea.

Precautions Contraindicated for abdominal distension due to excessive Dampness or food retention.

1. 7. Gan Cao (Radix Glycyrrhizae)

Description The dried root and rhizome of Glycyrrhiza uralensis Fisch., Glycyrrhiza inflata Bat., or Glycyrrhiza glabra L. Family Leguminosae.

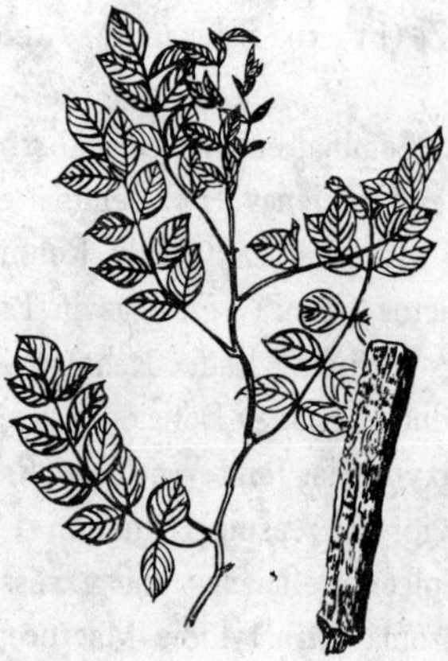

Characteristics Sweet in flavor, neutral in nature, acting on the Heart, Lung, Spleen and Stomach Channels.

Action Replenishing the Spleen-Qi, moisturizing the Lung to arrest cough, relieving spasm and pain, detoxicating and moderating the properties of other drugs.

Indications

(1) Deficiency of Spleen and Stomach, insufficiency of Qi of the Middle-jiao, poor appetite, loose stools, short breath and lassitude. For treatment, it is usually used with Ren Shen (Radix Ginseng), Bai Zhu (Rhizoma Atractylodis Macrocephalae), Fu Ling (Poria), etc., as in Sijunzi Tang (Decoction of Four Noble Drugs); in the case of Deficiency of Qi with insufficiency of Blood marked by palpitation, spontaneous sweating, irregular-interval pulse, used with Sheng Di (Radix Rehmanniae), Mai Dong (Radix Ophiopogonis), Ren Shen (Radix Ginseng), etc., as in Zhi Gancao Tang (Decoction of Radix Glycyrrhizae Praeparata).

(2) Cough and dyspnea. For cough induced by pathogenic Wind-Cold, used with Ma Huang (Herba Ephedrae) and Xing Ren (Semen Armeniacae Amarum), as in Sanao Tang (Decoction of Three Crude Drugs); for cough due to pathogenic Wind-Heat, used with Sang Ye (Folium Mori) and Jie Geng (Radix Platycodi), as in Sang Ju Yin

(Decoction of Folium Mori and Flos Chrysanthemi); for cough due to Lung-Heat, used with Sheng Shi Gao (Gypsum Fibrosum), Xing Ren (Semen Armeniacae Amarum) and Ma Huang (Herba Ephedrae), named Ma Xing Shi Gan Tang (Decoction of Herba Ephedrae, Semen Armeniacae Amarum, Gypsum Fibrosum and Radix Glycyrrhizae).

(3) Spasm and pain in the Stomach, abdomen and four limbs. For epigastric and abdominal pain due to Deficiency-Cold of the Stomach and Spleen, it is used with Gui Zhi (Ramulus Cinnamomi), Bai Shao (Radix Paeoniae Alba), etc., as in Xiao Jianzhong Tang (Minor Decoction for Strengthening the Middle-jiao); for spasm and pain of the four limbs due to impairment of the Ying and Blood, usually used with Shao Yao (Radix Paeoniae Alba), as in Shaoyao Gancao Tang (Decoction of Radix Paeoniae Alba and Radix Glycyrrhizae).

(4) Pyogenic skin infections, food or drug poisoning. For pyogenic skin infections, used with Jin Yin Hua (Flos Loniceae), Lian Qiao (Fructus Forsythiae), etc.; for sorethroat, used with Jie Geng (Radix Platycodi), as in Jiegeng Tang (Decoction of Radix Platycodi); for food or drug poisoning, used with mung beans and Fang Feng (Radix Ledebouriellae).

(5) Used in compound recipes to reduce the toxicity of other drugs or moderate the properties and coordinate the effects of different drugs.

Administration 2～10g, or 10～30g when used as a chief ingredient, for making a decoction. Unprocessed for clearing away Fire and toxin; processed for replenishing Spleen-Qi and relieving spasm.

Precautions Contraindicated for abdominal distension due to excessive Dampness, or vomiting. Antagonistic to Da Ji (Radix Euphorbiae Pekinensis), Yuan Hua (Flos Genkwa), Gan Sui (Radix Euphorbiae Kansui) and Hai Zao (Sargassum). Long time medication of large dosage may lead to edema, to which attention should be paid.

1.8. Da Zao (Fructus Ziziphi Jujubae)

Description The dried mature fruit of Ziziphus jujuba Mill.

Family Rhamnaceae.

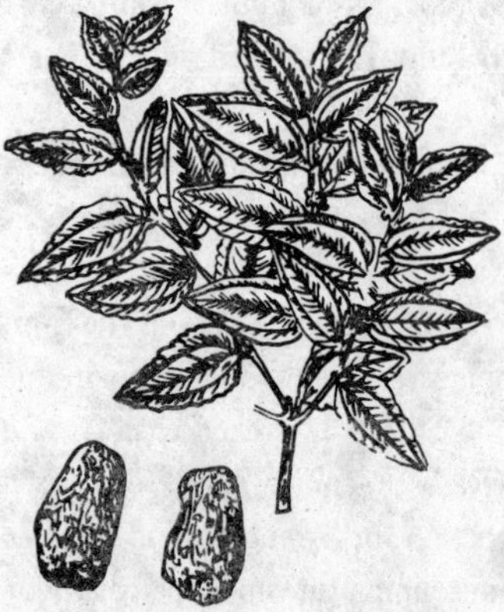

Characteristics Sweet in flavor, warm in nature, acting on the Spleen and Stomach Channels.

Action Invigorating the Spleen-Qi, tonifying Blood to calm the mind, and moderating the potency of drugs.

Indications

(1) Deficiency of both Spleen and Stomach, lassitude, poor appetite, loose stools, etc. For treatment, it is used with Dang Shen (Radix Codonopsis Pilosulae), Bai Zhu (Rhizoma Atractylodis Macrocephalae), etc.

(2) Sallow complexion due to Blood Deficiency, vexation and restlessness in women. For sallow complexion and emaciation, used with Shu Di (Radix Rehmanniae Praeparata) and Dang Gui (Radix Angelicae Sinensis); for vexation and restlessness in women due to Blood Deficiency, used with Gan Cao (Radix Glycyrrhizae) and Fu Xiao Mai (Fructus Tritici Levis), as in Dan Mai Dazhao Tang (Decoction of Radix Glycyrrhizae, Fructus Tritici Levis and Fructus Ziziphi Jujubae).

(3) Moderating the potency of some drugs. e.g. In Tingli Dazao Xiefei Tang (Decoction of Semen Lepidii seu Descurainiae and Fructus Ziziphi Jujubae for Removing Phlegm from the Lung), Da Zao (Fructus Ziziphi Jujubae) is used to moderate the potency of Ting Li Zi (Semen Lepidii seu Descurainiae) in order to protect Lung-Qi from being impaired while removing Phlegm from the Lung to relieve asthma; and in Shi Zao Tang (Decoction of Ten Chinese Dates), Da Zao (Fructus Ziziphi Jujubae) is used in combination with Da Ji (Radix Euphorbiae Pekinensis), Yuan Hua (Flos Genkwa) and Gan Sui (Radix Euphorbiae Kansui) to ensure the purgation without damaging the vital Qi. In addition, it is usually used with Sheng Jiang (Rhizoma Zingiberis Recens) to coordinate the function

of Ying and Wei, or to strengthen the action of tonics.

Administration 3～12 pieces, or 10～30g for making a decoction. Peeled and smashed for making boluses.

Precautions Not applied for distension of the Stomach and abdomen due to excessive Dampness.

2. Drugs for Strengthening Yang

Drugs for strengthening Yang are generally sweet or salty in flavor, warm in nature, and capable of supplememting and supporting Yang. They are indicated for Yang Deficiency syndromes including Deficiency of Heart-Yang, of Spleen-Yang and of Kidney-Yang. As the Kidney dominates the Yang of the whole body, various Deficiency syndromes of Yang are related to Deficiency of Kidney-Yang, therefore, the therapy of tonifying Yang chiefly refers to warming and tonifying the Kidney-Yang.

Drugs of this category function in reinforcing the Kidney-Yang, tonifying the essense of life and strengthening the tendons and bones and they are used for treating fatigue, chilliness, cold limbs, aching of the loins and knees, impotence, spermatorrhea, sterility due to uterine Coldness, watery leucorrhagia, frequent urination, enuresis, white tongue coat with deep pulse, etc. In addition, when there occurs failure of Kidney-Yang which cannot warm the Spleen-Yang, diarrhea may result; while insufficiency of Kidney-Yang which fails to receive Qi may give rise to short breath. For these reasons, some of these drugs can also be used for treating diarrhea induced by Deficiency of both Spleen and Kidney or short breath due to Deficiency of both Lung and Kidney.

Most drugs of this category are warm and dry in property and they are likely to impair Yin and enhance Fire and therefore they should not be used in cases of Yin Deficiency with excessive Fire.

2.1. Lu Rong (Cornu Cervi Pantotrichum)

Description The hairy, non-ossific young horn of a stag of

Cervus nippon Temminck or Cervus elaphus Linnaeus. Family Cervidae.

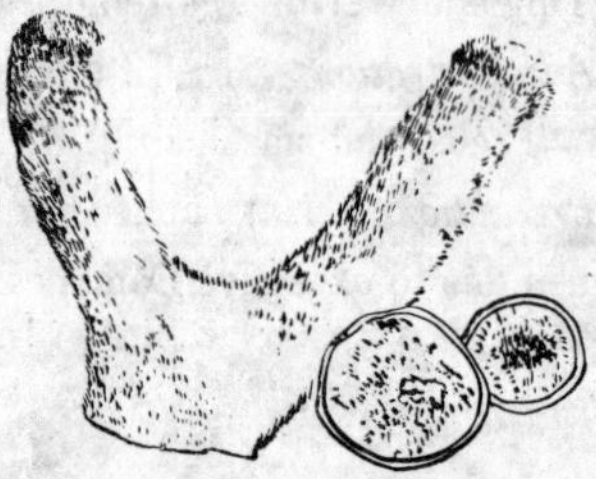

Characteristics Sweet and salty in flavor, warm in nature, acting on the Liver and Kidney Channels.

Action Tonifying Kidney-Yang, vital essence and Blood, and strengthening tendons and bones.

Indications

(1) Insufficiency of Kidney-Yang and consumption of the vital essence and Blood marked by chilliness, cold limbs, impotence, spermatorrhea, sterility due to uterine Coldness, frequent urination, aching of the loins and knees, dizziness, tinnitus, lassitude, etc. For treatment, it can be used either alone by grinding it into powder for oral administration or together with Ren Shen (Radix Ginseng), Shu Di (Radix Rehmanniae Praeparata), etc., as in Shen Rong Guben Wan (Bolus of Radix Ginseng and Cornu Cervi Pantorichum for Consolidating the Constitution).

(2) Insufficiency of vital essence and Blood marked by flaccidity of extremities, infantile maldevelopment with delayed walking and infantile metopism. Usually used together with Shu Di (Radix Rehmanniae Praeparata), Shan Zhu Yu (Fructus Corni), etc., as in Jiawei Dihuang Wan (Bolus of Radix Rehmanniae Praeparata with Additional Ingredients).

(3) Metrorrhagia, metrostaxis and profuse leucorrhea due to Coldness and Deficiency of the Chong and Ren Channels and inconsolidation of the Dai Channel. For treatment, usually used with Gou Ji (Rhizoma Cibotii), Bai Lian (Radix Ampelopsis), etc. In addition it can be used to treat non-healing carbuncles long after the rupture or deep-rooted carbuncles of Yin nature by warming and tonifying Yang and promoting pus discharge.

Administration 1～3g, ground into fine powder to be taken orally three times a day, or prepared in bolus and compound powder.

Precautions Being potent in tonification, it should not be given abruptly in large dosage. It is contraindicated in the following conditions: Yin Deficiency with Fire Excess, Heat in Blood, hyperactivity of Stomach-Fire, Phlegm-Heat in Lung as well as affection of epidemic febrile diseases caused by exopathogens.

2.2. Rou Cong Rong (Herba Cistanchis)

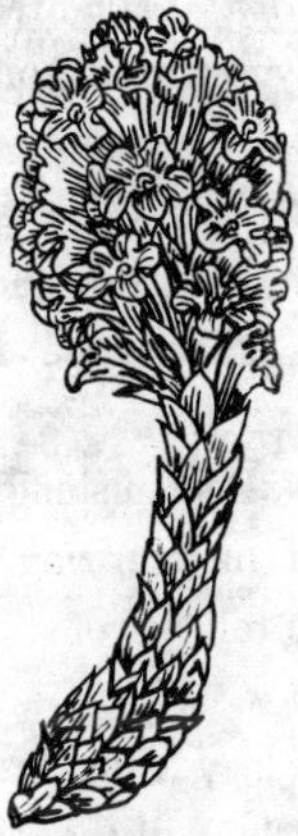

Description The fleshy stem with scales of Cistanche deserticola Y. C. Ma. Family Orobanchaceae.

Characteristics Sweet and salty in flavor, warm in nature, acting on the Kidney and Large Intestine Channels.

Action Replenishing Kidney and Yang, moisturizing the intestines to treat constipation.

Indications

(1) Kidney Deficiency characterized by impotence, cold pain in the loins and knees, sterility due to uterine Coldness, etc. For treating impotence due to insufficiency of Kidney-Yang and Deficiency of the vital essence induced by Kidney Deficiency, it is used together with Shu Di (Radix Rehmanniae Praeparata) and Tu Si Zi (Semen Cuscutae), as in Roucongrong Wan (Bolus of Herba Cistanchis); for sterility due to insufficiency of the vital essence and Blood, usually used with Lu Jiao Jiao (Colla Cornus Cervi) and Dang Gui (Radix Angelicae Sinensis); for cold pain in the loins and knees with flaccidity of the muscles, used with Ba Ji Tian (Radix Morindae Officinalis), Du Zhong (Cortex Eucommiae), etc., as in Jingang Wan (Pill for Treating Flaccidity due to Kidney Deficiency).

(2) Constipation due to Dryness of the Intestines and exhaustion of Body-Fluid. Used with Huo Ma Ren (Fructus Cannabis), Chen Xiang (Lignum Aquilariae Resinatum), etc., as in Runchang Wan

(Pill for Moisturizing Bowels).

Administration 10～20g for making a decoction.

Precautions As this drug is neither potent nor quick in action, a large dosage is necessary in application. It is contraindicated for Yin Deficiency with Fire Excess or loose stools.

2.3. Suo Yang (Herba Cynomorii)

Description The dried fleshy stem of Cynomorium songaricum Rupr. Family Cynomoriaceae.

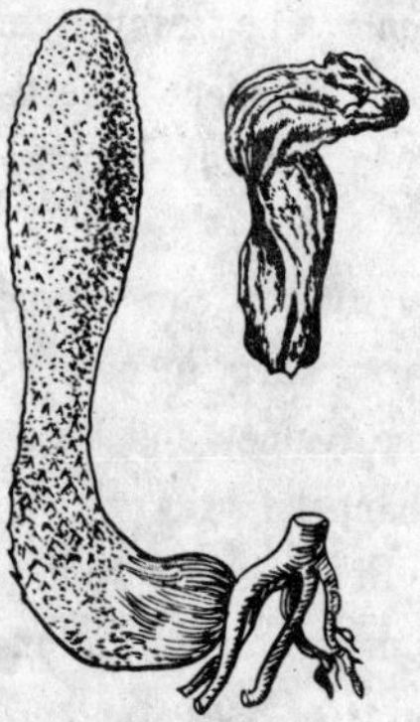

Characteristics Sweet in flavor, warm in nature, acting on the Liver and Large Intestine Channels.

Action Replenishing Kidney-Yang and moisturizing the Intestines to relieve constipation.

Indications

(1) Kidney-Yang insufficiency syndromes such as impotence, sterility, aching of the loins and knees and flaccidity of the muscles. For treatment, it is used with Shu Di (Radix Rehmanniae Praeparata), Gui Ban (Plastrum Testudinis), etc., as in Huqian Wan (Tiger Bone Pill for Checking Exuberance of Yang). As it is similar in function to Rou Cong Rong (Herba Cistanchis), Suo Yang is usually used in place of Rou Cong Rong (Herba Cistanchis) to treat impotence and sterility induced by insufficiency of Kidney-Yang, vital essence and Blood.

(2) Constipation due to exhaustion of Body-Fluid and dryness of intestines. It is used with Huo Ma Ren (Fructus Cannabis), Dang Gui (Radix Angelicae Sinensis), etc.

Administration 10～15g for making a decoction.

Precautions Contraindicated for Yin Deficiency with Fire Excess, diarrhea or constipation due to sthenic Heat.

2.4. Ba Ji Tian (Radix Morindae Officinalis)

Description The fleshy root of Morinda officinalis How. Family

Rubiaceae.

Characteristics Acrid and sweet in flavor, slightly warm in nature, acting on the Kidney Channel.

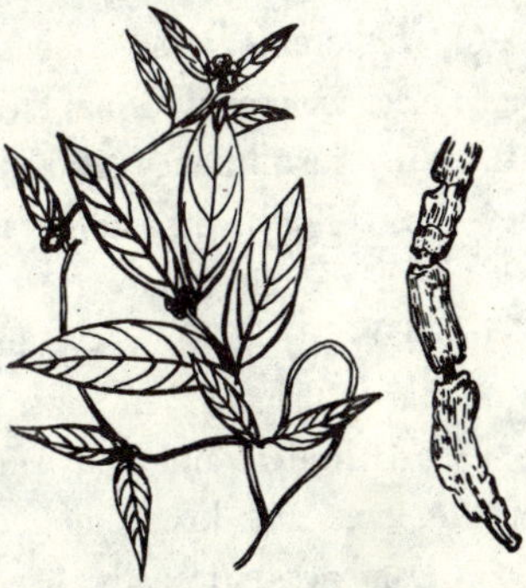

Action Tonifying the Kidney, strengthening Yang, eliminating pathogenic Wind and Dampness.

Indications

(1) Insufficiency of Kidney-Yang marked by impotence, frequent urination, sterility due to uterine Coldness, irregular menstruation and cold pain in the lower abdomen. For treating impotence and sterility, it is used together with Shu Di (Radix Rehmanniae Praeparata), Rou Gui (Cortex Cinnamomi), etc.; for frequent urination, enuresis, used with Fu Pen Zi (Fructus Bubi), Yi Zhi Ren (Fructus Alpiniae Oxyphyllae), etc.; for irregular menstruation, used with Gao Liang Jiang (Rhizoma Alpiniae Officinarum), Rou Gui (Cortex Cinnamomi), etc., as in Baji Wan (Pill of Radix Morindae Officinalis).

(2) Pain of the loins and knees or flaccidity of muscles caused by insufficiency of Kidney-Yang complicated by invasion of Wind-Dampness. For treatment, it is used with Du Zhong (Cortex Eucommiae), Bi Xie (Rhizoma Dioscoreae Hypoglaucae), etc., as in Jingang Wan (Pill for Treating Flaccidity due to Kidney Deficiency).

Administration 10~15g for making a decoction.

Precautions Contraindicated for Yin Deficiency with excessive Fire and for Damp-Heat syndromes.

2. 5. Xian Mao (Rhizoma Curculiginis)

Description The dried rhizome of Curculigo orchioides Gaertn. Family Amaryllidaceae.

Characteristics Acrid in flavor, hot in nature, toxic, and acting on the Kidney Channel.

Action Warming the Kidney-Yang and depriving the pathogenic Cold and Dampness.

Indications

(1) Impotence, seminal emission, incontinence of urine, etc. caused by insufficiency of Kidney-Yang. For treatment, it is used with Yin Yang Huo (Herba Epimedii), Ba Ji Tian (Radix Morindae Officinalis), etc.

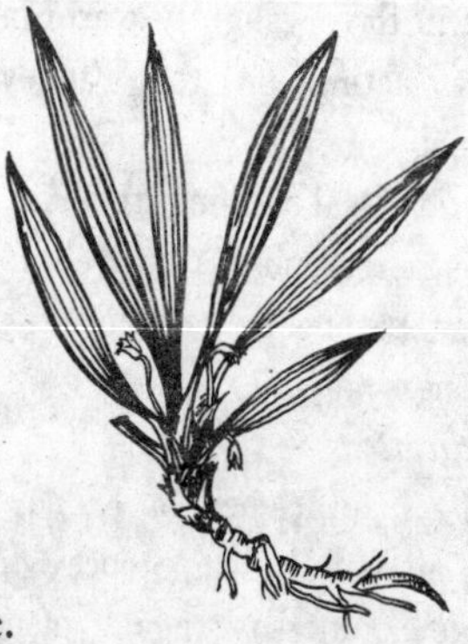

(2) Arthralgia and cold pain of the loins and knees due to Cold Dampness. Usually used with Gou Ji (Rhizoma Cibotii), Du Zhong (Cortex Eucommiae), etc.

Administration 3 ~ 10g for making a decoction or medicated wine. It can also be prepared into powder or pills.

Precautions Contraindicated for Yin Deficiency with Fire Excess.

2.6. Yin Yang Huo (Herba Epimedii)

Description The aerial part of Epimedium brevicornum Maxim., or Epimedium sagittatum (Sieb. et Zucc.) Maxim., or Epimedium pubescens Maxim., or Epimedium koreanum Nakai. Family Berberidaceae.

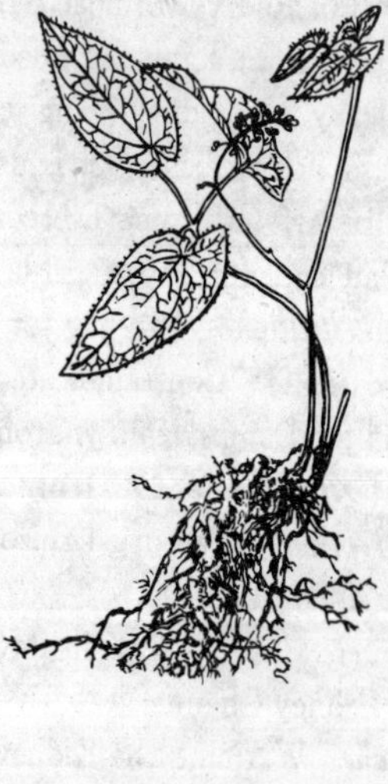

Characteristics Acrid and sweet in flavor, warm in nature, and acting on the Liver and Kidney Channels.

Action Tonifying the Kidney and strengthening Yang, eliminating pathogenic Wind and Dampness.

Indications

(1) Impotence, frequent urination, weakness of the loins and knees, etc. induced by insufficiency of Kidney-Yang. For treatment, it can be soaked in wine for oral administration, or used together with Shu Di (Radix Rehmanniae Praeparata), Xian Mao (Rhizoma Curculiginis), etc.

(2) Rheumatic arthritis or numbness of the limbs. Usually used with Wei Ling Xian (Radix Clematidis), Cang Er Zi (Fructus Xanthii), etc.

Administration 10～15g for making a decoction. It can also be soaked in wine for oral use or made into powder, pills or extract.

Precautions Contraindicated for Yin Deficiency with Fire Excess.

2.7. Du Zhong (Cortex Eucommiae)

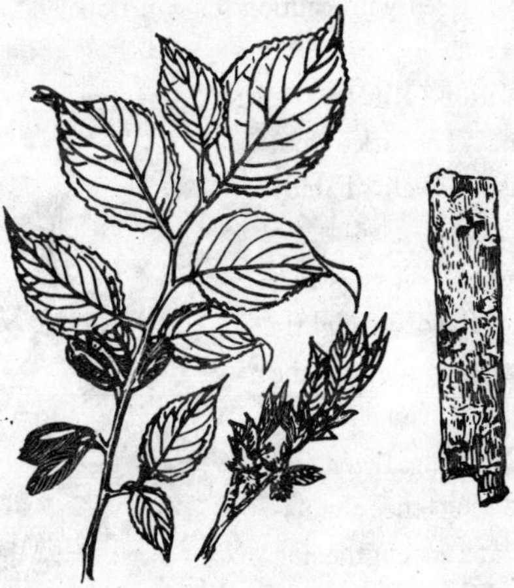

Description The dried trunk bark of Eucommia ulmoides Oliv. Family Eucommiaceae.

Characteristics Sweet in flavor, warm in nature, acting on the Liver and Kidney Channels.

Action Tonifying Liver and Kidney, strengthening the tendons and bones, and preventing miscarriage.

Indications

(1) Aching pain of the loins and knees, flaccidity of the muscles or

impotence, frequent urination, etc. caused by insufficiency of Liver and Kidney. For the former, it is used with Bu Gu Zhi (Fructus Psoraleae), Hu Tao Rou (Juglandis Regiae), etc., as in Qinge Wan (Pill for Lumbago due to Kidney Deficiency); for the latter, it is used with Shan Zhu Yu (Fructus Corni), Tu Si Zi (Semen Cuscutae), etc.

(2) Threatened abortion, vaginal bleeding during pregnancy, metrorrhagia, metrostaxis, etc. caused by insufficiency of Liver and Kidney and unconsolidation of the Chong and Ren Channels. Used with Xu Duan (Radix Dipsaci), etc. or with the flesh of Chinese dates to be made into bolus.

Administration 10～15g for making a decoction. Stir-fried Du Zhong (Cortex Eucommiae) has better effects than the unprepared one.

Precautions Used with caution for Yin Deficiency with Fire-Excess.

2. 8. Xu Duan (Radix Dipsaci)

Description The dried root of Dipsacus asper Wall. Family Dipsacaceae.

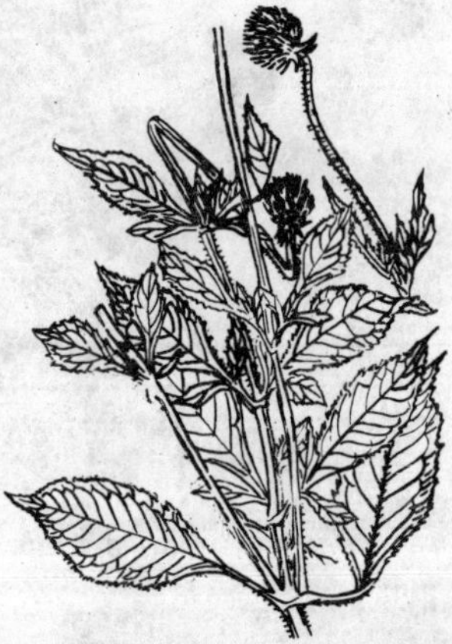

Characteristics Bitter, sweet and acrid in flavor, slightly warm in nature, acting on the Liver and Kidney Channels.

Action Tonifying Liver and Kidney, regulating the circulation of Blood and strengthening the tendons and bones.

Indications

(1) Insufficiency of Liver and Kidney with obstructed Blood flow manifested as aching of the loins and legs, weakness of the feet and knees, etc. For treatment, it is usually used together with Du Zhong (Cortex Eucommiae), Niu Xi (Radix Achyranthis Bidentatae), etc.

(2) Asthenia of Liver and Kidney, and unconsolidation of the

Chong and Ren Channels marked by metrorrhagia, metrostaxis, excessive fetus movement and threatened abortion. For metrorrhagia and metrostaxis, it is used with Shan Zhu Yu (Fructus Corni), E Jiao (Colla Corii Asini), etc., for excessive fetus movement and threatened abortion, used with Sang Ji Sheng (Ramulus Loranthi), Tu Si Zi (Semen Cuscutae), etc., as in Shoutai Wan (Bolus for Protecting Fetus).

(3) Traumatic injuries, bone fracture as well as suppurative skin infections. Xu Duan (Radix Dipsaci) is the key drug for treating traumatic injuries and it is usually used together with Gu Sui Bu (Rhizoma Drynariae), Zi Ran Tong (Pyritum), etc. For mastitis, used with Pu Gong Ying (Herba Taraxaci) and ground into powder for oral use.

Administration 10～20g for making a decoction. Stir-fried with salt water for tonifying Liver and Kidney, consolidating the Meridians and preventing miscarriage; stir-fried with wine for activating Blood circulation and treating traumatic injuries.

Precautions Used with caution for Yin Deficiency with Fire Excess.

2.9. Gou Ji (Rhizoma Cibotii)

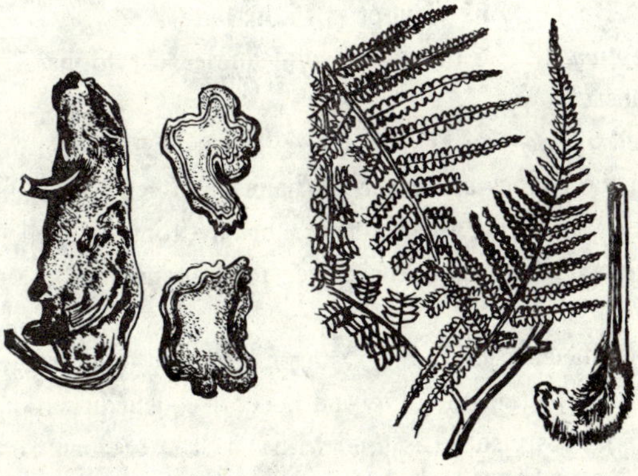

Description The rhizome of Cibotium barometz (L.) J Sm. Family Dicksoniaceae.

Characteristics Bitter and sweet in flavor, warm in nature, acting on the Liver and Kidney Channels.

Action Tonifying the Liver and Kidney, strengthening the loins and knees, and eliminating pathogenic Wind and Dampness.

Indications

(1) Insufficiency of Liver and Kidney complicated by affection of pathogenic Wind-Cold-Dampness manifested by lumbago, backache, limited movement of the back and flaccidity of the feet and knees. For treatment, it is usually used with Du Zhong (Cortex Eucommiae), Xu Duan (Radix Dipsaci), etc., as in Gouji Yin (Decoction of Rhizoma Cibotii).

(2) Inconsolidation due to Kidney Deficiency marked by incontinence of urine and profuse leucorrhea. For frequent urination with lumbago, used with Mu Gua (Fructus Chaenomelis) and Wu Jia Pi (Cortex Acanthopancis Radicis); for asthenic Cold of the Chong and Ren Channels marked by profuse leucorrhea, usually used with Lu Rong (Cornu Cervi Pantotrichum), Bai Lian (Radix Ampelopsis), etc.

Administration 10～15g for making a decoction.

Precautions Contraindicated for Kidney Deficiency with Heat pathogen or dribbling and painful micturition with dark urine.

2.10. Bu Gu Zhi (Fructus Psoraleae)

Description The dried fruit of Psoralea corylifolia L. Family Luguminosae.

Characteristics Bitter and acrid in flavor, very warm in nature, acting on the Kidney and Spleeen Channels.

Action Tonifying the Kidney-Yang, treating seminal emission and enuresis, and warming the Spleen to stop diarrhea.

Indications

(1) Insufficiency of Kidney-Yang marked by impotence, seminal emission, cold pain in the loins and knees, frequent urination, enuresis, etc. For treatment, it is used with Tu Si Zi (Semen Cuscutae), Ba Ji Tian (Radix Morindae Officinalis), etc. ; for lumbago due to Kidney Deficiency, usually used with Hu Tao Ren (Juglandis Regiae), Du Zhong (Cortex Eucommiae), etc., as in Qing'e Wan

(Pill for Treating Kidney Deficiency); for enuresis and frequent urination, used with Yi Zhi Ren (Fructus Alpiniae Oxyphyllae), Fu Pen Zi (Fructus Rubi), etc.

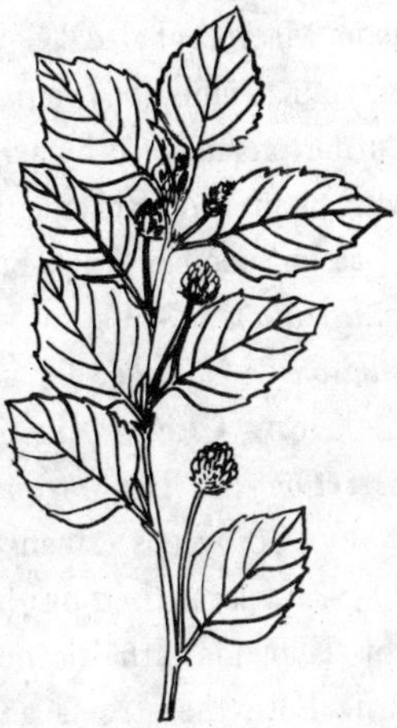

(2) Deficiency of both Spleen-Yang and Kidney-Yang marked by chronic diarrhea or diarrhea before dawn. Usually used with Rou Dou Kou (Semen Myristicae), Wu Wei Zi (Fructus Schisandrae) and Wu Zhu Yu (Fructus Euodiae), as in Sishen Wan (Pill of Four Miraculous Drugs).

Administration 5~10g for making a decoction.

Precautions Contraindicated for Yin Deficiency with excessive Fire and constipation.

2. 11. Yi Zhi Ren (Fructus Alpiniae Oxyphyllae)

Description The ripe fruit of Alpinia oxyphylla Miq. Family Zingiberaceae.

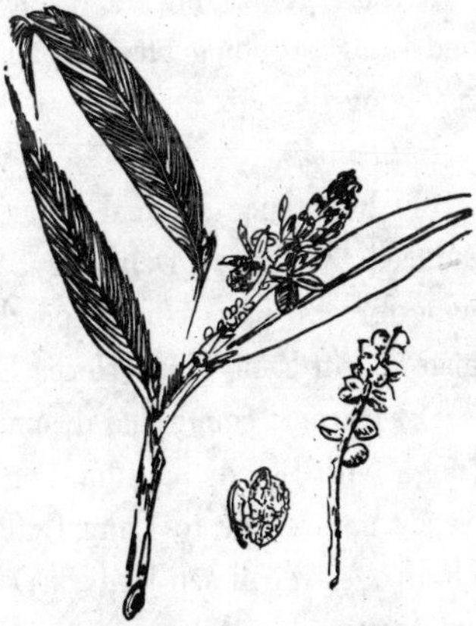

Characteristics Acrid in flavor, warm in nature, acting on the Spleen and Kidney Channels.

Action Warming the Spleen, improving the appetite and digestion, conserving saliva, warming the Kidney to keep the Kidney essence and reduce urination.

Indications

(1) Cold pain in the abdomen, vomiting, anorexia and profuse salivation caused by asthenc Cold of the Spleen and Stomach. For treatment, it is used together with

Dang Shen (Radix Codonopsis Pilosulae), Bai Zhu (Rhizoma Atractylodis Macrocephalae), Gan Jiang (Rhizoma Zingiberis), etc.

(2) Seminal emission, enuresis, frequent urination, whitish and turbid urine, etc. induced by asthenic Cold of the Kidney-Qi. Usually used with Shan Yao (Rhizoma Dioscoreae) and Wu Yao (Radix Linderae), as in Suoquan Wan (Pill for Decreasing Urination).

Administration 3～6g for making a decoction.

Precautions Not used for non-asthenic Cold syndromes.

2. 12. Dong Chong Xia Cao (Cordyceps)

Description The stroma formed by Cordyceps sinensis (Berk.) Sacc. parasitized on the larva of Hepialus armoricanus Oberthru. Both the stroma and the dead larva are used medicinally.

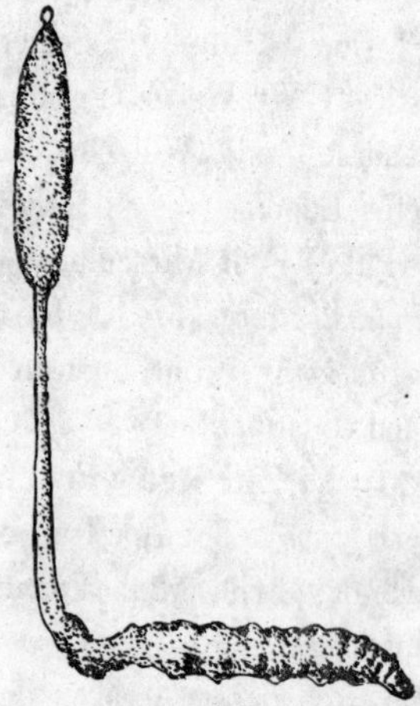

Characteristics Sweet in flavor, warm in nature, acting on the Kidney and Lung Channels.

Action Tonifying the Kidney and Lung, stopping bleeding and resolving Phlegm.

Indications

(1) Impotence, seminal emission, soreness of the loins and knees induced by Kidney Deficiency. For treatment, it can be soaked in wine for oral use, or used together with Du Zhong (Cortex Eucommiae), Yin Yang Huo (Herba Epimedii), etc.

(2) Chronic cough and dyspnea of Deficiency nature, consumptive cough with Bloody sputum. For chronic cough and dyspnea of Deficiency nature due to Lung Deficiency, usually used with Huang Qi (Radix Astragali seu Hedysari), Wu Wei Zi (Fructus Schisandrae), etc; for cough and dyspnea due to failure of Kidney in controlling Qi, used with Ge Jie (Gecko), Hu Tao Rou (Juglandis Regiae), etc. ; for consumptive cough with bloody sputum, used with Sha Shen (Radix

Adenophorae Strictae), E Jiao (Colla Corii Asini), etc. In addition, it is often used by stewing together with chicken, duck or port for treating general weakness after illness or spontaneous sweating with chilliness.

Administration 5～10g for making a decoction. It can be made into powder or bolus or stewed with meat.

Precautions Contraindicated for superficies-syndromes.

2. 13. Hu Tao Ren (Semen Juglandis)

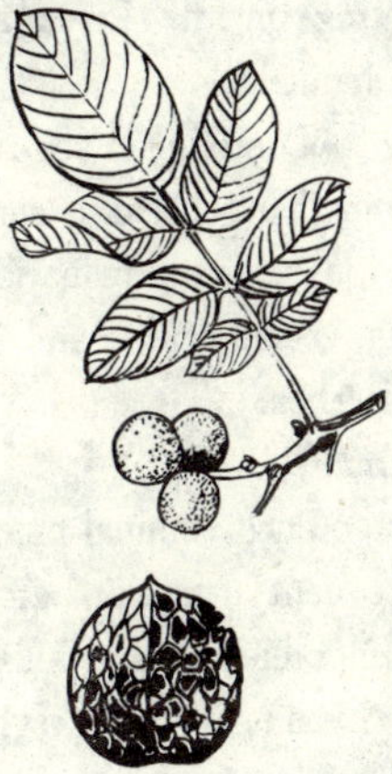

Description The dried ripe seed of Juglans regia. Family (Juglandaceae).

Characteristics Sweet in flavor, warm in nature, acting on the Kidney, Lung and Large Intestine Channels.

Action Tonifying the Kidney, warming the Lung and moiturizing the Intestines.

Indications

(1) Lumbago and weak feet due to Kidney Deficiency. For treatment, it is used together with Du Zhong (Cortex Eucommiae), Bu Gu Zhi (Fructus Psoraleae), etc., as in Qing'e Wan (Pill for Treating Kidney Deficiency).

(2) Asthma of Deficiency nature due to insufficiency of the Lung and Kidney. Usually used together with Ren Shen (Radix Ginseng) and Sheng Jiang (Rhizoma Zingiberis Recens), as in Renshen Hutao Tang (Decoction of Radix Ginseng and Semen Juglandis).

(3) Dryness of the bowels and constipation due to Deficiency of Blood and exhaustion of the Body-Fluid in old age or after an illness. Used either alone for oral intake after being chewed or together with Rou Cong Rong (Herba Cistanchis), Dang Gui (Radix Angelicae Sinensis), etc.

Administration 10～30g for making a decoction; 3～5 pieces for chewing. Unskinned for relieving cough and asthma, skinned for moisturizing the Intestines to treat constipation.

2.14. Tu Si Zi (Semen Cuscutae)

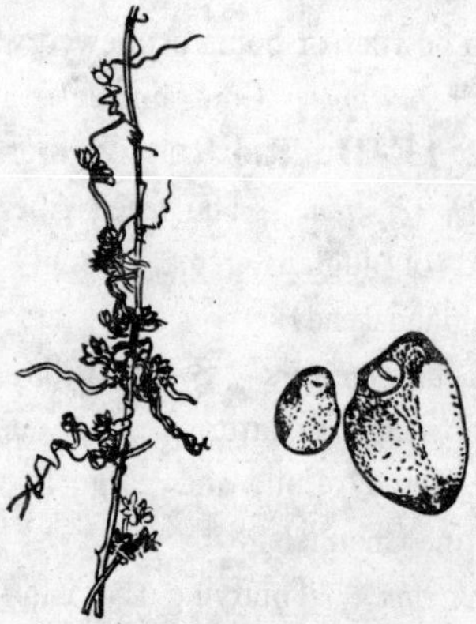

Description The dried seed of Cuscuta chinensis Lam. Family Convolvulaceae.

Characteristics Acrid and sweet in flavor, neutral in nature, acting on the Liver and Kidney Channels.

Action Tonifying Yang and invigorating Yin, checking seminal emission, reducing urination, improving visual acuity and relieving diarrhea.

Indications

(1) Impotence, seminal emission, tinnitus, aching of the loins and knees, frequent urination, etc. caused by Kidney Deficiency. For treating impotence and seminal emission, it is used with Gou Qi Zi (Fructus Lycii), Fu Pen Zi (Fructus Rubi), etc.; for aching of the loins and knees, used with Du Zhong (Cortex Eucommiae) of equal amount each and made into boluses with the paste of Shan Yao (Rhizoma Dioscoreae); for incontinence of urine, usually used with Lu Rong (Cornu Cervi Pantotrichum), Sang Piao Xiao (Oötheca Mantidis), etc.; for threatened abortion due to Kidney Deficiency, used with Xu Duan (Radix Dipsaci), Sang Ji Sheng (Ramulus Loranthi), etc.

(2) Blurring of vision due to insufficiency of Liver and Kidney and Deficiency of essence and Blood. Usually used with Shu Di (Radix Rehmanniae Praeparata), Che Qian Zi (Semen, Plantaginis), etc.

(3) Loose stools and anorexia due to Deficiency of both Spleen and Kidney. Used with Shan Yao (Rhizoma Dioscoreae), Dang Shen (Radix Codonopsis), etc.

Administration 10～15g for making a decoction.

Precautions Contraindicated for Yin deficiency with excessive Fire, constipation or dark and scanty urine.

2. 15. Sha Yuan Zi (Semen Astragali Complanati)

Description The dried ripe seed of Astragalus complanatus R. Br. Family Leguminosae.

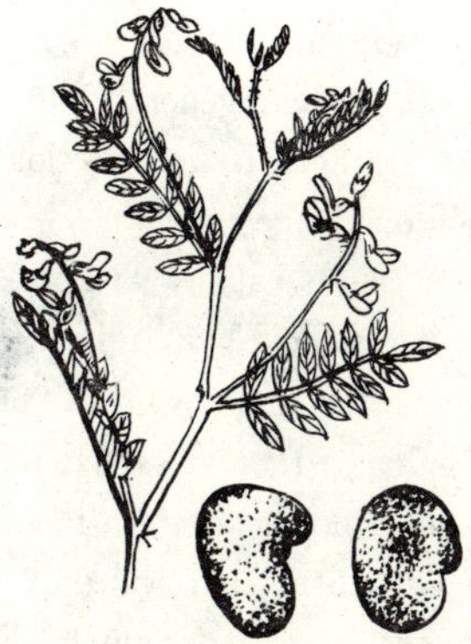

Characteristics Sweet in flavor, warm in nature, acting on the Liver and Kidney Channels.

Action Replenishing the Kidney to consolidate the vital essence, tonifying the Liver to improve visual acuity.

Indications

(1) Lumbago, seminal emission, prospermia, incontinence of urine, profuse leukorrhea, etc. caused by Kidney Deficiency. For treating emission and prospermia, it is used with Shan Yao (Rhizoma Dioscoreae), Qian Shi (Semen Euryales) etc., as in Jinsuo Gujing Wan (Gold Lock Pill for Keeping Kidney Essence); for enuresis and frequent urination, used with Fu Pen Zi (Fructus Bubi), Sang Piao Xiao (Oötheca Mantidis), etc.

(2) Vertigo, dizziness and blurred vision induced by insufficiency of the Liver and Kidney. Used either alone as a powder or together with Gou Qi Zi (Fructus Lycii), Shu Di (Radix Rehmanniae Praeparata), etc.

Administration 10～20g for making a decoction.

Precautions Contraindicated for Yin deficiency with excessive Fire and dysuria.

3. Drugs for Tonifying Blood

Drugs of this group are mostly sweet in flavor, warm in nature, and are capable of tonifying Blood. They are indicated for Blood Deficiency syndromes such as sallow complexion, pale lips and tongue, dizziness, palpitation, insomnia, as well as delayed menstruation with scanty and pale blood or even amenorrhea. Some of these drugs can also invigorate Yin and therefore they can be used for Yin Deficiency syndromes.

As "Qi can help generate Blood", so drugs for tonifying Qi can be used to strengthen the function of tonifying Blood; on the other hand, Blood Deficiency often leads to Yin Deficiency, and drugs for tonifying Yin is usually used in combination for treating Blood Deficiency complicated by Yin Deficiency.

Moiturizing and greasy in property, drugs for tonifying Blood could enhance Dampness and impede the Stomach, for this reason, they should not be used for retention of Dampness in the Middle-jiao marked by distension and stuffiness in the Stomach and abdomen with anorexia and loose stools. For asthenia of the Spleen and Stomach, drugs for strengthening the Spleen and Stomach and for digestion can be applied in small quantity in combination.

3. 1. Dang Gui (Radix Angelicae Sinensis)

Description The dried root of Angelica sinensis (oliv.) Diels. Family Umbelliferae.

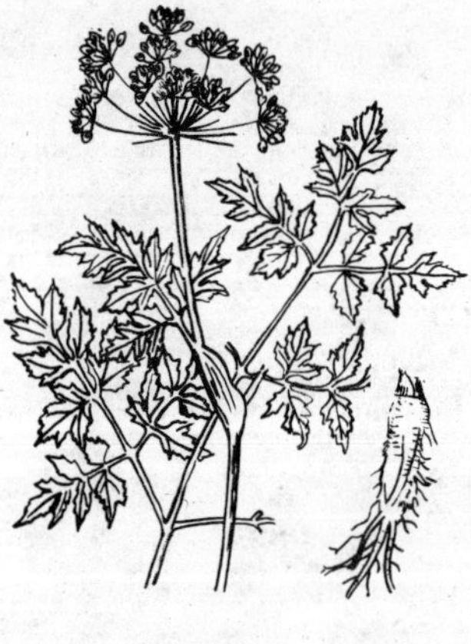

Characteristics Sweet and acrid in flavor, warm in nature, acting on the Heart, Liver and Spleen Channels.

Action Tonifying Blood, activating Blood circulation, relieving pain and moisturizing the bowels.

Indications

(1) Blood Deficiency marked by dizziness, palpitation, sallow complexion, pale lips and nails, etc. For treatment, it is used together with Shu Di (Radix Rehmanniae

Praeparata),Bai Shao (Radix Paeoniae Alba),etc. ,as in Siwu Tang (Decoction of Four Ingredients);for Blood Deficiency and Qi weakness, used with large amount of Huang Qi (Radix Astragali seu Hedysari) to promote Qi flow and generate Blood, as in Danggui Buxue Tang (Decoction of Radix Angelicae Sinensis for Tonifying Blood).

(2) Irregular menstruation, amenorrhea and menorrhalgia. In the case caused by Blood Deficiency, it is used with Shu Di (Radix Rehmanniae), Bai Shao (Radix Paeoniae Alba), etc. , as in Siwu Tang (Decoction of Four Ingredients);in the case due to Blood stasis, used with Tao Ren (Semen Persicae), Hong Hua (Flos Carthami),etc. ,as in Tao Hong Siwu Tang (Decoction of Four Ingredients plus Semen Persicae and Flos Carthami);in the case of accompanying Qi stagnation, used with Xiang Fu (Rhizoma Cyperi), Chai Hu (Radix Bupleuri),etc. ; in the case induced by Blood Deficiency with Cold invasion, used with Rou Gui (Cortex Cinnamomi), Pao Jiang (Rhizoma Zingiberis),etc. , as in Wenjing Tang (Decoction for Warming the Channels);in the case of accompanying Heat in the Blood, used with Mu Dan Pi (Cortex Moutan Radicis), Huang Qin (Radix Scutellariae),etc.

(3) Abdominal pain due to asthenic Cold, pain due to ecchymoma, traumatic injuries and rheumatic arthritis. For abdominal pain due to asthenic Cold, usually used with Gui Zhi (Ramulus Cinnamomi), Bai Shao (Radix Paeoniae Alba), Sheng Jiang (Rhizoma Zingiberis Recens), etc. , as in Danggui Jianzhong Tang (Decoction of Radix Angelicae for Strengthening the Middle-jiao);for limb pain due to Blood stasis, used with Ru Xiang (Olibanum), Mo Yao (Myrrha), etc. , as in Huoluo Xiaoling Dan (Effective Bolus for Activating Energy Flow in Channels) ; for traumatic injuries, usually used with Dai Huang (Radix et Rhizoma Rhei), Tao Ren (Semen Persicae), Hong Hua (Flos Carthami),etc. , as in Fuyuan Huoxue Tang (Decoction for Recovery and Activating Blood Circulation);for rheumatic arthralgia of the shoulders and arms, used with Qiang Huo (Rhizoma seu Radix Noto-pterygii), Fang Feng (Radix Ledebouriellae), Jiang Huang (Rhizoma Curcumae Longae), etc. , as in Juanbi Tang

(Decoction for Treating Rheumatic or Rheumatoid Arthritis).

(4) Suppurative skin infections. At the initial stage, used with Jin Yin Hua (Flos Lonicerae), Chi Shao (Radix Paeoniae Rubra), etc., as in Xianfang Huoming Yin (Fairy Decoction for Treating Cutaneous Infections); for non-rupture of the abscesses, used with Huang Qi (Radix Astragali seu Hedysari), Zao Jiao Ci (Spina Gleditsiae), etc., as in Tounong San (Powder for Promoting Discharge of Pus); for slow-healing ulcerations long after the rupture, used with Ren Shen (Radix Ginseng), Shu Di (Radix Rehmanniae Praeparata), etc., as in Shiquan Dabu Tang (Decoction of Ten Powderful Tonics).

(5) Constipation due to Blood Deficiency and Dryness of the Intestines. Usually used with Rou Cong Rong (Herba Cistanchis), Huo Ma Ren (Fructus Cannabis), etc.

Administration 5～15g for making a decoction. Unprocessed for tonifying Blood and moiturizing the Intestines; stir-fried with wine for regulating Meridians and activating Blood circulation.

Precautions Contraindicated for excessive Dampness in the Middle-jiao and loose stools.

3. 2. Shu Di (Radix Rehmanniae Praeparata)

Description The prepared root of Rehmannia glutinosa Libosch. Family Scrophulariaceae.

Characteristics Sweet in flavor, slightly warm in nature, acting on the Liver and Kidney Channels.

Action Tonifying the Blood and Yin, and replenishing the vital essence and marrow.

Indications

(1) Blood Deficiency marked by sallow complexion, irregular menstruation, palpitation, insomnia, metrorrhagia and metrostaxis. For treatment, it is used with Dang Gui (Radix Angelicae Sinensis), Bai Shao (Radix Paeoniae Alba), Chuan Xiong (Rhizoma Ligustici Chuanxiong), etc., as in Siwu Tang (Decoction of Four Ingredients).

(2) Insufficiency of Kidney-Yin marked by soreness and flaccidity of the loins and knees, hectic fever, night sweat, seminal emission or

diabetes. Usually used with Shan Yao (Rhizoma Dioscoreae), Shan Zhu Yu (Fructus Corni), etc., as in Liuwei Dihuang Wan (Bolus of Six Drugs Including Radix Rehmanniae Praeparata).

(3) Deficiency of the vital essence and Blood manifested by dizziness, blurred vision, tinnitus, deafness, premature grey hair, etc. Usually used with He Shou Wu (Radix Polygoni Multiflori), Nü Zhen Zi (Fructus Ligustri Lucidi), Han Lian Cao (Herba Ecliptae), Shan Zhu Yu (Fructus Corni), etc.

Administration 10～30g for making a decoction.

Precautions Contraindicated for Qi stagnation with profuse Phlegm, distending pain of the Stomach and abdomen, anorexia or loose stools.

3.3 He Shou Wu (Radix Polygoni Multiflori)

Description The root tuber of Polygonum multiflorum Thunb. Family Polygonaceae.

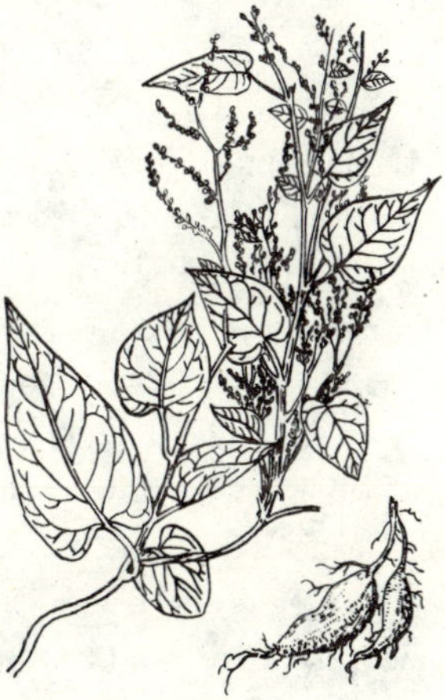

Characteristics Bitter, sweet and astringent in flavor, slightly warm in nature, acting on the Liver and Kidney Channels.

Action Tonifying the vital essence and Blood, arresting malaria, detoxicating and moisturizing the intestines to relieve constipation.

Indications

(1) Insufficiency of the Liver and Kidney, Deficiency of the vital essence and Blood manifested as dizziness, blurred vision, premature grey hair, aching of the loins with weakness of the feet, seminal emission, metrorrhagia, etc. For treatment, it is used with Dang Gui (Radix Angelicae Sinensis), Gou Qi Zi (Fructus Lycii), Tu Si Zi (Semen Cuscutae), etc., as in Qibao Meiran Dan (Hair Beauty Pill of Seven Precious Drugs).

(2) Intractable malaria. Used with Ren Shen (Radix Ginseng),

Dang Gui (Radix Angelicae Sinensis), etc., as in He Ren Yin (Decoction of Radix Polygoni Multiflori and Radix Ginseng).

(3) Scrofula and sores. For scrofula, used with Xia Ku Cao (Spica Prunellae), Tu Bei Mu (Bulbus Fritillariae Thunbergii), etc.; for pyogenic skin infections with swelling, pain and itching all over the body, used with Fang Feng (Radix Ledebouriellae), Ku Shen (Radix Sophorae Flavescentis), etc.

(4) Constipation due to Blood insufficiency and Dryness of the Intestines. Usually used with Dang Gui (Radix Angelicae Sinensis), Huo Ma Ren (Fructus Cannabis), etc.

Administration 10～30g for making a decoction. Processed for tonifying the vital essence and Blood; unprocessed for arresting malaria, detoxication and moisturizing the Intestines; fresh root is especially effective for detoxication and moisturizing the Intestines.

Precautions Not used for loose stools or severe Phlegm-Dampness.

3. 4. Bai Shao (Radix Paeoniae Alba)

Description The dried root of Paeonia lactiflora Pall. Family Ranunculaceae.

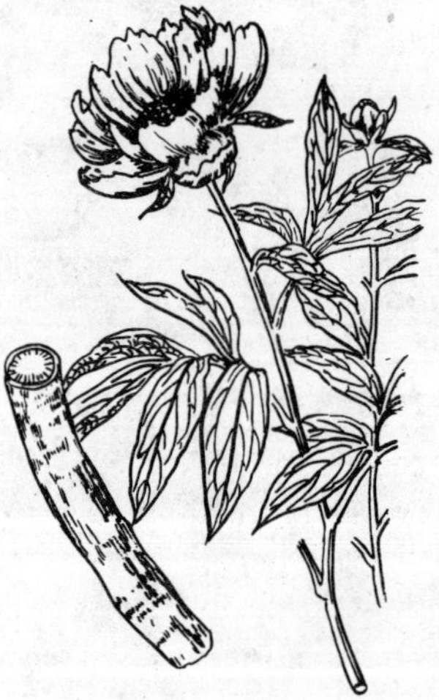

Characteristics Bitter and sour in flavor, slightly cold in nature, acting on the Liver and Spleen Channels.

Action Tonifying Blood, astringing Yin, nourishing Liver to relieve pain and suppressing the Liver-Yang.

Indications

(1) Blood Deficiency marked by irregular menstruation, dysmenorrhea, metrorrhagia, metrostaxis, etc. For treatment, it is used with Dang Gui (Radix Angelicae Sinensis), Chuan Xiong (Rhizoma Ligustici Chuanxiong), Shu Di

(Radix Rehmanniae Praeparata), etc., as in Siwu Tang (Decoction of Four Ingredients).

(2) Derangement of Ying and Wei marked by spontaneous sweating due to superficies Deficiency, or night sweat due to Yin Deficiency. For the former, it is used with Gui Zhi (Ramulus Cinnamomi), Sheng Jiang (Rhizoma Zingiberis Recens), Da Zao (Fructus Ziziphi Jujubae), etc. ; for the latter, it is used with Long Gu (Os Draconis), Mu Li (Concha Ostreae), etc.

(3) Pain of the chest, hypochondrium, Stomach and abdomen induced by disorder of Liver-Qi, or spasm and pain in the limbs. For treating hypochondriac pain due to Blood Deficiency and stagnation of the Liver-Qi, used with Dang Gui (Radix Angelicae Sinensis), Chai Hu (Radix Bupleuri), etc., as in Xiaoyao San (Ease Powder) ; for Stomachache, abdominal pain and spasm of the limbs caused by either disharmony between Liver and Spleen or lack of nutrients due to Blood Deficiency, used with Gan Cao (Radix Glycyrrhizae), as in Shaoyao Gancao Tang (Decoction of Radix Paeoniae Alba and Radix Glycyrrhizae); for abdominal pain with diarrhea, used together with Bai Zhu (Rhizoma Atractylodis Macrocephalae), Ju Pi (Pericarpium Citri Reticulatae) and Fang Feng (Radix Ledebouriellae), as in Tongxie Yaofang (Prescription of Importance for Diarrhea with Pain); for dysentery with abdominal pain, used with Mu Xiang (Radix Aucklandiae), Bing Lang (Semen Arecae), Huang Lian (Rhizoma Coptidis), etc., as in Shaoyao Tang (Decoction of Radix Paeoniae Alba).

(4) Headache, dizziness, etc. due to insufficiency of Liver-Yin and hyperactivity of Liver-Yang. Usually used with Sheng Di (Radix Rehmanniae), Niu Xi (Radix Achyranthis Bidentatae), Dai Zhe Shi (Ochra), etc., as in Jianling Tang (Sweeping Down Decoction for Hypertension).

Administration 5～10g, or 30g in a large dosage, for making a decoction. Unprocessed for astringing Yin and calming the Liver; stir-fried for nourishing Liver to relieve pain. When stir-fried with wine, it is less cold in nature.

Precautions Not used alone for Yang exhaustion with asthenic

Cold. Antagonistic to Li Lu (Radix Veratri).

3.5. E Jiao (Colla Corii Asini)

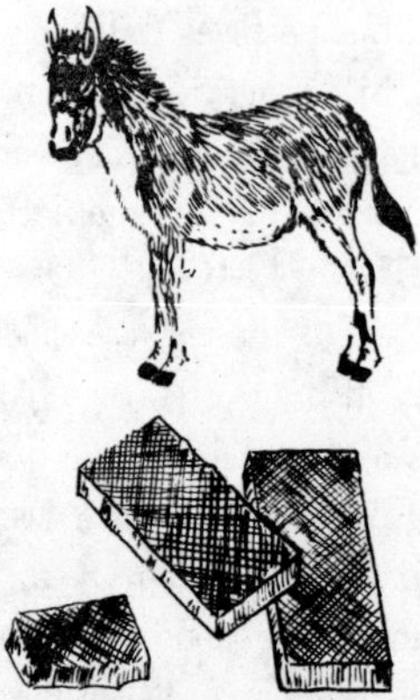

Description Donkey hide stewed and concentrated as gelatinous masses, of Equus asinus L. Family Equidae.

Characteristics Sweet in flavor, neutral in nature, acting on the Lung, Liver and Kidney Channels.

Action Tonifying the Blood, stopping bleeding, nourishing Yin and moisturizing the Lung.

Indications

(1) Vertigo, palpitation, etc. due to Blood Deficiency. This drug is very effective for tonifying Blood and it is usually used with Dang Shen (Radix Codonopsis Pilosulae), Dang Gui (Radix Angelicae Sinensis), etc.

(2) Loss of Blood due to Deficiency. This drug is very effective for bleeding complicated by Blood Deficiency and it can be used alone or in combination with other drugs. For treating hematemesis, epistaxis and hemoptysis due to Yin Deficiency and Blood Heat, it is used with Sheng Di (Radix Rehmanniae), Mai Dong (Radix Ophiopogonis), etc. ; for metrorrhagia and metrostaxis or profuse menstruation due to Deficiency and impairment of the Chong and Ren Channels, used with Ai Ye (Folium Artemisiae Argyi), Dang Gui (Radix Angelicae Sinensis), etc., as in Jiao Ai Tang (Decoction of Colla Corii Asini and Folium Artemisiae Argyi); for hematemesis, hemafecia, metrorrhagia and metrostaxis of asthenic Cold type, used with Zao Xin Tu (Terra Flava Usta), Fu Zi (Radix Aconiti Praeparata), etc., as in Huangtu Tang (Decoction of Baked Yellow Earth).

(3) Vexation and insomnia due to Yin Deficiency with excessive Fire. Usually used with Huang Lian (Rhizoma Coptidis), Bai Shao

(Radix Paeoniae Alba), etc., as in Huanglian Ejiao Tang (Decoction of Rhizoma Coptidis and Colla Corii Asini).

(4) Cough due to either Yin Deficiency or Lung Dryness. For cough, dyspnea, dry throat, scanty or bloody sputum due to Lung Deficiency and Fire Excess, used with Ma Dou Ling (Fructus Aristolochiae), Xing Ren (Semen Armeniacae Amarum), etc., as in Bufei Ejiao Tang (Decoction of Colla Corii Asini for Replenishing the Lung); for impairment of the Lung-Yin by Dryness manifested as dry cough without sputum, asthma, vexation, thirst, dry nose and throat, used with Sheng Shi Gao (Gypsum Fibrosum), Sang Ye (Folium Mori), etc., as in Qingzao Jiufei Tang (Decoction for Moisturizing Dryness in the Lung).

Administration 5～10g dissolved in boiled hot water or millet wine for oral intake. Unprocessed for tonifying Yin and moisturizing Dryness; stir-fried with Pu Huang (Pollen Typhae) for arresting bleeding; stir-fried with the powder of clam shell for moisturizing the Lung.

Precautions As it is sticky and greasy in property, this drug is likely to impede digestion and therefore, it should not be used for Spleen Deficiency with anorexia or vomiting and diarrhea. In addition, bleeding of the sthenic Heat type or bleeding with stagnation or stasis of Blood can not be applied to.

4. Drugs for Tonifying Yin

Drugs of this group are mostly sweet in flavor, cold or cool in nature, and capable of tonifying Yin and Body-Fluid, promoting the production of Body-Fluid to moisturize the Dryness, etc. They are indicated for dry cough with little sputum, Dryness of the mouth and tongue due to Deficiency of Lung-Yin; dry throat and thirst with red tongue and scanty tongue coat due to insufficiency of Stomach-Yin; blurred vision and xenophthalmia of the eyes, dizziness and tinnitus due to insufficiency of Liver-Yin; soreness and lassitude of the loins and knees, seminal emission and night sweat, etc. due to insufficiency of Kidney-Yin.

As these drugs are usually sweet, cold, moisturizing and greasy in property, and therefore they should not be used for asthenic Cold of the Spleen and Stomach, retention of the Phlegm-Dampness in the interior or abdominal distension with loose stools.

4. 1. Bei Sha Shen (Radix Glehniae)

Description The root of Glehnia littoralis Fr. Schmidt ex Miq. Family Umbelliferae.

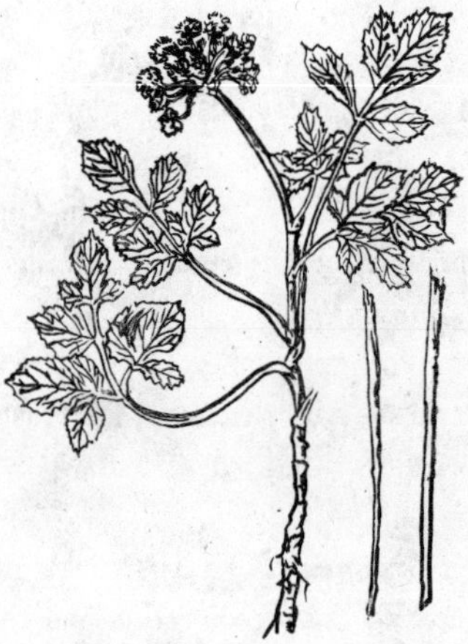

Characteristics Sweet in flavor, slightly cold in nature, acting on the Lung and Stomach Channels.

Action Clearing away Heat from the Lung, tonifying Yin, reinforcing the Stomach and promoting the production of Body-Fluid.

Indications

(1) Yin Deficiency and Heat in the Lung marked by dry cough with little sputum, or phthisical cough and hemoptysis. For the treatment of the former, it is used together with Mai Dong (Radix Ophiopogonis), Yu Zhu (Rhizoma Polygonati Odorati), Sang Ye (Folium Mori), etc., as in Shashen Maidong Tang (Decoction of Radix Glehniae and Radix Ophiopogonis); for the latter, used with Zhi Mu (Rhizoma Anemarrhenae), Mai Dong (Radix Ophiopogonis), Bie Jia (Carapax Trionycis), etc.

(2) Dry throat and thirst due to impairment of Yin by febrile diseases. Usually used with Mai Dong (Radix Ophiopogonis), Sheng Di (Radix Rehmanniae), etc., as in Yiwei Tang (Decoction for Replenishing Stomach).

Administration 10～15g for making a decoction.

Precautions Contraindicated for asthenic Cold syndromes. Antagonistic to Li Lu (Radix Veratri).

4.2. Mai Men Dong (Radix Ophiopogonis)

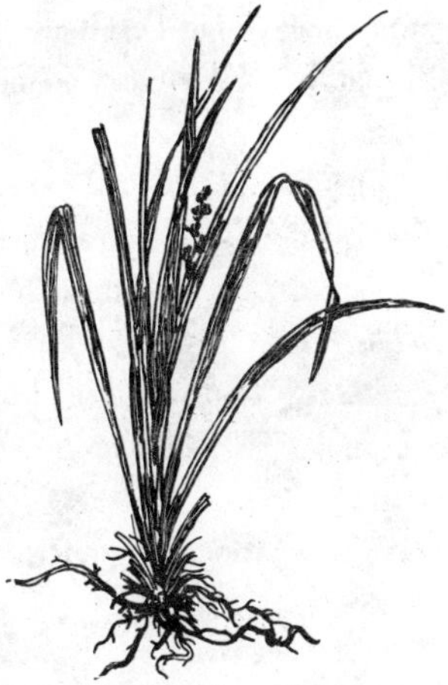

Description The root tuber of Ophiopogon japonicus (Thunb.) Ker-Gawl. Family Liliaceae.

Characteristics Sweet and slightly bitter in flavor, slightly cold in nature, acting on the Lung, Heart and Stomach Channels.

Action Moisturizing the Lung and tonifying Yin, replenishing the Stomach, promoting the production of fluid, clearing away Heart-Fire to relieve vexation.

Indications

(1) Insufficiency of Lung-Yin marked by dry cough with thick sputum, or phthisical cough with hemoptysis, etc. For treating Yin Deficiency with Heat invasion marked by dry cough with little sputum, it is used with Sang Ye (Folium Mori), Xing Ren (Semen Armeniacae Amarum), etc., as in Qingzao Jiufei Tang (Decoction for Relieving Dryness of the Lung); for Deficiency of Lung-Yin marked by phthisical cough with hemoptysis, used with Tian Men Dong (Radix Asparagi), as in Erdong Gao (Extract of Radix Ophiopogonis and Radix Asparagi).

(2) Dry tongue and thirst due to insufficiency of Stomach-Yin. Usually used with Sha Shen (Radix Glehniae), Sheng Di (Radix Rehmanniae), etc., as in Yiwei Tang (Decoction for Replenishing Stomach).

(3) Vexation and insomnia. In case they are induced by invasion of the Heart and Ying system by Heat, it is used with Huang Lian (Rhizoma Coptidis), Dan Shen (Radix Salviae Miltiorrhizae), Dan Zhu Ye (Herba Lophatheri), etc, as in Qingying Tang (Decoction for

Clearing Away Heat in the Ying System); for those induced by Yin Deficiency with Heat in the interior, used with Xuan Shen (Radix Scrophulariae), Sheng Di (Radix Rehmanniae), Suan Zao Ren (Semen Ziziphi Spinosae), etc., as in Tianwang Buxin Dan (Cardiotonic Pill).

(4) Constipation due to Dryness in the intestines. Usually used with Sheng Di (Radix Rehmanniae) and Xuan Shen (Radix Scrophulariae), named Zengye Tang (Fluid-increasing Decoction).

Administration 10～15g for making a decoction.

Precautions Contraindicated for cough due to either affection of exopathogenic Wind-Cold or retention of Phlegm-Dampness in the Lung.

4.3. Tian Men Dong (Radix Asparagi)

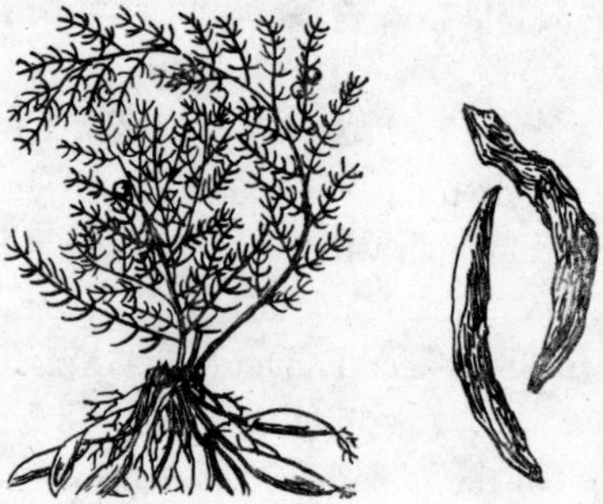

Description The dried root tuber of Asparagus cochinchinensis (Lour.) Merr. Family liliaceae.

Characteristics Sweet and bitter in flavor, extremely cold in nature, acting on the Lung and Kidney Channels.

Action Clearing away Fire in the Lung, nourishing Yin and moisturizing the Dryness.

Indications

(1) Dry cough with thick sputum and difficult expectoration due to Heat in the Lung, or phthisical cough with hemoptysis. For treatment, it is used with Mai Men Dong (Radix Ophiopogonis), as in Erdong Gao (Extract of Radix Asparagi and Radix Ophiopogonis).

(2) Dry tongue and thirst induced by consumption of Yin by febrile diseases and Deficiency of Body-Fluid. Used with Ren Shen (Radix Ginseng) and Sheng Di (Radix Rehmanniae), named Sancai Tang (Decoction of Three Drugs for Increasing Body-Fluid).

(3) Yin Deficiency with Excessive Fire, tidal fever and night sweat, seminal emission, etc. Used with Shu Di (Radix Rehmanniae Praeparata) and Huang Bo (Cortex Phellodendri), as in Sancai Fengsui Dan (Bolus of Three Drugs for Consolidating the Essence).

(4) Constipation due to Dryness of the Intestines. Usually used with Sheng Di (Radix Rehmanniae), Dang Gui (Radix Angelicae Sinensis), etc.

Administration 6～15g for making a decoction.

Precautions Contraindicated for asthenic Cold of the Spleen and Stomach, anorexia and loose stools.

4. 4. Yu Zhu (Rhizoma Polygonati Odorati)

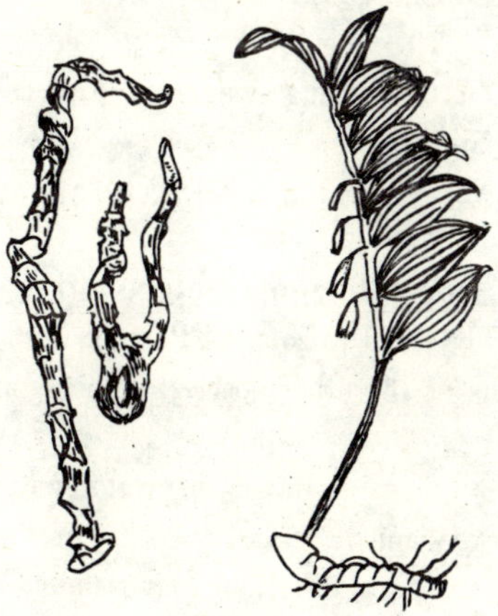

Description The dried rhizome of Polygonatum odoratum (Mill.) Druce. Family Liliaceae.

Characteristics Sweet in flavor, neutral in nature, acting on the Lung and Stomach Channels.

Action Nourishing Yin and moisturizing the Lung, promoting the production of Body-Fluid to replenish Stomach.

Indications

(1) Consumption of Lung-Yin and Stomach-Yin, cough induced by Dryness and Heat, dry tongue and thirst. For treatment, it is used together with Sha Shen (Radix Glehniae), Mai Dong (Radix Ophiopogonis), etc., as in Yuzhu Maidong Tang (Decoction of Rhizoma Polygonati Odorati and Radix Ophiopogonis); for late-stage epidemic diseases, when consumption of Stomach-Yin leads to Dryness of the mouth and tongue and anorexia, usually used together with Sha Shen (Radix Glehniae), Mai Dong (Radix Ophiopogonis) and Sheng Di (Radix Rehmanniae), as in Yiwei Tang (Decoction for Replenishing Stomach).

(2) Yin Deficiency with affection of Wind-Heat marked by headache, fever, cough, dry and sore throat, etc. Used with Bai Wei (Radix Cynanchi Atrati), Jie Geng (Radix Platycodi), Bo He (Herba Menthae), etc., as in Jiajian Weirui Tang (Modified Decoction of Rhizoma Polygonati Odorati).

Administration 10～15g for making a decoction. Unprocessed for replenishing Yin by clearing away Heat; processed for replenishing Yin by tonification.

Precautions Not used for Spleen Deficiency with Phlegm-Dampness.

4. 5. Huang Jing (Rhizoma Polygonati)

Description The dried rhizome of Polygonatum sibiricum Red., P. cyrtonema Hua or the other species of the same genus. Family Liliaceae.

Characteristics Sweet in flavor, neutral in nature, acting on the Spleen and Kidney Channels.

Action Moisturizing the Lung, nourishing Yin, replenishing Spleen and activating Qi circulation.

Indications

(1) Soreness and weakness of the loins and knees, dizziness and tinnitus, premature grey hair, etc. due to Deficiency of Kidney and consumption of the vital essence. For treatment, it is usually used with Shu Di (Radix Rehmanniae Praeparata), Gou Qi Zi (Fructus

Lycii),etc.

(2) Deficiency and weakness of the Spleen and Stomach with lassitude, anorexia, weak pulse, etc. Usually used with Dang Shen (Radix Codonopsis Pilosulae) and Fu Ling (Poria). In the case of Deficiency of Spleen-Yin and Stomach-Yin with dry mouth and anorexia, constipation and red tongue without tongue coat, used with Sha Shen (Radix

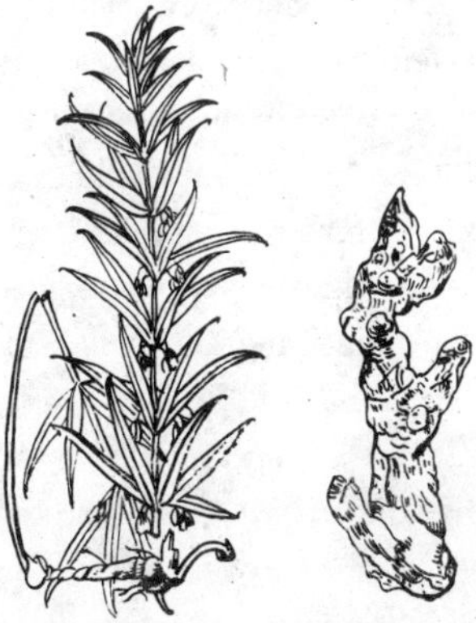

Glehniae), Mai Dong (Radix Ophiopogonis), etc. In addition, this drug can be used to treat diabetes by adding Huang Qi (Radix Astragali seu Hedysari), Tian Hua Fen (Radix Trichosanthis), etc.

Administration 10～20g, or 30～60g of fresh rhizome, for making a decoction.

Precautions Not applied to Spleen Deficiency with Dampness, cough with profuse sputum or loose stools due to Cold invasion of the Middle-jiao.

4.6. Bai He (Bulbus Lilii)

Description The scale leaf of the bulb of Lilium lancifolium Thunb. or several species of the same genus. Family Liliaceae.

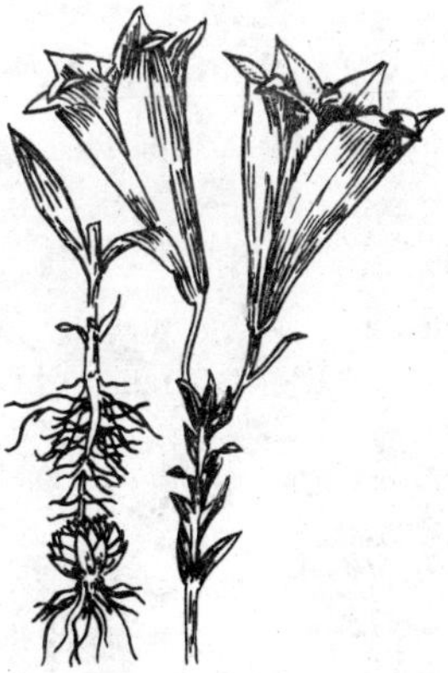

Characteristics Sweet in flavor, slightly cold in nature, acting on the Lung and Heart Channels.

Action Moisturizing the Lung to relieve cough, clearing away Heart-Fire to tranquilize the mind.

Indications

(1) Cough due to Heat in the Lung, phthisical cough with hemoptysis, etc. For chronic cough with bloody sputum due to Heat in the Lung, it is used with Kuan Dong Hua (Flos Farfarae), named Bai Hua Gao (Extract of Bulbus Lilii and Flos Farfarae); for phthisical cough with hemoptysis and sore throat, used together with Sheng Di (Radix Rehmanniae), Xuan Shen (Radix Scrophulariae), etc., as in Baihe Gujin Tang (Decoction of Bulbus Lilii for Strengthening the Lung).

(2) Late-stage febrile diseases with lingering fever, fidgetiness due to Deficiency, fright-induced palpitation, insomnia and dreaminess. Used with Zhi Mu (Rhizoma Anemarrhenae) or Sheng Di (Radix Rehmanniae), as in Baihe Zhimu Tang (Decoction of Bulbus Lilii and Rhizoma Anemarrhenae) and Baihe Dihuang Tang (Decoction of Bulbus Lilii and Radix Rehmanniae).

Administration 10～30g for making a decoction. Unprocessed for clearing away Heart-Fire; processed for moisturizing the Lung.

Precautions Not applied to cough due to Wind-Cold or loose stools due to Cold in the Middle-jiao.

4.7. Gou Qi Zi (Fructus Lycii)

Description The dried ripe fruit of Lycium barbarum L. Family Solanaceae.

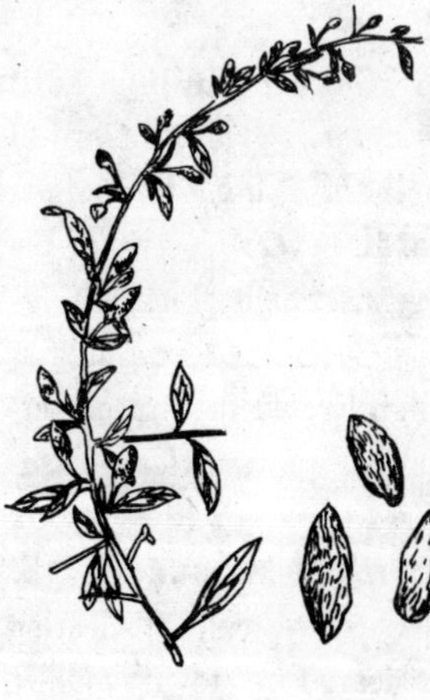

Characteristics Sweet in flavor, neutral in nature, acting on the Liver, Kidney and Lung Channels.

Action Replenishing the Liver and Kidney, moisturizing the Lung and improving the acuity of vision.

Indications

(1) Deficiency of Liver-Yin and Kidney-Yin marked by lassitude of the loins and knees, dizziness, tinnitus, seminal emission, diabetes, etc. For treatment, it is

used either alone by chewing and eating the steamed fruit or together with Sheng Di (Radix Rehmanniae), Shu Di (Radix Rehmanniae Praeparata), Tian Men Dong (Radix Asparagi), etc.

(2) Insufficiency of Liver and Kidney marked by dizzinesss and blurred vision. Usually used with Ju Hua (Flos Chrysanthemi), Shu Di (Radix Rehmanniae Praeparata), etc., as in Qi Ju Dihuang Wan (Bolus of Fructus Lycii, Flos Chrysanthemi and Radix Rehmanniae Praeparata).

(3) Phthisical cough due to Yin Deficiency. Usually used with Mai Dong (Radix Ophiopogonis), Zhi Mu (Rhizoma Anemarrhenae), etc.

Administration 5～10g for making a decoction.

Precautions Not applied to Spleen Deficiency with loose stools.

4.8. Gui Ban (Plastrum Testudinis)

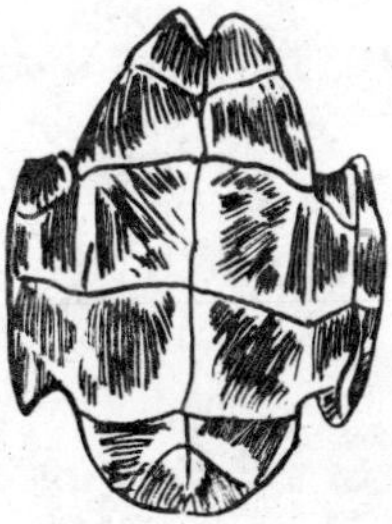

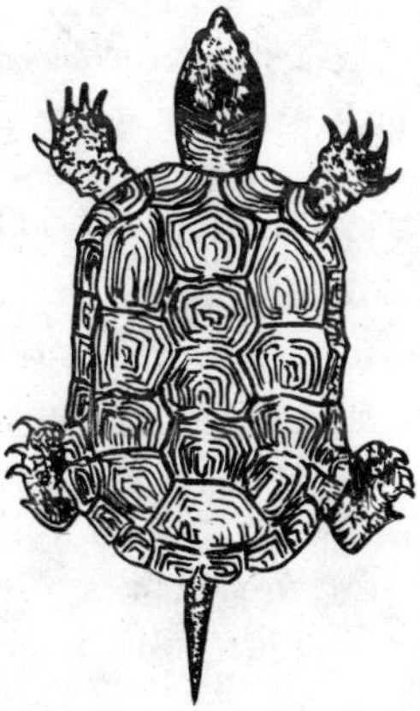

Description The plastron of Chinemys reevesii (Gray). Family Testudinidae.

Characteristics Sweet and salty in flavor, cold in nature, acting on the Liver, Kidney and Heart Channels.

Action Nourishing Yin and suppressing Yang, replenishing the Kidney, strengthening the bones, tonifying Blood and Heart, regulating menstruation and relieving metrorrhagia.

Indications

(1) Yin Deficiency and Yang Excess, Yin Deficiency with excessive Fire or consumption of Yin by febrile diseases and up-stirring of asthenic Wind. For treating Yin Deficiency and Yang Excess manifested as dizziness and vertigo, it is used with Tian Dong (Radix Asparagi), Xuan Shen (Radix Scrophulariae), Long Gu (Os Draconis), Mu Li (Concha Ostreae), etc., as in Zhengan Xifeng Tang (Decoction for Tranquilizing Liver-Wind); for Yin Deficiency with excessive Fire marked by hectic fever and night sweat, used with Zhi Mu (Rhizoma Anemarrhenae), Huang Bo (Cortex Phellodendri), etc., as in Da Buyin Wan (Major Bolus for Replenishing Yin); for consumption of Yin by Heat and up-stirring of asthenic Wind in the interior marked by convulsion of the extremities, usually used with Bai Shao (Radix Paeoniae Alba), Bie Jia (Carapax Trionycis), etc., as in Da Dingfeng Zhu (Great Pearl for Wind Syndrome).

(2) Deficiency of Kidney-Yin marked by flaccidity of the loins and feet, weakness of the tendons and bones and infantile metopism. For treatment, it is used with Shu Di (Radix Rehmanniae Praeparata), Suo Yang (Herba Cynomorii), etc., as in Huqian Wan (Tiger Bone Pill for Checking Exuberance of Yang).

(3) Yin Deficiency and Heat in the Blood marked by profuse menstruation, metrorrhagia, metrostaxis, leucorrhagia, etc. Usually used with Bai Shao (Radix Paeoniae Alba), Huang Bo (Cortex Phellodendri), etc., as in Gujing Wan (Pill for Checking Menorrhagia).

(4) Deficiency of Heart marked by palpitation induced by fright, insomnia and forgetfulness. Usually used with Long Gu (Os Draconis), Yuan Zhi (Radix Polygalae), etc.

Administration 10～30g for making a decoction, crushed and decocted prior to other drugs.

Precautions Contraindicated for Deficiency of Spleen-Yang and Stomach-Yang. Used with caution for pregnant women.

4.9. Bie Jia (Carapax Trionycis)

Description The shell of Trionyx sinensis (Wiegmann). Family Trionychidae.

Characteristics Salty in flavor, cold in nature, acting on the Liver

Channels.

Action Nourishing Yin and suppressing Yang, softening hard masses and resolving lumps.

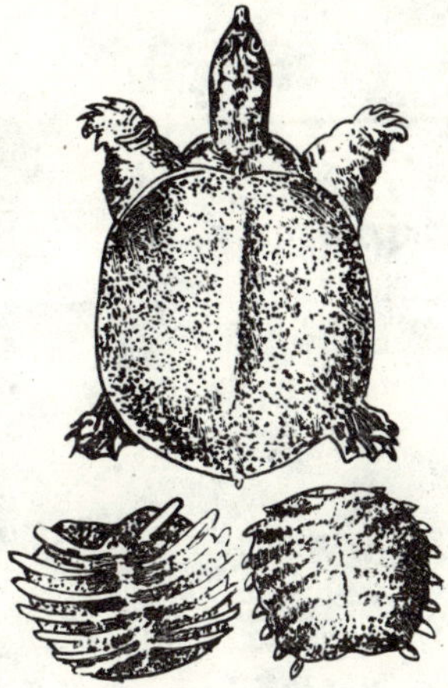

Indications

(1) Syndromes induced by Yin Deficiency and up-stirring of Wind. For treatment, it is used together with Mu Li (Concha Ostreae), Sheng Di (Radix Rehmanniae), etc., as in Erjia Fumai Tang (Pulse-restoring Decoction of Two Kinds of Shells).

(2) Fever due to Yin Deficiency. For treating Yin Deficiency with Heat in the interior marked by hectic fever and night sweat, used with Yin Chai Hu (Radix Stellariae), Di Gu Pi (Cortex Lycii Radicis), etc., as in Qinggu San (Powder for Clearing Away Internal Heat); for impairment of Yin by febrile diseases marked by night fever, red tongue with scanty tongue coat, used with Qing Hao (Herba Artemisiae Annuae), Sheng Di (Radix Rehmanniae), etc., as in Qinghao Biejia Tang (Decoction of Herba Artemisiae Annuae and Carapax Trionycis).

(3) Long-term malaria leading to splenomegaly, amenorrhea and mass in the abdomen. For malaria with splenomegaly, and costal pain, used with Chai Hu (Radix Bupleuri), Zhe Chong (Eupolyphaga seu Steleophaga), etc., as in Biejia Jian Wan (Pill of Carapax Trionycis).

Administration 10～30g for making a decoction, crushed and decocted prior to other drugs. Unprocessed for nourishing Yin and suppressing Yang; processed for softening the hard mass and resolving the lumps; scalded with sand for making pills or a powder.

Precautions Contraindicated for asthenic Cold of the Spleen and Stomach, poor appetite with loose stools or during pregnancy.

Astringents

Drugs whose principal action is arresting or reducing the excessive loss of the vital essence and Body-Fluid are referred to as astringents.

Most drugs of this category are sour or astringent in flavor and capable of strengthening the superficies to stop sweating, astringing the intestines to arrest diarrhea, keeping the Kidney essence to reduce urination, astringing the Lung to relieve cough, arresting bleeding and checking leucorrhagia, etc. They are chiefly indicated for weak constitution after long-term illness, spontaneous perspiration and night sweat, protracted diarrhea or dysentery, seminal emission, enuresis, frequent urination, metrorrhagia, metrostaxis, leucorrhagia, intractable cough and asthma of Deficiency nature, etc. induced by inconsolidation of the vital Qi.

As the root cause of the syndromes of incessant and excessive loss of the Body-Fluid and vital essence is Deficiency of the vital Qi, and prolonged illness will further consume Body-Fluid, vital essence and Blood and render the vital Qi more deficient, and therefore corresponding tonics should be applied in combination with astringents, so that the principal and secondary aspects can be treated at the same time. For example, Qi Deficiency with spontaneous perspiration should be treated by adding drugs for reinforcing Qi; Yin Deficiency with night sweat should be treated by adding drugs for tonifying Yin; Spleen Deficiency with chronic diarrhea should be treated by adding drugs for replenishing Spleen; while Kidney Deficiency with seminal emission should be treated by adding drugs for strengthening Kidney.

Astringents have the side effects of retaining the pathogenic factors, and for this reason, they should not be used alone for superficies-syndromes, retention of Dampness in the interior or lingering fever.

0. 1. Wu Wei Zi (Fructus Schisandrae)

Description The dried mature fruit of Schisandra chinensis (Turcz.) Baill., or Schisandra sphenanthera Rehd. et Wils. Family Magnoliaceae.

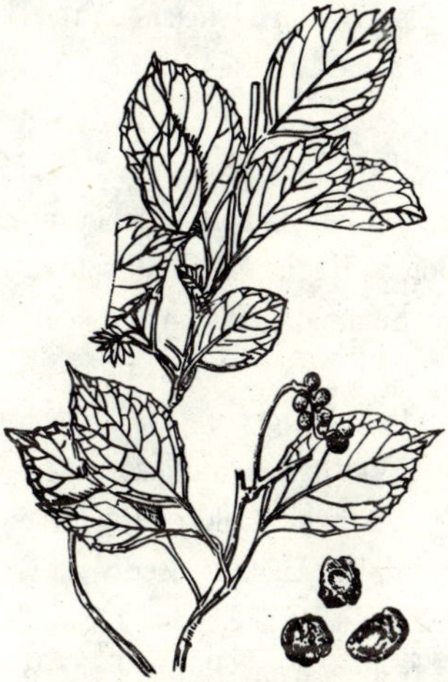

Characteristics Sour in flavor, warm in nature, acting on the Lung, Stomach and Heart Channels.

Action Astringing the Lung, tonifying the Kidney, promoting the production of Body-Fluid, arresting sweating, seminal emission and diarrhea, and tranquilizing the mind.

Indications

(1) Intractable cough and asthma of Deficiency nature. This drug is most effective for treating chronic cough and asthma of Deficiency nature induced by Deficiency of Lung and Kidney. For treating chronic cough due to Lung Deficiency, it is used together with Ying Su Ke (Pericarpium Papaveris), Wu Mei (Fructus Mume), etc; for dyspnea due to Kidney Deficiency, used with Shan Zhu Yu (Fructus Corni), Shu Di (Radix Rehmanniae Praeparata), etc., as in Douqi Wan (All converging Pill); for retention of Cold with affection of

pathogenic Wind-Cold, asthmatic cough, short breath and consumption of Lung, used with Xi Xin (Herba Asari), Gan Jiang (Rhizoma Zingiberis), etc., as in Xiao Qinglong Tang (Minor Decoction of Green Dragon).

(2) Thirst due to consumption of Body-Fluid, spontaneous sweating and night sweat. For treating impairment of Qi and Yin by Heat manifested as palpitation, weak pulse, thirst and profuse sweat, it is used with Ren Shen (Radix Ginseng) and Mai Dong (Radix Ophiopogonis), named Shengmai San (Pulse-activating Powder); for incessant sweating due to debility, used with Bai Zi Ren (Semen Biotae), Ren Shen (Radix Ginseng), Ma Huang Gen (Radix Ephedrae), Mu Li (Concha Ostreae), etc., as in Baiziren Wan (Semen Biotae Pill); for diabetes, used with Huang Qi (Radix Astragali seu Hedysari), Sheng Di (Radix Rehmanniae), Mai Dong (Radix Ophiopogonis), Tian Hua Fen (Radix Trichosanthis), etc., as in Huangqi Tang (Decoction of Radix Astragali seu Hedysari).

(3) Seminal emission and spermatorrhea due to Deficiency of Kidney. Used either alone or together with Sang Piao Xiao (Oötheca Mantidis), Long Gu (Os Draconis), etc., as in Sangpiaoxiao Wan (Pill of Oötheca Mantidis).

(4) Asthenic Cold of the Spleen and Kidney marked by diarrhea before dawn. Usually used with Bu Gu Zhi (Fructus Psoraleae), Wu Zhu Yu (Fructus Euodiae), Rou Dou Kou (Semen Myristicae), etc., as in Sishen Wan (Pill of Four Wonderful Drugs).

(5) Insufficiency of the Heart-Fire and Deficiency of the Kidney-Yin marked by fidget, palpitation, insomnia and dreaminess. For treatment, it is used with Sheng Di (Radix Rehmanniae), Mai Dong (Radix Ophiopogonis), Dan Shen (Radix Salviae Miltiorrhizae), Suan Zao Ren (Semen Ziziphi Spinosae), etc., as in Tianwang Buxin Dan (Cardiotonic Pill).

Administration 2～6g for making a decoction; 1～3g for taking as a powder.

Precautions Not applied to lingering superficies-syndromes, sthenic Heat in the interior, beginning of cough or onset of measles without complete eruption.

0.2. Wu Mei (Fructus Mume)

Description The smoked immature fruit (green plum) of Prunus mume (Sieb.) Sieb. et Zucc. Family Rosaceae.

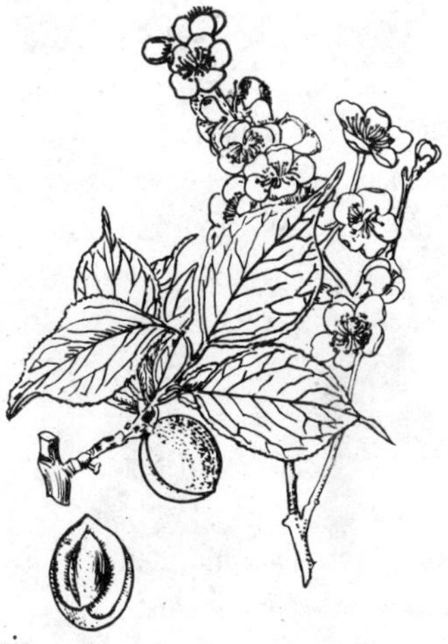

Characteristics Sour in flavor, neutral in nature, acting on the Liver, Spleen, Lung and Large Intestine Channels.

Action Astringing the Lung to relieve cough, astringing the Intestines to stop diarrhea, promoting the production of Body-Fluid to quench thirst, and normalizing the function of Stomach to alleviate colic caused by ascariasis.

Indications

(1) Chronic cough due to Deficiency of the Lung. For treatment, it is used with Ying Su Ke (Pericarpium Papaveris), Ban Xia (Rhizoma Pinelliae), Xing Ren (Semem Armeniacae Amarum), E Jiao (Colla Corii Asini), etc., as in Yifu San (Only One Dose Powder).

(2) Prolonged diarrhea and dysentery. Usually used with Rou Dou Kou (Semen Myristicae), Dang Shen (Radix Codonopsis Pilosulae), He Zi (Fructus Chebulae), etc., as in Guchang Wan (Pill for Consolidating the Intestines).

(3) Diabetes due to asthenic Heat. Usually used with Tian Hua Fen (Radix Trichosanthis), Mai Dong (Radix Ophiopogonis), Ge Gen (Radix Puerariae), Ren Shen (Radix Ginseng), etc., as in Yuquan Wan (Jade Spring Pill).

(4) Abdominal pain and vomiting induced by ascariasis. Usually used with Xi Xin (Herba Asari), Hua Jiao (Pericarpium Zanthoxyli), Gan Jiang (Rhizoma Zingiberis), Huang Lian (Rhizoma Coptidis), etc., as in Wumei Wan (Fructus Mume Bolus). In addition, oral use of this drug can stop bleeding and it is used for metror-

rhagia and metrostaxis; external use of it can subdue swellings and cure ophthalmic pterygium.

Administration 3~10g, 30g in a large dosage, for making a decoction; q. s. for external application. Carbonized for arresting bleeding and relieving diarrhea; unprocessed for promoting the production of Body-Fluid and relieving colic due to ascariasis.

Precautions Contraindicated for superficies-syndromes, sthenic Heat or stagnation in the interior.

0. 3. Shan Zhu Yu (Fructus Corni)

Description The dried ripe pulp of Cornus officinalis Sieb. et Zucc. Family Cornaceae.

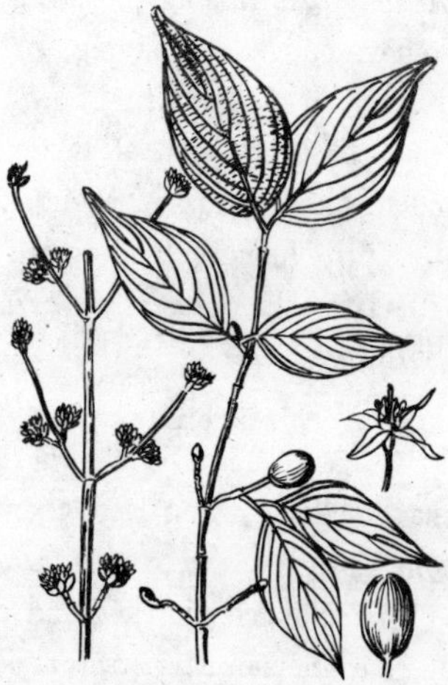

Characteristics Sour in flavor, slightly warm in nature, acting on the Liver and Kidney Channels.

Action Tonifying the Liver and Kidney and inducing astringency.

Indications

(1) Insufficiency of the Liver and Kidney marked by dizziness, lassitude of the loins and knees, impotence, seminal emission, incontinence of urine, etc. For treating Deficiency of the Liver-Yin and Kidney-Yin marked by dizziness and lassitude of the loins and knees, it is usually used together with Shu Di (Radix Rehmanniae Praeparata), Shan Yao (Rhizoma Dioscoreae), etc., as in Liuwei Dihuang Wan (Bolus of Six Ingredients Including Radix Rehmanniae Praeparata); for insufficiency of Kidney-Yang marked by impotence and seminal emission, used with Bu Gu Zhi (Fructus Psoraleae), Dang Gui (Radix Angelicae Sinensis), etc., as in Caohuan Dan (Pill for Treating Deficiency of Both the Liver and Kidney); for incontinence of urine, used with Sang Piao Xiao (Oötheca Mantidis), Fu Pen Zi (Fructus Rubi), etc.

(2) Profuse and incessant perspiration, severe dibility with impending collapse. Usually used with Ren Shen (Radix Ginseng), Fu Zi (Radix Aconiti Praeparata), Long Gu (Os Draconis), Mu Li (Concha Ostreae), etc.

(3) Profuse menstruation, metrorrhagia and metrostaxis. Used with Wu Zei Gu (Os Sepiae), Qian Cao Tan (Radix Rubiae Carbonisatus), Zong Lü Tan (Trachycarpi Carbonisatus), etc., as in Guchong Tang (Decoction for Reinforcing the Chong Channel).

Administration 5～10g, or 30g in a large dosage, for making a decoction.

Precautions Not used for hyperactivity of Liver-Yang, constitution of Damp-Heat or difficult micturition.

0. 4. Ma Huang Gen (Radix Ephedrae)

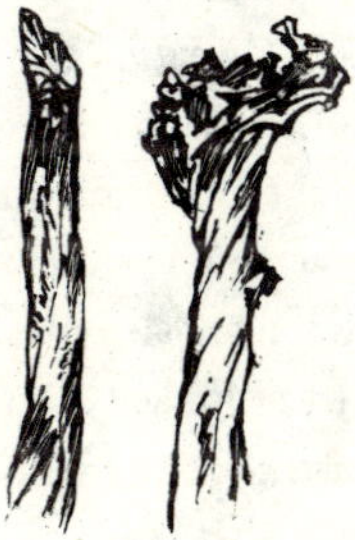

Description The dried root of Ephedrae sinica Stapf and E. intermedia Schrenk et C. A. Mey. Family Ephedraceae.

Characteristics Sweet in flavor, neutral in nature, acting on the Lung Channel.

Action Arresting sweating.

Indications All kinds of sweating of Deficiency nature. This drug is the key drug for relieving sweating. For treating spontaneous and incessant sweating, it is used with Dang Gui (Radix Angelicae Sinensis), Huang Qi (Radix Astragali seu Hedysari), etc., as in Mahuanggen San (Powder of Radix Ephedrae); for spontaneous sweating due to Yang Deficiency, usually used with Ren Shen (Radix Ginseng) and Fu Zi (Radix Aconiti Praeparata); for night sweat due to Yin Deficiency, used with Shu Di (Radix Rehmanniae Praeparata), Shan Zhu Yu (Fructus Corni), Long Gu (Os Draconis), Mu Li (Concha Ostreae), etc.; for postpartum sweating due to Deficiency, used with Huang Qi (Radix Astragali seu Hedysari) and Dang Gui (Radix Angelicae Sinensis).

Administration 3～10g for making a decoction; q. s. for external use as a powder.

Precautions Not used for superficies-syndromes.

0.5. Fu Xiao Mai (Fructus Tritici Levis)

Description The unripe caryopsis of Triticum aestivum L. Family Gramineae.

Characteristics Sweet in flavor, cool in nature, acting on the Heart Channel.

Action Activating Qi flow, clearing away Heat and arresting sweating.

Indications

(1) Spontaneous sweating and night sweat. It can be taken frequently after it is baked brown and ground to powder. It can also be used together with other drugs, e.g. used with Huang Qi (Radix Astragali seu Hedysari) and Wu Wei Zi (Fructus Schisandrae) for spontaneous sweating due to Deficiency of the superficies; used with Shan Yao (Rhizoma Dioscoreae), Shan Zhu Yu (Fructus Corni), etc. for night sweat due to Yin Deficiency.

(2) Hectic fever and consumptive fever. Used with Sheng Di (Radix Rehmanniae), Mai Dong (Radix Ophiopogonis), Di Gu Pi (Cortex Lycii Radicis), etc.

Administration 15～30g for making a decoction; 3～6g for making a powder after it is baked brown.

Precautions Not applied to superficies-syndromes.

0.6. He Zi (Fructus Chebulae)

Description The dried ripe fruit of Terminalia chebula Retz. or T. chebula Retz. var. tomentella Kurt. Family Combretaceae.

Characteristics Sour, bitter and astringent in flavor, neutral in nature, acting on the Lung and Large Intestine Channels.

Action Astringing the Intestines to stop diarrhea, astringing the Lung to relieve cough and lowering the adverse flow of Qi to ease the throat.

Indications

(1) Chronic diarrhea and dysentery. For treating long-term dysentery with abdominal pain and fever, it is used with Huang Lian (Rhizoma Coptidis), Mu Xiang (Radix Aucklandiae) and Gan Cao (Radix

Glycyrrhizae), as in Hezi San (Powder of Fructus Chebulae); for prolonged diarrhea due to asthenic Cold or prolapse of anus, used with Gan Jiang (Rhizoma Zingiberis), Ying Su Ke (Pericarpium Papaveris), etc.

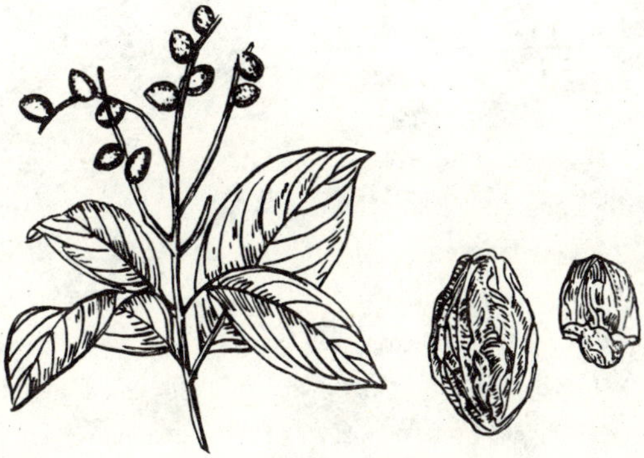

(2) Chronic cough due to Lung Deficiency or hoarseness. For cough and dyspnea due to Lung Deficiency, it is used with Dang Shen (Radix Codonopsis Pilosulae), Wu Wei Zi (Fructus Schisandrae), etc.; for stagnation of Phlegm-Fire in the Lung marked by chronic cough with loss of voice, used with Jie Geng (Radix Platycodi) and Gan Cao (Radix Glycyrrhizae), as in Hezi Tang (Decoction of Fructus Chebulae).

Administration 3～10g for making a decoction. Unprocessed for astringing the Lung to eliminate Fire; roasted for astringing the Intestines to arrest diarrhea.

Precautions Contraindicated for superficies-syndromes or Damp-Heat in the interior.

0.7. Rou Dou Kou (Semen Myristicae)

Description The dried seed of Myristica fragrans Houtt. Family Myristicaceae.

Characteristics Acrid in flavor, warm in nature, acting on the Spleen, Stomach and Large Intestine Channels.

Action Warming the Middle-jiao to activate the circulation of Qi, astringing the Intestines to arrest diarrhea.

Indications

(1) Prolonged and incessant diarrhea of asthenic Cold nature. For that induced by asthenic Cold in the Spleen and Stomach, it is used with Ren Shen (Radix Ginseng), Bai Zhu (Rhizoma Atractylodis Macrocephalae), Rou Gui (Cortex Cinnamomi), etc., as in Yangzang Tang (Decoction for Tonifying the Viscera); for chronic diarrhea, diarrhea before dawn due to Deficiency of the Spleen-Yang and Kidney-Yang, used with Bu Gu Zhi (Fructus Psoraleae), Wu Wei Zi (Fructus Schisandrae) and Wu Zhu Yu (Fructus Euodiae), named Sishen Wan (Pill of Four Wonderful Drugs); for long-term and incessant diarrhea accompanied with Qi stagnation and abdominal distension, used with Mu Xiang (Radix Aucklandiae), etc.

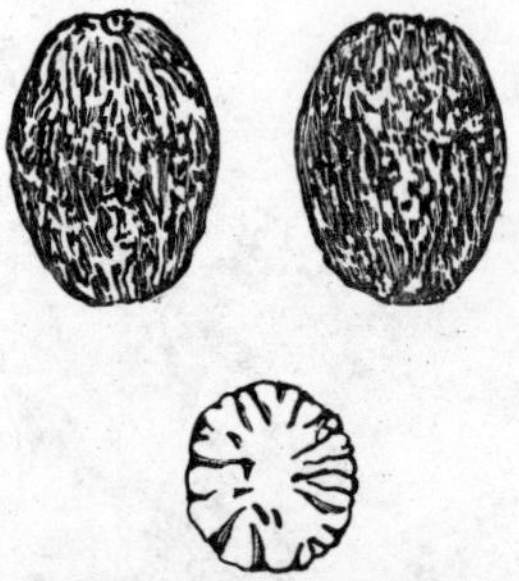

(2) Distending pain of the Stomach and abdomen, anorexia, vomiting, etc. induced by asthenic Cold and Qi stagnation. Usually used with Mu Xiang (Radix Aucklandiae), Gao Liang Jiang (Rhizoma Alpiniae Officinarum), etc.

Administration 3～10g for making a decoction; 1.5～3g for making a powder or pills. When processed, it can strengthen the function of warming the Middle-jiao to stop diarrhea.

Precautions Contraindicated for diarrhea and dysentery due to Damp-Heat.

0.8. Lian Zi (Semen Nelumbinis)

Description The dried ripe seed of Nelumbo nucifera Gaertn. Family Nymphaeaceae.

Characteristics Sweet and astringent in flavor, neutral in nature, acting on the Spleen, Kidney and Heart Channels.

Action Replenishing the Spleen to arrest diarrhea, tonifying the Kidney to control seminal emission, and nourishing the Heart to tranquilize the mind.

Indications

(1) Chronic diarrhea with anorexia due to Spleen Deficiency. For treatment, it is used together with Ren Shen (Radix Ginseng), Bai Zhu (Rhizoma Atractylodis Macrocephalae), etc., as in Shen Ling Baizhu San (Powder of Radix Ginseng, Poria and Rhizoma Atractylodis Macrocephalae).

(2) Seminal emission and spermatorrhea due to Kidney Deficiency. Used with Sha Yuan Zi (Semen Astragali Complanati), Long Gu (Os Draconis), etc., as in Jinsuo Gujing Wan (Golden Lock Pill for Keeping the Kidney Essence).

(3) Incoordination between the Heart and Kidney marked by palpitation and insomnia. Used with Mai Dong (Radix Ophiopogonis), Fu Ling (Poria), etc. In addition, it can be used for metrorrhagia, metrostaxis and leucorrhagia in women.

Administration 6～15g for making a decoction.

Precautions Not applied to dry stool or constipation.

0.9. Sang Piao Xiao (Oötheca Mantidis)

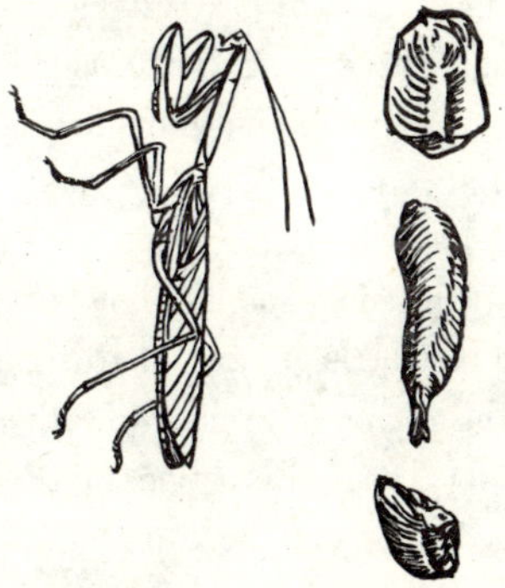

Description The dried oötheca of Tenodera sinensis Saussure. Family Mantidae.

Characteristics Sweet and salty in flavor, neutral in nature, acting on the Kidney Channel.

Action Tonifying the Kidney, strengthening Yang, preserving the essence and reducing urination.

Indications

(1) Enuresis, frequent urination, seminal emission due to inconsolidation of Kidney-Qi. For treating frequent urination, enuresis and seminal emission, it is used with Ren Shen (Radix Ginseng), Long Gu (Os Draconis), etc., as in Sangpiaoxiao San (Powder of Oötheca Mantidis); for seminal emission and whitish and turbid urine, used

with Long Gu (Os Draconis) (both powdered) and taken with salt water.

(2) Impotence. Usually used with Lu Rong (Cornu Cervi Pantotrichum), Tu Si Zi (Semen Cuscutae), etc.

Administration 3~10g for making a decoction.

Precautions Contraindicated for Yin Deficiency with excessive Fire or frequent urination due to Heat in the urinary bladder.

0. 10. Wu Zei Gu (Os Sepiella seu Sepiae)

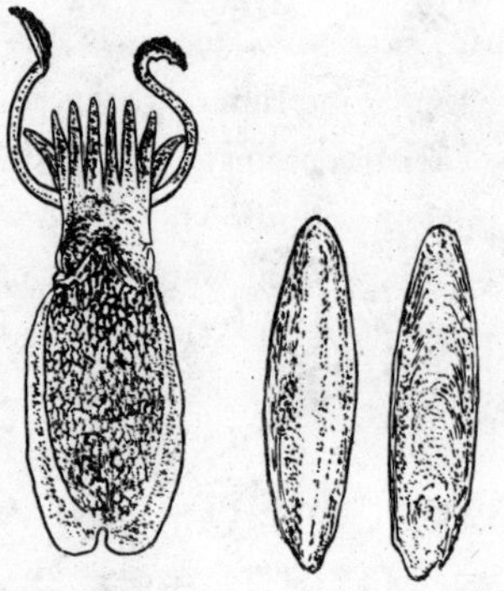

Description The bone of Sepiella maindroni de Rochebrune, or Sepia esculenta Hoyle. Family Sepiidae.

Characteristics Salty and astringent in flavor, slightly warm in nature, acting on the Liver, Kidney and Stomach Channels.

Action Inducing astringency to stop bleeding, preserving the Kidney essence to arrest leucorrhagia, decreasing the production of gastric acid to relieve stomachache, eliminating Dampness to heal wounds.

Indications

(1) Various bleedings such as metrorrhagia, metrostaxis, traumatic bleeding and bleedings from the Lung and Stomach. For treating metrorrhagia and metrostaxis, it is used with Qian Cao (Radix Rubiae), Zong Lü Tan (Trachycarpi Carbonisatus), etc., as in Guchong Tang (Decoction for Reinforcing the Chong Channel); for bleedings from the Stomach and Lung, used together with Bai Ji (Rhizoma Bletillae), etc., named Wu Ji San (Powder of Os Sepiae and Rhizoma Bletillae); for traumatic bleeding, used alone as a powder for external application.

(2) Seminal emission and leucorrhagia. For treating seminal emission, used with Shan Zhu Yu (Fructus Corni), Tu Si Zi (Semen Cuscutae), etc.; for leucorrhagia with red and white vaginal dis-

charge, used with Bai Zhi (Radix Angelicae Dahuricae) and Xue Yu Tan (Crinis Carbonisatus), as in Baizhi San (Powder of Radix Angelicae Dahuricae).

(3) Stomachache with acid regurgitation. Usually used with Bei Mu (Bulbus Fritillariae Cirrhosae), named Wu Bei San (Powder of Os Sepiae and Bulbus Fritillariae Cirrhosae).

(4) Exudative skin infections, eczema or slow-healing ulcerations. For treatment, it can be used alone as a powder for external application or used together with calcined Shi Gao (Gypsum Fibrosum), Ku Fan (Alumen), Huang Bo (Cortex Phellodendri), Qing Dai (Indigo Naturalis), etc.

Administration 6～12g for making a decoction; 1.5～3g for making a powder; q.s. for external application.

Precautions Contraindicated for Yin Deficiency with Heat in the interior.

简明中药学

编　　著　郑贵力
　　　　　张成博
译　　者　杨慧琴
责任编辑　马万年

*

山东科学技术出版社出版
济南市玉函路 16 号　邮政编码　250002
山东滨州新华印刷厂印刷
中国国际图书贸易总公司发行
中国北京车公庄西路 35 号
北京邮政信箱第 399 号　邮政编码　100044

*

1997 年(大 32 开)　1 版 1 次
ISBN 7－5331－1841－3
R·533
07200
14－E－3023P